AF181582

Recent Results in Cancer Research 111

Founding Editor
P. Rentchnick, Geneva

Managing Editors
Ch. Herfarth, Heidelberg · H. J. Senn, St. Gallen

Associate Editors
M. Baum, London · V. Diehl, Köln
C. von Essen, Villigen · E. Grundmann, Münster
W. Hitzig, Zürich · M. F. Rajewsky, Essen

Recent Results in Cancer Research

Volume 101: Locoregional High-Frequency Hyperthermia and Temperature Measurement
Edited by G. Bruggmoser, W. Hinkelbein, R. Engelhardt, M. Wannenmacher
1986. 96 figures, 8 tables. IX, 143. ISBN 3-540-15501-5

Volume 102: Epidemiology of Malignant Melanoma
Edited by R. P. Gallagher
1986. 15 figures, 70 tables. IX, 169. ISBN 3-540-16020-5

Volume 103: Preoperative (Neoadjuvant) Chemotherapy
Edited by J. Ragaz, P. R. Band, J. H. Goldie
1986. 58 figures, 49 tables. IX, 162. ISBN 3-540-16129-5

Volume 104: Hyperthermia and the Therapy of Malignant Tumors
Edited by C. Streffer
1987. 52 figures, 63 tables. IX, 207. ISBN 3-540-17250-5

Volume 105: Breast Cancer
Edited by S. Brünner and B. Langfeldt
1987. 59 figures, 43 tables. IX, 132. ISBN 3-540-17301-3

Volume 106: Minimal Neoplasia
Edited by E. Grundmann and L. Beck
1988. 128 figures, 61 tables. IX, 194. ISBN 3-540-18455-4

Volume 107: Application of Hyperthermia in the Treatment of Cancer
Edited by R. D. Issels and W. Wilmanns
1988. 118 figures, 56 tables. XII, 277. ISBN 3-540-18486-4

Volume 108: Supportive Care in Cancer Patients
Edited by H.-J. Senn and L. Schmid
1988. 62 figures, 97 tables. XII, 342. ISBN 3-540-17150-9

Volume 109: Preclinical Hyperthermia
Edited by W. Hinkelbein, G. Bruggmoser, R. Engelhardt
1988. 182 figures, 40 tables. XI, 261. ISBN 3-540-18487-2

Volume 110: Combined Modality Therapy of Gastrointestinal Tract Cancer
Edited by P. Schlag, P. Hohenberger, U. Metzger
1988. 105 figures, 122 tables. XVII, 301. ISBN 3-540-18610-7

H. Scheurlen R. Kay M. Baum (Eds.)

Cancer Clinical Trials: A Critical Appraisal

With 37 Figures and 53 Tables

Springer-Verlag
Berlin Heidelberg New York
London Paris Tokyo

Dr. Hans Scheurlen
Institut für Medizinische Biometrie und Informatik
Universität Heidelberg
Im Neuenheimer Feld 325, 6900 Heidelberg, FRG

Dr. Richard Kay
Department of Probability and Statistics
University of Sheffield
Sheffield S3 7RH, Great Britain

Professor Dr. Michael Baum
King's College, School of Medicine and Dentistry
CRC Clinical Trials Centre, Rayne Institute
123 Coldharbour Lane, London SE5 9NU, Great Britain

ISBN-13: 978-3-642-83421-9 **e-ISBN-13: 978-3-642-83419-6**
DOI: 10.1007/978-3-642-83419-6

This work is subject to copyright. All rights are reserved, whether the whole or part of the material is concerned, specifically the rights of translation, reprinting, reuse of illustrations, recitation, broadcasting, reproduction on microfilms or in other ways, and storage in data banks. Duplication of this publication or parts thereof is only permitted under the provisions of the German Copyright Law of September 9, 1965, in its version of June 24, 1985, and a copyright fee must always be paid. Violations fall under the prosecution act of the German Copyright Law.

© Springer-Verlag Berlin Heidelberg 1988
Softcover reprint of the hardcover 1st edition 1988

The use of registered names, trademarks, etc. in this publication does not imply, even in the absence of a specific statement, that such names are exempt from the relevant protective laws and regulations and therefore free for general use.

Product Liability: The publisher can give no guarantee for information about drug dosage and application thereof contained in the book. In every individual case the respective user must check its accuracy by consulting other pharmaceutical literature.

Typesetting, printing, and binding: Appl, Wemding
2125/3140-543210

Preface

The controlled clinical trial has become an essential part of the clinician's decision-making process. Clinical trials, however, still raise methodological problems that are important and at the same time controversial: subgroup analysis and interactions, meta-analysis of similar trials, consideration of subjective clinical opinions and those of the public at large, assessment of quality of life, prevention trials, and so on. In February 1987 we took our third step along the road to evaluating these issues in dialogues between clinicians, psychologists, legal experts, and statisticians. The talks presented at the meeting were revised by the authors afterwards and have been rearranged by the editors to form a strictly organized book. The two preceding meetings in 1978[1] and 1981[2] focused strongly on adjuvant therapy in primary breast cancer, but this topic served merely as a nucleus in the third meeting.

This meeting, although called the Third Heidelberg Symposium was forced to leave Heidelberg and in fact was held in Freiburg. Without the interest and enthusiasm of Professor Martin Schumacher and his colleagues in Freiburg the meeting would never have taken place. The meeting was generously supported again by the Federal Ministry of Research and Technology *(Bundesministerium für Forschung und Technologie, BMFT)* within the framework of the West German BMFT Breast Cancer Study Group. We are grateful, in particular, to Mr. Hans W. Herzog for his personal involvement.

Juni 1988 H. Scheurlen, R. Kay, M. Baum

---

[1] Scheurlen H, Weckesser G, Armbruster I (eds) (1979) Clinical trials in early breast cancer. Methodological and clinical aspects of treatment comparisons. Proceedings of a symposium, Heidelberg, Germany, 4th to 8th December, 1978.

[2] Baum M, Kay R, Scheurlen H (eds) (1982) Clinical trials in early breast cancer. 2nd Heidelberg symposium, 1981. Experiencia [Suppl] 41.

Contents

We would like to inform our readers that the correct sequence of the authors of the contribution "New Drug Development in Gastrointestinal-Tract Cancer" in *Recent Results in Cancer Research, Vol. 110* (P. Schlag, P. Hohenberger, and U. Metzger, Eds., Combined Modality Therapy of Gastrointestinal Tract Cancer) is

F. T. Garzon, M. R. Berger, H. Bischoff, and D. Schmähl.

Owing to an unfortunate oversight on the part of the publisher, F. T. Garzon was erroneously listed as the second author of this contribution. We apologize both to the authors of this contribution and to our readers for this regrettable error.

Springer-Verlag GmbH & Co. KG

*List of Contributors**

---

* The address of the principal author is given on the first page of each contribution.

[1] Page on which contribution begins.

Scientific Fundamentals

The Crooked Path Toward the Objectivation of Therapeutic Experience

U. Tröhler

Abteilung für Medizingeschichte, Universität Göttingen, Nikolausberger Weg 7b, 3400 Göttingen, FRG

The notion of objective evaluation of therapy is closely linked today to that of the clinical trial. Although we are in fact living in an age of clinical trials, they are still controversial in both lay and even medical circles, particularly because of the use of the techniques of randomization and masked assessment, often with the help of a placebo, and because these trials deal with groups of patients rather than with individuals. In order to understand our present situation, it might be helpful to survey the historical development of clinical trials and to consider what was the basis for decisions in therapeutics before, or still is concomitant with, the introduction of such clinical trials.

If we return for a moment to the cradle of Western scientific medicine, we learn from the medical texts of Greek and Roman antiquity that there were two basic approaches to therapeutics. For the *dogmatic* approach it was essential to know the cause of disease in order that therapy be derived rationally. If correctly done it had to succeed and therefore did not need to be validated. Equally, a failure could be explained away rationally, e.g., the therapy was applied too late or not in the proper manner. For the strictly *empirical* approach, on the other hand, clinical symptoms led directly to practical therapy, regardless of any theoretical considerations. Success alone was the decisive criterion, and to assess it the ancients described the classical empirical triad of observation, comparison of data with the literature, and conclusion by analogy. They further held that observations must be repeated several times in order to yield valuable experience and that negative results must be considered as well (Ackerknecht 1969). Most of us today prefer a middle way between, or, more precisely, follow the sequence of, a purely dogmatic and an empirical approach: The clinical trial is in fact a modern refinement of the latter designed to test the rationally derived hypotheses of the former.

We must not forget, however, that until fairly recently our knowledge of the causes of disease was very speculative - which indeed still is the case in some fields. In addition, the sage empirical precepts were only rarely observed even in antiquity, routine and experience based on post hoc, ergo propter hoc impressions carrying the day instead. Moreover, the empirical approach, being purely practical, fell into general discredit in all the learned disciplines during the Middle Ages, for dogmatism underpinned by scholastic deductive logic had the advantage of

Recent Results in Cancer Research, Vol. 111
© Springer-Verlag Berlin · Heidelberg 1988

providing "certain" knowledge, in agreement with the wisdom of the ancients and with divine revelation. It was not until the seventeenth century that a shift from the emphasis on learned dogmatism to a more practical empirical attitude took place, not only in medicine but in the other academic fields as well. Henceforth, experience, much maligned before, became the core of a new empiricism, once it was augmented by experimentation according to Baconian inductive logic. This modern empiricism has since become the pearl in the epistemological oyster. At the same time, it was realized that it could give no certain knowledge but only yielded probable results.

In medicine, and particularly in therapeutics, this change took longer than in other fields. For a learned doctor of the seventeenth century, concentrating as he was on the welfare of individuals, it was difficult to think in terms of groups of patients, let alone to experiment with them. Furthermore, the notion of therapeutic "experience" still meant many things, for instance, adherence to mere routine, or falling into the trap of the post hoc, ergo propter hoc fallacy. How could we otherwise explain the everlasting praise of panaceas, old and new, or of bloodletting vampirism and secret medicines, or the recommendation of contradicting therapies in the name of "experience"? This confusion was finally realized in the eighteenth century: an elite of authors started to differentiate such "pseudo experience," as they called it, from real experience in therapeutics (Ackerknecht 1962). In practice, the determination of success rates of surgical operations such as lithotomy against bladder stones and amputation of limbs was a start, the parameters being simple and objective: success or death (Tröhler 1978, 1987). As for cancer surgery, Alexander Monro I of Edinburgh (1697–1767) kept statistics on his mastectomies for cancer, which show that he did not neglect long-term observations. He told his students that:

> "Of nearly fifty, which I have been present at the extirpation of, only four patients remained free of the disease for two years. ... This disease does not always return to the part where the former tumour was taken away; but more frequently in the neigbourhood and sometimes at considerable distance. Upon a relapse, the disease in those I saw was more violent, and much quicker in progress than in others on whom no operation had been performed."
>
> (Quoted by Wright St. Clair 1964)

We also owe many of our modern concepts to eighteenth-century military and naval medicine, where a soldier counted less as an individual than as "a life," i.e., as part of a group. James Lind (1716–1794), for instance, is rightly famous for a planned trial which he conducted on board ship in 1747, involving six concomitantly treated groups of two scurvy patients each. His work in the second half of the century, done at Haslar Naval Hospital, was also very important. He had more than a thousand beds at his disposal and used this opportunity for therapeutic experimentation in particular wards. From his works can be drawn a true research program containing the following main points: (a) A series of nonselected observations made during a given time should be the basis for decision in therapeutics: in this we see the dawn of the idea of randomization. (b) Lind fought "the habit of publishing individual successful cases only." (c) Accurate notes must be taken, for memory alone cannot be trusted. (d) One should compare the results of treatment to the unassisted efforts of nature in comparable patients.

Lind understood the placebo effect; he knew of "the role of faith" in therapeutics. He furthermore presented his results statistically, often in terms of relative fatality. From such data he meant to derive a standard plan for treating specific diseases, which could, however, not be infallible in every case, for, as he put this probalistic view: "Yet more enlarged experience must ever evince the fallacy of all positive assertions in the healing art." (Tröhler 1981).

In the British literature of the late eighteenth century many more reports of therapeutic evaluation using observational and experimental methods ranging from the analysis of statistical returns via "historical controls" to planned single-blind placebo studies can be found (Tröhler 1978). Recent historical studies suggest that they were less frequent on the Continent (Herzog 1983; Molinari 1987; Zatka 1984). Yet it would be erroneous to believe that dogmatism had vanished by 1800, even in Britain, for in fact Europe then saw once again the heyday of rational systems such as those of John Brown and Anton Mesmer, or those of German romantic medicine as well as of homeopathy (Risse 1971; Schott 1985; Schwanitz 1983).

Formal opposition to the empirical and at the same time to the probabilistic approach did not manifest itself in Britain, but it can be found in Paris in the 1830s, where it had meanwhile become known as the "methode numérique" championed by Pierre Charles Alexandre Louis (1787-1872). In the Académie Royale des Sciences and the Académie Royale de Médecine, two formal debates took place on the issue around 1835. The arguments in favor of statistics in clinical medicine being the same as those advanced for example by Lind in the eighteenth century, those of the opponents are of particular interest to us. They were of two kinds. The first type, which we may call the "old school," wondered whether the old certainty could possibly ever be replaced by probability. Would this not mean that medicine would become a gambling place? It was further held that by administering the same therapy indiscriminately to groups of patients, one deprived the single patient of his individuality. How could the variability of biological phenomena be rendered by the constancy of figures which, moreover, would never be able to take into account the "art of medicine"?

The second kind of arguments were "modern" ones: Some were pragmatic: for example, that two sufficiently large groups of comparable patients would never be found. It was also said that such trials were clinically inadequate, inasmuch as they did not reflect the daily reality of the doctor who always faced an individual rather than a group of patients. For this reason, also, it was felt that trials were ethically disputable insofar as the doctors organizing them were interested only in the outcome of the majority. To ignore the minority seemed to show a completely anti-medical attitude. Finally, mathematicians also advanced theoretical criticism: Doctors used simple arithmetic comparisons in trials which required the application of the calculus of probability.

The discussions on clinical statistics were resumed in Paris in the middle of the nineteenth century. A sort of compromise was reached: Statistics with their probabilities were correct for hygiene, epidemiology, or preventive medicine (Murphy 1981). But these relatively recent disciplines were seen quite separate from "real" clinical medicine, which was just about to embark on claims to new dogmatic certainty by advances in pathophysiology and bacteriology, by the introduction of new diagnostic tools (such as the stethoscope, the optical "scopes," and later the ECG and X-rays) and of therapeutic possibilities (such as painless antiseptic surgery; Reiser 1978).

Comparative therapeutic experimentation was for the most part forgotten (Piquemal 1974; Cassedy 1984). Statistics were being used, but in a one-sided way. Increasing the numbers increased the impression of certainty - a technique which spread particularly among surgeons in the rapidly growing area of modern aseptic surgery (Tröhler 1984; Voumard 1987). This type of statistics became a way to quantify prejudice.

The notion of the need of proper methodology for therapeutic evaluation did not come up again until the present century, particularly in the Anglo-Saxon countries. The first randomization was actually performed in Britain in 1923 in an agricultural field experiment, the first group randomization in a clinical trial in the United States in 1931. The first individual randomization was done in the British Medical Research Council's streptomycin trial in 1948. This also was the first trial strictly conducted according to the double-blind technique (Lilienfeld 1982; Armitage 1983).

This chronology of events raises three questions. (a) How did the quest for validation come about in the 18th Century? (b) How can we explain the stagnation in the nineteenth century and (c) the unfolding of the methodological fan again in the twentieth? The answers can be found within medicine itself, i.e., in medical inventions, medical philosophy, and sociology (Tröhler 1978, 1988), but there are also nonmedical explanations such as the state of statistics: In the nineteenth century, they were concerned chiefly with mass phenomena, with correlations and regressions rather than with the determination of the significance of differences between groups. All the relevant tests were developed in England in the early twentieth century only.

In conclusion, if we consider the present-day controversy over clinical trials in the light of historical evidence, it might be maintained that we should attempt to overcome our methodological shortcomings and ethical reservations by improving scientific skills, for the alternative historical pattern seems in fact a fall back into an age of dogmatic pseudo experience, which for such a long time has dominated Western scientific medicine.

References

Ackerknecht EH (1962) Aspects of the history of therapeutics. Bull Hist Med 36: 389-419

Ackerknecht EH (1969) Die therapeutische Erfahrung und ihre allmähliche Objektivierung. Gesnerus 26: 26-35

Armitage P (1983) Trials and errors: the emergence of clinical statistics. J R Stat Soc Ser A (General) 146: 321-334

Cassedy JH (1984) American medicine and statistical thinking 1800-1860. Harvard University Press, Cambridge, MA

Herzog D (1983) Zahlenmäßige Grundlagen in der medizinischen Fachliteratur Frankreichs um 1760. M D thesis, University of Basel

Lilienfeld AM (1982) Ceteris paribus: the evolution of the clinical trial. Bull Hist Med 56: 1-18

Molinari M (1987) Die Bedeutung numerischer Evaluation in der Klinik in Frankreich zwischen 1774 und 1793. M D thesis, University of Basel
Murphy TD (1981) Medical knowledge and statistical methods in early nineteenth-century France. Med Hist 25: 301-319
Piquemal J (1974) Succès et décadence de la méthode numérique en France à l'époque de Pierre-Charles Alexandre Louis. Méd de France, no 250 pp 11-22, 59-60
Reiser SJ (1978) Medicine and the reign of technology. Cambridge University Press, Cambridge
Risse GB (1971) The quest for certainty in medicine: John Brown's system of medicine in France. Bull Hist Med 45: 1-12
Schott H (ed) (1985) Franz Anton Mesmer und die Geschichte des Mesmerismus. Steiner, Wiesbaden
Schwanitz HJ (1983) Homöopathie und Brownianismus. Fischer, Stuttgart
Tröhler U (1978) Quantification in British medicine and surgery 1750-1830, with special reference to its introduction into therapeutics. University College, London
Tröhler U (1981) Towards clinical investigation on a numerical basis: James Lind at Haslar hospital 1758-1783. In: Danon J, Cid R (eds) Proceedings of the 27th int congr hist med, Barcelona 1980, vol 1. Academia de Ciències Mediques de Catalunya i Balears, Barcelona, pp 414-419
Tröhler U (1984) Auf dem Wege zur physiologischen Chirurgie. Der Nobelpreisträger Theodor Kocher 1841-1917. Birkhäuser, Basel
Tröhler U (1987) Die Gewißheit der Chirurgie? Auf dem Weg zur Objektivierung der klinisch-therapeutischen Erfahrung um 1750. Schweiz Rundsch Med Prax 76: 958-961
Tröhler U (1988) The history of therapeutic evaluation between dogmatic certainty and empiric probability. J R Soc Med (in print)
Voumard P-A (1987) L'approche statistique en France vue à travers les Archives Générales de Médecine de 1860 à 1875. M D thesis, University of Basel
Wright St, Clair RE (1964) Doctors Monro. A medical saga. Wellcome Historical Medical Library, London
Zatka L (1984) Zur Bedeutung numerischer Evaluation in der Klinik zwischen 1801 und 1836 anhand des Archivs für medizinische Erfahrung. M D thesis, University of Basel

Randomised Trials: The Case for Science in Medicine

M. Baum

King's College School of Medicine and Dentistry, CRC Clinical Trials Centre, Rayne Institute, 123 Coldharbour Lane, London SE5 9NU, Great Britain

Introduction

It is quite apparent to me that very few people understand the meaning of the word "epistemology". It may be difficult to pronounce but it is quite easy to understand. Epistemology is the study of the growth of knowledge, or "how do we know what we think we know"? What I would now like to try to get across is that scientific philosophy is not a rarefied activity indulged in by retired physicians who have nothing better to do with the remainder of their lives; rather, it is a very important aspect of medical education and medical practice. I will illustrate this by describing aspects of the growth of philosophy and how this has an impact on our everyday practice. I would like to start off with Aristotle, the Greek philosopher who was the father of inductivism. Inductivism is another word that is frequently used but not clearly understood. Simply put, inductivism is the process by which you generate a hypothesis and then seek corroborative evidence to prove that your hypothesis is an expression of the truth. The history of medicine is littered with the tragic failures of this philosophical approach. Galen, a second-century physician, was the master of inductivism in medical practice and his malign influence led to 1600 years of sterility. This sterility was not merely an inhibition of medical progress; it also included the perpetuation of barbaric and useless treatments such as that of bleeding and cupping, the panacea approaches for most ills up until the early years of the past century. To this day, you will meet contemporary inductivists pacing the marble corridors of ultramodern high-technology hospitals, introducing and perpetuating dangerous therapies without having the intellectual honesty to seek anything other than corroborative evidence in support of their ideas. I would now like to take you 1000 years further, to the birth of the deductive process in medical science. William of Okam was a thirteenth-century English monk, and his famous aphorism "Entiae non multiplicandum necessitatum" describes the philosophical underpinning of the modern approach to medical diagnosis. A loose translation of the Latin would be that on observing multiple phenomena you should try to explain your observations in terms of the simplest underlying cause. Thus, the whole process of diagnosis is the eliciting of symptoms and signs from the patient, and instead of coming up with multiple explana-

Recent Results in Cancer Research, Vol. 111
© Springer-Verlag Berlin · Heidelberg 1988

tions for them we apply Okam's razor to postulate a single causal explanation with multiple epiphenomena.

We can now move on approximately 100 years, to the birth of the hypothetico-deductive scientific process. Again, do not be frightened off by the jargon. Philosophers, just like medical practitioners, have their own language, and their words are chosen carefully to have specific meanings. A good way of understanding the early concepts of deductive scientific empiricism is to remember Francis Bacon's maxim: "If you start with certainties you will surely finish with doubt, whereas if you are prepared to start with doubts, you may yet finish with certainties." Thus, Francis Bacon implied for the first time that it was laudable to have doubts and that dogma and certainty did not apply in the area of science, which needed to be clearly separated from the domain of metaphysics and religion. A good way of illustrating this approach is to consider the history of our understanding of the circulation of blood. Galen taught that the blood ebbed and flowed throughout the body via pores between the ventricles of the heart, but he made no attempt to investigate this hypothesis. The great Vesalius, after carrying out his anatomical dissections, described his failure to observe Galen's proposed channels through the ventricular septum. Everyone rejected the observations of Vesalius because they refuted the teachings of Galen, and Galen could never be wrong! Eventually, along came the English physician William Harvey, who used very simple clinical observations to deduce that the blood flowed from the arteries into the veins via an as yet undiscovered series of channels joining these vascular structures. It was 100 years later that there was a spectacular corroboration of this hypothesis, when Anthon van Leeuwenhoek of Amsterdam designed the first microscope and saw for the first time the vascular capillaries predicted by William Harvey. Sir John Corrigan, in his biography of William Harvey, described how, following the publication of his revolutionary concepts, Harvey was considered a subversive and lost his medical practice. In fact, most of the great revolutionary scientists in the world were considered subversives in their time, but beware of the logical syllogism that all subversives must be great scientists, unrecognised in their time. In other words, just because Harvey ultimately achieved a spectacular corroboration of what was thought a subversive idea, this does not mean that every subversive idea has to be considered a scientific revolution. Another important aspect of this history of the discovery of circulation of the blood is that many of the quantum leaps in scientific progress depended on the description and design of instrumentation that extended the scope of human senses, like Gallileo's telescope or, more recently, the Nobel-prize winner Caesar Milstein's description of monoclonal antibodies, which now allow us to see proteins on the surface of cells that we have never been able to observe before.

The first major breakthrough in the control of the natural history of any disease concerns the prevention of smallpox following the invention of vaccination by Edward Jenner. John Hunter, a famous London surgeon, was a friend of Edward Jenner, and in a letter that Hunter wrote in 1777 in reply to Jenner's enquiries, he stated: "I think your solution is just but why think, why not try the experiment?" And so Jenner conducted the first series of human experiments and, as a result of those experiments, smallpox, one of the greatest scourges of humanity, was eradicated from the world. Asking questions, challenging dogma and conducting experiments are all expressions of the dominant scientific philosophy of today, and it was the work of Sir Karl Popper, the greatest living scientific philosopher, who pulled all these threads together in his famous book *The Logic of Scientific Discovery* (Popper 1959). He clearly defined the demarcation between that which was science and that which was nonscience. Science is the study of theories that are subject to falsifiability, whereas nonscience concerns aspects of our life where beliefs are not subject to the laws of falsification; thus, astronomy is science whilst astrology is nonscience. And orthodox medicine, if it refuses to be considered a science, will become nothing other than quackery. Popper extended the Baconian view on scientific deductivism by teaching that we never arrive at certainty. One's search for the truth is always an approximation. One travels hopefully but never arrives, and it is precisely this Popperian view of science which is the underlying philosophy of the randomised controlled clinical trial. I happen to believe that the statisticians who invented the mathematics governing the conduct of clinical trials have developed a new instrument to allow us to see things which exist in reality that we would not otherwise see. These statisticians, therefore, are revolutionary scientists and innovators of the same importance in the history of science as Galileo and Anthon van Leeuwenhoek. To understand their importance, you have to appreciate that if we were able to wave a magic wand and cure every single case of non-Hodgkin's lymphoma in the world, it would have a trivial impact on mortality statistics, whereas if we could improve the death rate from the common cancers, such as lung cancer, gastric cancer, and breast cancer or reduce mortality from ischemic heart disease by as little as 3%, that would have an enormous medical and sociological impact.

It is extremely difficult, and I suspect extremely boring, to consider these philosophical issues in the abstract. The beauty of the hypothetico-deductive method of science is that it is a very practical philosophy that sees its expression in our day-to-day activities and with every exchange between patient and doctor. I therefore propose to illustrate all these concepts with a short review of the history of the development of treatment for carcinoma of the breast, which remains the most common malignancy of women in Europe and North America and is still the most common cause of death for women in the 35- to 60-year age-group.

The History of the Treatment of Breast Cancer

Breast cancer has been recognised as a clinical entity from before the time of Hippocrates. An ancient Egyptian papyrus clearly described the disease and its demarcation from acute inflammatory mastitis (Breasted 1930). The ancient Egyptian physicians wisely advised a noninterventional approach. In fact, one of the greatest tragedies in the history of this subject has been the persistent error in confusing activity with progress. Mastectomy of a kind was introduced by the surgeons of the Graeco-Roman period, but probably the first clearly defined hypothesis concerning the nature of the disease and its appropriate treatment can be attributed to Galen. He preached that breast cancer was a systemic disorder due to the retention and excess of black bile (melancholia). As inductive support for this hypothesis, he pointed out that the disease was more common in postmenopausal women, who cease their monthly menstrual loss, and that the menstrual periods were a natural mechanism for clearing the body of excess black bile (De Moulin 1983). The therapeutic consequences, therefore, were self-evident, and for the next 1600 years, women were treated by purgation and bleeding to rid the body of the putative excess of black bile. Local therapy consisted predominantly of cautery and noxious topical applications for the management of offensive and bleeding ulcers. It goes without saying that nothing other than anecdotal support for these remedies existed in the literature. The first conceptual and, hence, therapeutic revolution dates from the time of Virchow in the 1860s. He demonstrated, by anatomical dissections of cadavers of women who had died of untreated advanced breast cancer, that the disease was commonly seen plugging the lymphatic channels and replacing the regional lymph nodes. He deduced, therefore, that the disease was not a systemic disorder but a localised abnormality, with the spread of the disease along tissue planes via columns of cancer cells growing along the lymph channels. The cancer was then temporarily arrested in the lymph nodes which were thought to act as filter traps. With exhaustion of the proximal lymph node barriers the more distal lymph node barriers became infected and, ultimately, the disease gained access to the vital organs by a centrifugal extension of this process. The therapeutic consequences of this biological model were taken up by William Halsted in America, Willhelm Meyer in Germany and Samson Handley (Halsted 1898) in the United Kingdom, all within a few years of each other. All three of these great and influential surgeons developed a radical type of mastectomy, which attempted to rid the body of the primary focus and all surgically accessible lymph node deposits, whilst avoiding cutting across infected lymphatic channels. There was never any prima facie evidence that the introduction of this radical approach improved on the more conservative type of surgery or, for that matter, the systemic therapy prevalent until the 1880s. On the contrary, publications exist demonstrating that throughout the first 30 years of this century the best result achieved by the radical approach was approximately a 10% 10-year survival, which is almost identical to that achieved by Gross in Philadelphia in the 1880s (Gross 1880). In fairness to Halsted, it must be recognised that he successfully reduced the operative mortality and improved the local control of the disease. It also has to be remembered that the majority of the cases they were treating in that era would be considered locally advanced today and would be excluded from trials of primary local therapy. Surgeons became very frustrated with the failure of the Halsted radical mastectomy to cure breast cancer, but instead of questioning the underlying hypothetical model, improvements were sought by extending the concept to its logical conclusion, leading to the surgical barbarity of extended radical mastectomies and even forequarter amputations. Inevitably, there was a reaction against such barbarity, and we should never forget the contributions of the great and distinguished British surgeon Sir Geoffrey Keynes; in the face of all established surgical dogma, Keynes introduced a conservative mode of treatment for this disease in the early 1930s, eventually publishing a historical paper in the *British Medical Journal* demonstrating that the results of local excision plus radium-needle insertion were equal to any published data advocating the use of the radical approach (Keynes 1937). Perhaps as a result of the intervening war years and Sir Geoffrey Keynes' retirement, this conservative approach never achieved popularity. On the contrary, Sir Stanford Cade, summing up a debate on the merits of the treatment of early breast cancer at the Royal Society of Medicine in 1947, sanctioned the radical mastectomy as the appropriate treatment for stage I of the disease (Cade 1948). We thus have the prospect of two great surgical names advocating diametrically opposed therapies. If the big men could not agree, what were the little men to do? As is the case throughout the history of our subject, the little men followed the dictates of the authority with the highest profile and the greatest charisma. This can hardly be considered science of any description, but is more akin to the behaviour of the faithful within a religious cult. The appropriate scientific response to such a clash of convictions is neatly summed up in the words of Sir Karl Popper:

"Instead of discussing the probability of the hypothesis, we should try to assess what trials it has withstood and how far it has been able to prove its fitness to survive" (Popper 1959).

Randomised Controlled Trials of Locoregional Therapy

The first truly randomised trials for the treatment of early breast cancer can be credited to the Manchester Christie group, headed by Paterson and Russell (Paterson and Russell 1959). Since then a host of complementary studies have been completed, with mature follow-up data available for between 10 and 30 years. These studies have compared, in a strictly scientific manner, treatments varying from extended radical mastectomy on the one hand to local excision, with or without radiotherapy, at the most conservative extreme. In retrospect, the trials of this period were really addressing themselves to two different questions. Firstly, would the use of radical radiotherapy provide the same degree of local control and the same cure rate as radical surgery? In other words, was radiotherapy as effective as surgery in ablating cancer from the regional nodes? The second set of trials was asking a more interesting biological question concerning the relevance of the regional lymph nodes in the putative immunosurveillance of cancer. Thus, procedures that preserved the axillary nodes intact were compared with surgical or radiotherapeutic techniques aimed at total destruction of these nodes (Berstock et al. 1985). Observed in toto, we can now say with the greatest of statistical confidence that although the degree of local control varies directly with the magnitude of the treatment field, no important differences in survival have been detected. Biological extrapolations from these data might suggest one of three conclusions:

1. Untreated lymph node metastases do not act as a source of tertiary spread.
2. The immunosuppressive effects of radical surgery or regional radiotherapy are of no clinical relevance.
3. The metastasising capacity of involved nodes is balanced by the immunosurveillance mediated in some way by the intact uninvolved lymph nodes.

Whatever the explanation, these accumulated data support the concept of biological predeterminism, and further analyses of subgroups suggest that those patients with lymph nodes invaded by cancer at the time of diagnosis are those most often predetermined to die (Fisher 1970). As a result of this experience, all but a few die-hards amongst surgeons and radiotherapists experienced a paradigm shift. The lymph node status of the patient is now looked upon as an expression rather than a determinant of prognosis. It is an amusing pastime to study the attitudes of the die-hards amongst the medical profession and their attempts to rationalise away the failures of the radical approach. Firstly, it has been argued that if the patients were diagnosed early as a result of screening programmes, then the radical mastectomy would cure them all. Secondly, the failure of radical surgery and radical radiotherapy within randomised controlled trials represents the failure of the surgeons and radiotherapists to deliver the treatment correctly. The therapeutic inductivists still point to the uncontrolled data sets from the great radical surgeons and the centres of radiotherapeutic excellence. Finally, those women who have suffered radical mastectomy and are alive and well to tell their tale 30 years later are once again paraded as a living tribute to the perfection of the treatments they received. To my mind, this type of conceptual rationalisation is no different from the logic adduced by proponents of fringe medicine (Baum 1983).

The Quality of Life After the Treatment of Early Breast Cancer

It is reasonable for members of the lay public to ask whether there is life after mastectomy. The pioneering work of Peter Maguire has clearly demonstrated that about one third of patients treated for breast cancer by some form of mastectomy will suffer serious and debilitating psychosexual morbidity (Maguire 1982). Of course, the other side of the coin must not be overlooked. Seventy percent of women provided with a modest amount of rehabilitation and prosthetic advice can enjoy a fulfilling and normal life by drawing on their natural reserves to cope with one of life's major crises. It is a reasonable assumption that the loss of the breast contributes the major component to the psychosexual morbidity of the treatment, but, like all medical assumptions, this needs challenging. In 1981, the Cancer Research Campaign launched a trial to compare mastectomy with breast conservation for women diagnosed as suffering from early breast cancer. The study was conducted with informed consent, and is unique in having a built-in formal assessment of the psychosexual morbidity in both arms of the trial. The results of this study are, to say the least, counterintuitive, suggesting that the major contribution to the psychosexual morbidity is not so much the treatment as the diagnosis of the disease itself (Fallowfield et al. 1986). This should not suggest for a moment a return to the bad old days of radical mastectomy, but should redirect our attention to the development of counselling services, to enable women to come to terms with their diagnosis and the inevitable threat to their life that this poses.

Trials of Adjuvant Systemic Therapy

If the majority of patients with early breast cancer and positive axillary nodes die, however perfect the locoregional therapy, then surely they carry occult micrometastases present at the time of diagnosis. As that must be the case, then cure can result only from the addition of an effective systemic therapy. Experience with advanced breast cancer demonstrates an objective response rate of the order of 60%, with prolonged cyclical combination therapy, which is twice that expected with an endocrinological approach. Ipso facto, node-positive patients should be cured by adjuvant systemic chemotherapy. So compelling were these arguments and so beautiful the new hypothesis, that many medical oncologists felt it unethical to do randomised trials and, like all inductivists, they soon found sufficient corroborative evidence to satisfy themselves. To my mind, such individuals are as guilty as those who uncritically accepted the Halstedian dogma 70 years ago, particularly as some of these chemotherapeutic excesses can be considered the medical equivalent of a forequarter amputation! A recent review of the results of randomised controlled trials of adjuvant chemotherapy has arrived at the following general conclusions (Goldhirsch et al. 1986):

1. Whatever combination regimen is used, there is likely to be a significant delay in the time to first relapse.
2. Although many individual trials have yet to show an improvement in crude survival, a statistical overview of all the available data suggests that a 30% reduction in the risk of dying over the first 5 years may be achieved following the treatment of premenopausal women with node-positive disease. The benefits for postmenopausal women are, to say the least, marginal.

What, therefore, are the biological implications of these results? Firstly, there is little doubt that the natural history of early breast cancer has been perturbed, lending support to the deterministic model. Whether this perturbation will translate itself into a useful therapeutic advantage for groups other than premenopausal node-positive patients remains to be seen. Secondly, the intriguing difference between the behaviour of pre- and postmenopausal women deserves some explanation. The chemotherapy lobby is not short of inductivists, and much support has been generated for the concept that the effect of adjuvant systemic chemotherapy is dose related (Bonadonna and Valagusa 1981). Postmenopausal women seem incapable of tolerating the maximal (?optimal) doses prescribed. This suggestion requires further exploration, with trials of high-dose v. low-dose chemotherapy. To accept the suggestion without prospective studies is to be guilty of a tautology, yet, at the same time, if older women are incapable of tolerating high-dose chemotherapy, then this surely is an inherent defect of the treatment unless one is prepared to push the drugs beyond the tolerance of the patient, surely a dangerous and inhumane policy. An alternative explanation for this differential effect might be that the cytotoxic drugs mediate their effect by a chemical castration. This hypothesis has already won some support, following studies of ovarian and pituitary function in women receiving adjuvant chemotherapy (Rose and Davis 1977). It follows, therefore, that to test the hypothesis generated by the trials of adjuvant chemotherapy, one should conduct trials of adjuvant endocrine therapy investigating prophylactic castration and the use of adjuvant tamoxifen.

Trials of prophylactic castration following local treatment for cancer are not new but have suffered in the past from inadequate sample size, leaving uncertainty as to its potential benefit. This subject has recently been reviewed, suggesting that such an approach might indeed produce results of the same order achieved by polychemotherapy for premenopausal women but at the great expense of inducing a premature menopause in young women already facing the threat of loss of the breast (Cole 1970). For the purpose of this paper, though, I wish to concentrate on the trial of tamoxifen therapy, which can be judged to have had the most profound effect on our biological thinking about the disease. The Nolvadex Adjuvant Trial Organisation (NATO) launched a study in 1977 to investigate whether the anti-oestrogen tamoxifen (Nolvadex) would have any benefit for women undergoing mastectomy for early breast cancer (NATO 1983). Approximately 1300 patients were recruited over a period of 2 and a half years. These consisted of premenopausal node-positive cases and postmenopausal node-positive and -negative cases. Following local therapy, women were randomised to the group receiving tamoxifen, 10 mg twice daily for 2 years, or to an untreated control group. A second-order hypothesis suggested that the women most likely to benefit were those whose primary tumour was rich in oestradiol receptor (E2R) content. Therefore, as a parallel study, attempts were made to collect samples of the tumours from all patients entered into the trial. However, for logistic reasons, this was possible in only about 50% of the cases. The published data have demonstrated a significantly prolonged disease-free interval in the treated group as a whole, which has recently been translated into a 30% reduction in the risk of dying within the first 5 years following treatment (NATO 1985 a). Support for the fact that this result was not a statistical fluke has emerged from the statistical overview conducted by Mr. Richard Peto and his colleagues and presented at the Consensus Development Conference at the National Cancer Institute in Washington, USA, in September 1985 (UK Breast Cancer Trials Cancer Coordinating Committee/UICC 1984). Following this presentation, the NCI sanctioned the use of tamoxifen as monotherapy for the majority of women over the age of 50 at the time of diagnosis. Paradoxically, a Cox's multi-variant regression analysis within the NATO trial has failed to demonstrate any interaction between the treatment and subgroups divided according to menopausal, nodal or E2R status.

Biological Fall-out from Trials of Adjuvant Tamoxifen

If the survival advantage of patients treated for 2 years with tamoxifen persists over the long term then this would suggest that the anti-oestrogen has a tumoricidal capacity for the putative micrometastases present at the time of the diagnosis. This in itself would be interesting, suggesting that subclinical tumour deposits are biologically different from overt metastatic disease. Of potentially greater interest is the suggestion that the oestrogen-receptor status of the primary tumour does not predict the likelihood of response to adjuvant tamoxifen. As such an outcome fails to reinforce popular prejudice, there would naturally be the temptation to ignore or reject these data. It has already been suggested that the measurement of E2R in a multicentre trial with inter- and intralaboratory variation will produce many false-negative results. This may indeed be the case, but it remains unquestionable that the assay of E2R in this study has told us something of biological relevance about the primary cancers, as there is a powerful correlation between the E2R status and prognosis, irrespective of primary or adjuvant therapy (NATO 1985b). Rather than ignore these data out of hand, I believe it will be more fruitful to try to incorporate them within a modified hypothesis that can explain previous observations about the behaviour of breast cancer whilst at the same time incorporating the new and apparently irreconcilable observation. There is little doubt that the major pathway mediating the anti-tumour effect of tamoxifen in advanced breast cancer is via the oestradiol receptor; however, the observations from the NATO trial raise the question as to whether tamoxifen exerts some of its effect on microscopic foci of the disease by another pathway. Recently, a ubiquitous tamoxifen-binding protein has been discovered in tissues, which is unrelated to E2R (Kon 1983). Furthermore, tamoxifen in sufficiently high concentrations can inhibit the growth of both oestrogen-receptor-positive and oestrogen-receptor-negative human breast cancer cell lines (Lippman and Bolan 1975). Perhaps tamoxifen binding to this cytosolic protein can interfere with another fundamental biochemical pathway upon which the continued growth of the cancer cell is dependent.

Exciting new discoveries concerning the nature of oncogenes and the relationship between oncogenic sequences in the cellular genome, and the production of specific growth factors or the expression of growth factor receptors, could easily be incorporated with these observations into a new biological model concerning the nature of breast cancer (Dunn 1986). If tamoxifen can inhibit the cellular cascade of biochemical reactions which are a consequence of the activation of the epidermoid growth factor receptor, then this might suggest that the oestradiol-receptor status of the breast cancer is merely an epiphenomenon of cellular differentiation, indirectly reflecting the rate of inappropriate growth factor activation. Thus, the E2R serves as a prognostic indicator, reflecting the growth rate of the cancer, rather than simply as an expression of endocrine sensitivity. With this model, the oestrogen receptor could act as an amplifying mechanism concentrating the tamoxifen within the cancer cell, where it can act as an anti-growth factor. This would then explain the apparent selectivity of tamoxifen for advanced breast cancer amongst the oestrogen-receptor-positive cells, whilst at the same time explaining why it retains modest activity against microscopic deposits of oestrogen-receptor-negative cancer cells. Further support of the idea that the E2R is an indirect expression of the rate of growth factor production comes from the following observations: E2R-positive cancers are predominantly well differentiated on histological grading (Fisher et al. 1980). The E2R status of breast cancers is inversely correlated with the rate of replication of cells in vitro (Meyer et al. 1977). Growth factors are known to potently attract monocytes (Waterfield et al. 1983); a monocytosis is a recognised response to an actively growing tumour, and a heavy stromal round-cell infiltrate is associated with a negative E2R status (Steele 1983). Finally, two recent pieces of work have shown an inverse correlation between the oestrogen receptor content of a breast cancer and the expression of epidermoid growth factor receptors (EGFr) using specific monoclonal antibodies raised against EGFr (Sainsbury et al. 1985; Trivedi 1986).

To summarise, therefore, at one extreme we might have a breast cancer with a very high rate of expression of EGFr, where the rate of replication and protein synthesis does not allow sufficient time or amino acids for the assembly of E2R, whilst at the other extreme of EGFr expression, E2R assembly precedes the completion. This then raises the intriguing possibility that tamoxifen may slow the tumour via an anti-growth factor pathway until E2R is reassembled, and the cancer cell is re-differentiated, as a result of which the tamoxifen is further concentrated, exhibiting its secondary effect along the classical pathway.

All the predictions of this hypothesis are eminently testable, guaranteeing its refutation or elaboration with time.

Prevention of Breast Cancer

Following the recruitment into the NATO trial, the Cancer Research Campaign launched a large multicentre trial to study in greater depth the potential benefits of adjuvant tamoxifen. Over 2000 patients were recruited into this study before the undoubted benefits of adjuvant tamoxifen were published by the NATO group. At a maximum of 5 years of follow-up in this new trial, the same differences in favour of tamoxifen are emerging. An unexpected and exciting spin-off from this second major study concerned the appearance of contralateral breast cancers (Cuzick et al. 1985). Women with primary breast cancer may expect to develop a contralateral tumour at the rate of approximately 0.7%–1% per year. Within 3 years of

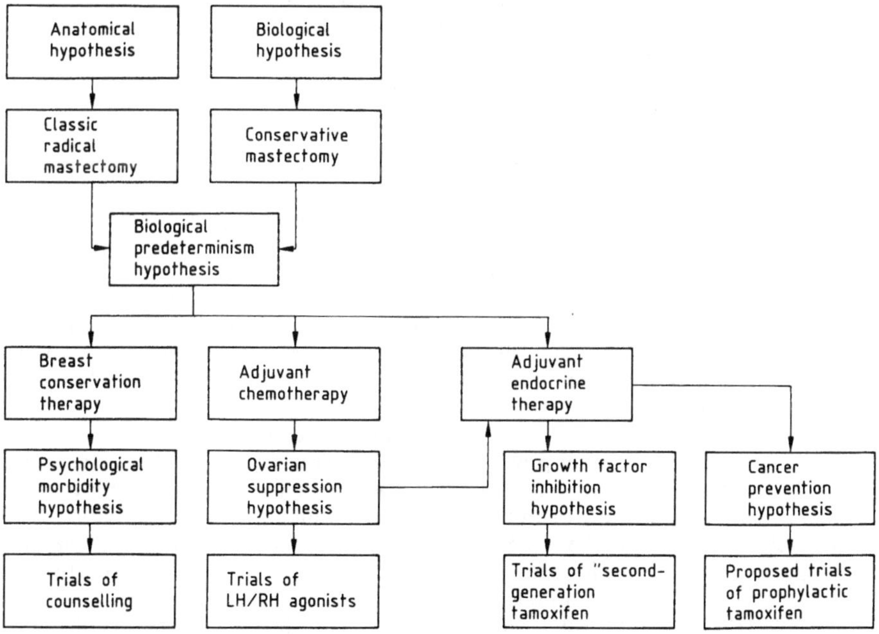

Fig. 1. The hypothetico-deductive cascade in the development of treatment of breast cancer

follow-up, approximately 3% of the untreated control group had already developed their contralateral cancer, as expected. However, those women exposed to adjuvant tamoxifen showed a significantly reduced rate of developing the second breast cancer. Of course, it is likely that these women had subclinical, synchronous contralateral cancers all the time, which had merely been inhibited as a result of exposure to the drug; but if this difference persists, we then have additional, powerful ammunition for those advocating an intervention trial for the prophylaxis of breast cancer in the population at risk within the community at large. A recent review paper in *The Lancet* has explored this possibility in detail (Cuzick et al. 1986).

Conclusion

Figure 1 illustrates the hypothetico-deductive cascade that has originated from the time that clinicians had the courage to challenge the therapeutic dogma of the surgical management of early breast cancer. Had it not been for the randomised controlled trial, women would still be subjected to Halsted radical mastectomies or even more aggressive local therapy, and the prospects for future cure or control would be grim indeed.

References

Baum M (1983) Quack cancer cures or scientific remedies? Clin Oncol 9: 275-280

Berstock DA, Houghton J, Haybittle J, Baum M (1985) The role of radiotherapy following total mastectomy for patients with early breast cancer. World J Surg 667-670

Bonadonna G, Valagusa P (1981) Dose-response effect of adjuvant chemotherapy in breast cancer. N Engl J Med 30: 10-15

Breasted JH (1930) The Edwin Smith papyrus. University of Chicago Press, Chicago, pp 403-406

Cade Sir S (1948) Discussion: the treatment of cancer of the breast. Proc R Soc Med 41: 129

Cole MP (1970) Prophylactic compared with therapeutic X-ray artificial menopause, 2nd Tenovus Workshop on Breast Cancer. Alpha-Omega, Cardiff, pp 2-11

Cuzick J, Baum M (1985) Tamoxifen and contralateral breast cancer. Lancet ii: 282

Cuzick J, Wang DY, Bulbrook RD (1986) The prevention of breast cancer. Lancet i: 83-86

De Moulin D (1983) In: A short history of cancer. Nyhoff, Boston

Dunn AR (1986) Viral and cellular oncogenes a molecular basis for breast and other cancers. In: Forbes JF (ed) Breast disease, vol 5. Churchill Livingstone, Edinburgh, pp 59-68

Fallowfield L, Baum M, Maguire GP (1986) The effects of breast conservation on the psychological morbidity associated with the diagnosis and treatment of early breast cancer. Br Med J (In press)

Fisher B (1970) The surgical dilemma in the primary therapy of invasive breast cancer. A critical appraisal. In: Current problems in surgery. Year Book Publishers, Chicago

Fisher B, Redmond C, Fisher ER (1980) The contribution of recent NSABP trials of primary breast cancer therapy to an understanding of tumour biology. Cancer 46: 1009

Goldhirsch A, Gelber RD, Davis BW (1986) Adjuvant chemotherapy trials in breast cancer: an appraisal and lessons for patient care outside the trials. In: Forbes JF (ed) Breast disease, vol 10. Churchill Livingstone, Edinburgh, pp 123-138

Gross SW (1880) A practical treatise of tumours of the mammary gland. Appleton, New York

Halsted WS (1898) The radical operation for the cure of carcinoma of the breast. Johns Hopkins Hospital reports, no 28, p 557

Keynes G (1937) Conservative treatment of cancer of the breast. Br Med J 643-647

Kon OL (1983) An antiestrogen-binding protein in human tissues. J Biol Chem 258: 3173

Lippman ME, Bolan G (1975) Oestrogen-responsive human breast cancer in long-term tissue culture. Nature 256: 592-593

Maguire P (1982) Psychiatric morbidity associated with mastectomy. In: Baum M, Kay R, Scheurlen H (eds) Clinical trial in early breast cancer, 2nd Heidelberg symposium. Birkhäuser, Basel, pp 373-380

Meyer JS, Rao BR, Stevens SC, White WL (1977) Low incidence of oestrogen receptors in breast carcinoma with rapid rates of cellular replication. Cancer 40: 2290

Nolvadex Adjuvant Trial Organisation (NATO) (1983) Controlled trial of tamoxifen as single adjuvant agent in management of early breast cancer. Interim analysis at 4 years by NATO. Lancet i: 257-261

Nolvadex Adjuvant Trial Organisation (NATO) (1985a) Controlled trial of tamoxifen as single adjuvant agent in management of early breast cancer. Analysis at 6 years by NATO. Lancet i: 836-840

Nolvadex Adjuvant Trial Organisation (NATO) (1985b) Six-year results of a controlled trial of tamoxifen as single adjuvant agent in management of early breast cancer. World J Surg 9: 756-764

Paterson RP, Russell MH (1959) Clinical trials in malignant disease. J Fac Radiol (Lond) 10: 130

Popper KR (1959) The logic of scientific discovery. Hutchinson, London

Rose DP, Davis TE (1977) Ovarian function in patients receiving adjuvant chemotherapy for breast cancer. Lancet i: 1174

Sainsbury JRC, Farndon JR, Sherbet GV, Harris AL (1985) Epidermal-growth factor receptors and oestrogen receptors in human breast cancer. Lancet i: 364-366

Steele RJC (1983) Clinical, histological and immunological studies in human breast cancer. MD thesis, University of Edinburgh

Trivedi D (1986) Antigenic profile of human breast tumours. PhD thesis, University of London

UK Breast Cancer Trials Cancer Coordinating Committee/UICC (1984) Review of mortality results in randomised trials in early breast cancer. Lancet ii: 1205

Waterfield MD, Scrace GT, Whittle N, et al (1983) Platelet-derived growth factor is structurally related to the putative transforming protein p28 of simian sarcoma virus. Nature 304: 34

A Critical Assessment of Approaches to Improving the Efficiency of Cancer Clinical Trials

R. Simon

National Cancer Institute, Landow Building, Room 4B06, Bethesda, MD 20892, USA

Introduction

There are many reasons for focusing attention on the efficiency of clinical trials. First, improving the efficiency of clinical trials may expedite the finding of improved treatments. Developing an effective treatment may be a multistep process involving failures and partial successes along the way. Improving the efficiency of each component clinical trial expedites the entire process. The proliferation of new treatments derived from an improved understanding of tumor biology provides an additional inducement to improve the efficiency by which we screen and evaluate treatments. There are also often strong ethical motivations for conducting each clinical trial as efficiently as possible. If one treatment is more effective than the other, then certainly one wishes to expose as few patients as possible to the inferior treatment. If the treatments are of equivalent antitumor efficacy but the new experimental therapy is more toxic, as is often the case, then one would like to discard the new treatment as soon as possible. In addition to the opportunity cost and the ethical cost, there is also a monetary cost providing an incentive to improving efficiency.

Many aspects of clinical trials are related to efficiency. I will attempt to comment here on several aspects that seem particularly important, timely, or relevant to this symposium.

Ask an Important Question

Obviously, the value of a clinical trial is determined in large part by the importance of the question addressed. The most elegantly conducted trial of a mundane or redundant question is of little value. So if we are critically assessing the efficiency of the process of identifying improved treatments, the way to start is by determining whether the most important clinical trials are being conducted. Unfortunately, the most important clinical trials are often the most difficult to organize. This is due to strongly held, but weakly supported, beliefs about the relative merits of the competing treatments. Another common difficulty is redundancy of the

Recent Results in Cancer Research, Vol. 111
© Springer-Verlag Berlin · Heidelberg 1988

concepts tested by different trials. Some degree of redundancy is desirable, but too often there is an excess of similar but different trials, each too small to provide a reliable answer. In such circumstances a meta-analysis of the trials is generally not satisfying, and the field would have been better served by the planning of fewer and larger trials.

The unconditional "power" calculation of Spiegelhalter et al. (1986) provides a way of quantifying the prior probability that a planned trial will demonstrate that an experimental treatment is superior to a control. I dislike the use of the therm "power" in this context, since the probability of obtaining a statistically significant result is averaged over the null hypothesis as well as alternative hypotheses. But the prior distribution for the true treatment difference provides a potentially useful measure of whether the clinical trial is worth doing.

There are, of course, other ways in which defects in the question asked may limit the importance of the clinical trial. For example, the target population may be inappropriately narrow or broad and the endpoint may be wrong. In some cases, tumor response rate is used as the primary endpoint when survival and quality of life are what matter.

Get a Reliable Answer

Getting a reliable answer is second in importance only to asking an important question. Although there is an important role for pilot and exploratory investigations, adding to the literature of inadequate and unreliable comparative trials does not represent efficient use of resources or of the goodwill of patients who wish to participate and contribute to the improvement of therapy. There are many components which influence the reliability of clinical trial results and there is insufficient time to review them here. Nine major components are covered by the Methodologic Guidelines for Clinical Trial Reports (Simon and Wittes 1985) that were developed for Cancer Treatment Reports and have now been adopted by most major cancer journals. Some of the key aspects of reliability are use of randomized treatment assignment, adequate sample size, good data quality, protocol adherence, sufficient follow-up, avoidance of exclusions, appropriate analysis, and lack of data dredging.

Large Simple Trials

Peto and his colleagues have emphasized the importance of very large sample size for identifying treatment improvements that are small to moderate (Yusuf et al. 1984). In the United States there has been a trend toward use of larger sample sizes in the major clinical trials conducted by the cooperative groups. These larger sample sizes are likely to be important for the identification of improved treatments. In some cases, however, the sample sizes advocated by Peto and colleagues are an order of magnitude greater than that used in major cancer clinical trials. In such circumstances they recommend drastic simplification of the logistic apparatus of conventional clinical trials in order to reduce cost per patient and to facilitate the participation of more physicians. Drastic simplification or elimination of data collection, treatment monitoring, pathology review, radiotherapy quality control, and informed consent would be required.

This proposal clearly has some merit. The amount of data collected in some clinical trials is excessive and is a barrier to physician participation. It also adds to the cost of clinical trials. Pathology review is sometimes extraneous, and some policies for the protection of patients from research risks seem unnecessarily bureaucratic and redundant. There are, however, two substantive limitations to the broad adoption of Peto's approach in cancer therapeutics. The first is that some degree of quality control of treatment delivered seems necessary, and such quality control requires more detailed data collection than is employed in Peto's studies of cardiovascular disease. Unless investigators and practitioners have some confidence that the treatment was delivered in reasonable accordance with the protocol, the meaning of a negative result will be ambiguous. Most cancer treatment is more complex or of longer duration than cardiovascular treatments and hence questions of protocol compliance are of more concern. The second issue, somewhat related to the first, is that some cancer treatments are complex or intensive or require special technology and cannot be delivered on a very broad scale by community physicians.

I believe that we should simplify our procedures for conducting clinicals trials to an extent that does not interfere with the principal objectives of the trials. There is resistance to such simplification on the part of some study chairpersons, but the importance of simplification for improving the efficiency of clinical trials means that careful review of procedures and data forms employed by each clinical trial organization is warranted.

Sequential Analysis

For many years there has been an obvious gap between the large volume of statistical literature on sequential analysis and the limited number of applications of the theory. Within the past few years this gap has narrowed, due to developments of the theory that make the methods more applicable to real clinical trials. Consequently, today sequential design and analysis is a meaningful method for improving the efficiency of clinical trials. There are, however, important limitations to the use of this tool. Some of these limitations are the following.

Data Quality

Interim analysis is dangerous unless the data on which it is based are reliable. Data collection in clinical trials is generally complex and involves many individuals. Bringing the data base up to date and verifying its accuracy is a prerequisite for an interim analysis. Consequently, proper interim analyses are themselves expensive and cannot be performed too often.

Survival Data

Survival or disease-free survival is the key endpoint for most cancer studies. In many cases survival times are commensurate with the accrual period of the trial. Consequently, by the time there is a sufficient number of events on which to perform an interim analysis, most of the patients to be accrued will already have been entered. The extent to which this is a limitation depends on the target sample size, the accrual rate, and the survival distributions, but it is a meaningful limitation to the potential value of sequential analysis in many cancer clinical trials. Sequential analysis can, however, facilitate the design of a follow-on study even if it does not substantially reduce the number of patients required for the original trial.

Another difficulty is that the early part of a survival curve, the part available at the time of interim analysis, provides little or no information about the later parts of the curve. We might assume that the two distributions being compared have proportional hazards. Under such an assumption, the relationship between the early parts of the two survival curves determines the relationship between the later parts, but we must remember that this is only an assumption that cannot be tested from the data at hand. In this sense, sequential analysis of survival data is "hazardous" unless the forms of the survival curves are known or the probability of survival beyond a meaningful time point on the plateau of the curve is used as the endpoint.

Multiple Endpoints and Subsets

In many clinical trials there are several endpoints of interest and several subsets of patients included. Interim analysis is often a nonalgorithmic process whose complexity is much greater than that which is incorporated in the statistical design.

The Need for a Replacement Study

If one treatment is found convincingly superior to the other in an interim analysis, there is an ethical need to terminate the trial. This rarely happens in cancer trials. Treatment differences are usually not large and the statistical power of interim analyses of survival data is usually low. It is more common to find that an interim analysis reveals that current results are inconsistent with the treatment difference targeted in planning the study. The method of stochastic curtailment (Lan et al. 1982) was originally developed for evaluating such a circumstance. The method of sequential confidence limits of Jennison and Turnbull (1984) and the two-stage designs of Ellenberg and Eisenberger (1985) and of Thall et al. (1988a) also provide useful sequential designs for early termination when the experimental treatment is not doing sufficiently well. Although such designs provide a potential enhancement to the efficiency of cancer clinical trials, they are sometimes not used because of the unavailability of a replacement study. Clinical trial organizations are often reluctant to terminate a study without starting another unless there is an ethical need to do so. This limitation to improvement in efficiency can be avoided with better planning.

Complexity of the Sequential Analysis Literature

The literature on sequential analysis is voluminous and complex. This in itself forms a barrier to the use of sequential designs. There are, however, simple designs that are easy to use and provide much of the potential efficiency of the more complex methods. The methods of Peto (1978), O'Brien and Fleming (1979), Ellenberg and Eisenberger (1985), Thall et al. (1988a), Lan et al. (1982), and Jennison and Turnbull (1984) are of this type. Peto's method permits continuous or sporadic monitoring and involves early termination to reject the null hypothesis only if the significance level is less than 0.001 (0.002 for one-sided tests). If early rejection does not occur, then the final analysis is essentially unaffected by interim monitoring. O'Brien and Fleming provided a similarly conservative method for group-sequential monitoring. It also has the property that if early rejection of the null hypothesis does not occur, then final analysis is unaffected by the interim monitoring. Thall, Simon, and Ellenberg developed a two-stage design for comparing an experimental treatment with a control, in which one may accept the null hypothesis of equivalence at the end of the first stage. Their design is based on a previous design of Ellenberg and Eisenberger. They also indicated how this can be used in conjunction with the O'Brien and Fleming upper boundary for early rejection of the null hypothesis. The design of Thall, Simon, and Ellenberg is optimal among two-stage designs in that the average expected sample size (averaged over the null and alternative hypotheses) is minimum subject to the specified type-one and -two errors. Lan, Simon, and Halperin developed the method of stochastic curtailment by which a trial can be terminated early, with either acceptance or rejection of the null hypothesis, if the probability of falling in the fixed sample size rejection region is sufficiently small or large respectively. These probabilities are calculated conditional on the data available at the time of interim analysis and under the alternative and null hypotheses respectively. The methods of Peto, O'Brien and Fleming, Ellenberg and Eisenberger, and that of Lan, Simon, and Halperin can all be used for monitoring a trial in which the target sample size was determined using a standard fixed sample size formula. The method of Thall, Simon, and Ellenberg requires a small increase in maximum sample size in order to maintain statistical power at the desired level.

Jennison and Turnbull (1984) provided a simple method for calculating sequential confidence limits for the difference in treatment efficacy. Confidence limits are very useful for interpreting interim results, as they indicate clearly what size effects are consistent with the data at hand (Simon 1986). The use of sequential confidence intervals and stochastic curtailment together provides a very powerful approach to interim monitoring. In some studies the rate of patient accrual is much less than expected. Consequently, although interim results are not definitive, the calculations of stochastic curtailment may reveal that the conditional power by the end of a fixed accrual period will be so low that one may wish to terminate the trial prematurely.

Factorial Designs

Peto (1978) and Byar and Piantadosi (1985) have suggested that factorial designs provide great potential for improving the efficiency of clinical trials. They asserted that one can answer two questions for about the price (sample size) of one. Since Peto's initial claim was made, statisticians have been looking for opportunities to apply factorial designs in cancer clinical trials but have found relatively few appropriate situations (Crowley 1985). I believe that there are two main limitations to the applicability of factorial designs to cancer clinical trials. First, many types of therapy have overlapping toxicity, so the level of one factor (e.g., drug) influences the timing or dose of the other factor. Proper factorial designs cannot be used in such situations. The second limitation is that the results of a 2×2 factorial trial can be unambiguously interpreted only if one assumes that there is no interaction between the factors and response, i.e., that the effect of one factor on response does not depend on the level of the other factor. Proponents of factorial designs sometimes claim as a strength the opportunity to discover such interactions. But it is easily shown that the statistical power for discovering such interactions is very low if the experiment has been designed to "answer two questions for the price of one." Are such interactions likely? The answer depends on the type of trial. If the factors represent the presence or absence of drugs, and if it is unlikely that both drugs are effective by themselves, then one might consider an interaction unlikely. But this would not be a reasonable assumption for biochemical modulation studies where an ineffective drug modulates the activity of another drug which may or may not be effective by itself. Most combination chemotherapy or combined chemotherapy-radiotherapy studies involve combining factors which themselves may very well be effective. It would be hazardous to assume, however, that if both factors are effective then the combination is more effective that either factor alone. Factorial analysis is based on such an assumption. Proponents of factorial designs sometimes say that the ambiguity of interpretation is unimportant unless there is a qualitative interaction between the effect of one factor and the level of the other. A qualitative interaction would correspond to a situation where the effect of factor A is positive at level zero of factor B, but the effect of factor A is negative at level one of factor B. When dealing with toxic or expensive treatments, however, changes in the magnitude of effects can be as important as qualitative interactions. Suppose chemotherapy is effective in the absence of radiotherapy but is not beneficial in the presence of radiotherapy. Analysis should determine whether this is the case, not assume it away because it is not a "qualitative interaction."

Factorial designs are clearly appropriate in some situations and are probably worth trying in some others. Although their realm of applicability seems limited in cancer clinical trials, statisticians should bear them in mind since they can be very useful.

Selection Designs

Classical experimental designs tend to require large numbers of patients because we require a small type-one error for testing the null hypothesis of equivalence. Why do we require this? Regulatory requirements that new treatments be demonstrated to be effective are sometimes a reason. We also want to know the truth about whether one treatment is more effective. The treatments often differ in cost and toxicity, and so selection of one treatment over another is a complex and subjective matter. Some situations, however, are simpler. If the treatments are similar in cost, toxicity, and complexity of administration, then choice among them may be based on a clinical trial designed using selection theory. There is a large amount of literature on ranking and selection theory, and the use of this theory in phase-2 trials is described by Simon et al. (1985). The design constraint usually employed is that if one treatment is superior by a specified amount d, then the probability of selecting it at the end of the trial must be at least some large constant P. For binary responses d may be a difference of 15 percentage points and P may be 0.90 or 0.95. It is assumed that one treatment will always be selected, regardless of how similar the final results are.

Thall et al. (1988b) have recently used selection ideas in the design of phase-3 trials. Their designs are of the two-stage type in which K experimental treatments are compared in the first stage. One experimental treatment is then selected to be compared with a control during the second stage. They employ a classical type-one error constraint for rejecting the null hypothesis that no experimental treatments are superior to the control. They also utilize a power constraint and determine the designs that minimize average expected sample size. Their design also has the property that no second stage is conducted if results for the experimental treatments in the first stage are unsatisfactory. Thall et al. (1988c) have also developed a similar design that uses the control treatment in both the first and second stage. This permits the first-stage data to be employed in the final analysis comparing the selected experimental treatment with the control. These designs were developed for situations with binary response, where there are too few patients to fully compare all candidate experimental treatments with the control. The objective of these designs is to identify one experimental treatment which is substantially better than the control and to provide conventionally strong evidence, a small type-one error, that an experimental treatment is in fact superior to the control.

Selection designs have also been studied by Whitehead (1985, 1986) for phase-2 and phase-3 trials. Whitehead takes a Bayesian approach, and his designs are directed to the situation where there is a large number of candidate experimental treatments. Both Whitehead's designs and those of Thall, Simon, and Ellenberg represent attempts to improve the efficiency of a program of treatment development when more than one new treatment is available. These designs can in some sense be viewed as alternatives to the conventional use of uncontrolled pilot studies for determining what regimen to test in a phase-3 trial. With the proliferation of interesting biological therapies available for evaluation, such designs warrant careful consideration in the design of clinical trials.

Response Surface Designs

Carter et al. (1983) have urged that response surface designs be used more often in cancer clinical trials. In a response surface design for two drugs, response as a function of the dosages of the two drugs would be explored. Alternatively, the time between administrations of the two drugs could be one of the dimensions instead of dose. With binary response, Carter et al. generally use a logit model with a quadratic function of the doses. After fitting the model, they determine confidence regions for the optimal dose vector and for the response at the optimum. The former confidence region permits them to determine whether there is "therapeutic synergism." Synergism in this context means that the response at the optimum is significantly greater than the best response that can be achieved with either single agent. Response surface designs could also be contemplated with survival as endpoint. But since it would be unethical to explore the region of the parameter space in which survival decreased because of treatment-related mortality, one would have to optimize along the boundary subject to constraints on toxicity. This approach has not been well explored.

With response surface designs the patients are allocated among a large number of "dose" combinations. Typically, five to ten patients per design point are used and many design points are included. This approach is conducive to fitting the response surface and evaluating the adequacy of fit. It is, of course, a very unconventional way of conducting a clinical trial and introduces many logistical and statistical complexities. For example, can the participating physicians reliably administer therapy in so many different ways? Do you fit the response surface using the doses assigned or the doses actually used? How do you stratify effectively with so many dosage groups? And there are many other challenging issues (Crowley 1985).

Response surface designs have been used very little in cancer clinical trials. Perhaps one of the main reasons is that they do not seem to fit into the conventional phase 1, 2, 3 framework. They require large sample sizes but are not conventional phase-3 trials. They should be considered, however, for optimizing combinations of proven effectiveness.

Prognostic Factors

The identification of important prognostic factors can improve the efficiency of clinical trials. Although many "statistically significant" prognostic factors are known, they generally explain a very small proportion of the variability in outcome among patients (Simon 1984). If a substantial portion of the variability in outcome can be accounted for by known factors, then treatment effects can be estimated more precisely and sample sizes reduced. Identification of major prognostic factors also permits the targeting of trials to more appropriate patient populations. For example, reduction of morbidity may be studied in good-risk patients and improvement of antitumor effect in poor-risk patients. This has been the successful course of research for several pediatric malignant diseases. Major improvement of prognostic prediction requires collaboration with investigators who utilize the most current biological assays, collection of large data bases, and improvement of statistical methodology for identifying and validating prognostic indicators.

References

Byar DP, Piantadosi S (1985) Factorial designs for randomized clinical trials. Cancer Treat Rep 10: 1055-1062
Carter WH Jr, Wampler GL, Stablein DM (1983) Regression methods in the analysis of survival data in cancer combination chemotherapy. Dekker, New York
Crowley J (1985) Discussion. Cancer Treat Rep 10: 1079-1080
Ellenberg SS, Eisenberger MA (1985) An efficient design for phase-III studies of combination chemotherapies. Cancer Treat Rep 10: 1147-1152
Jennison C, Turnbull BW (1984) Repeated confidence intervals for group sequential clinical trials. Controlled Clin Trials 5: 33-45
Lan KKG, Simon R, Halperin M (1982) Stochastically curtailed tests in long-term clinical trials. Commun Stat Sequential Anal 1: 207-219
O'Brien PC, Fleming TR (1979) A multiple testing procedure for clinical trials. Biometrics 35: 549-556
Peto R (1978) Clinical trial methodology. Biomedicine (Paris) 28: 24-36
Simon R (1984) The importance of prognostic factors in cancer clinical trials. Cancer Treat Rep 68: 185-192
Simon R (1986) Confidence intervals for reporting clinical trial results. Ann Intern Med 105: 4429-4435
Simon R, Wittes RE (1985) Methodologic guidelines for clinical trial reports. Cancer Treat Rep 69: 1-3
Simon R, Wittes RE, Ellenberg SS (1985) Randomized phase-II clinical trials. Cancer Treat Rep 69: 1375-1381
Spiegelhalter DJ, Freedman LS, Blackburn PR (1986) Monitoring clinical trials: conditional or predictive power? Controlled Clin Trials 7: 8-17
Thall PF, Simon R, Ellenberg SS (1988a) Optimal two-stage designs for clinical trials with binary response. Stat Med (in press)
Thall PF, Simon R, Ellenberg SS (1988b) A two-stage design for choosing among several experimental treatments and a control in phase-III clinical trials.
Thall PF, Simon R, Ellenberg SS (1988c) Two-stage selection and testing designs for comparative clinical trials. Biometrika (in press)
Yusuf S, Collins R, Peto R (1984) Why do we need some large, simple randomized trials? Stat Med 3: 409-420
Whitehead J (1985) Designing phase-II studies in the context of a programme of clinical research. Biometrics 41: 373-383
Whitehead J (1986) Sample sizes for phase-II and phase-III clinical trials: an integrated approach. Stat Med 5: 459-464

Statistical Standards for Protocols and Protocol Deviations

J. A. Lewis*

ICI Pharmaceuticals, Alderley Park, Macclesfield, Cheshire SK10 4TG, Great Britain

Introduction

Any pharmaceutical company involved in drug research in a major way is likely to develop internal standards for its clinical trial work. This is particularly so as the number of staff increases because of the need to control standards and to maintain consistent approaches. Statistical work is no exception, whether concerned with the design or the analysis of clinical trials.

Within ICI, the statisticians are in the process of developing a series of written guidelines for the statistical aspects of clinical trial work. The first two topics tackled have been 'The Protocol' and 'Protocol Deviations', and preliminary drafts of these have been produced. They are presented here not as polished finished articles, but as working documents which will undoubtedly develop further with experience.

The Protocol

The protocol of a clinical trial normally contains two sections which are the specific responsibility of the appropriate statistician: (a) the justification of the number of patients, and (b) the proposed methods of statistical analysis.

Under special circumstances the statistician also writes sections on the following topics: (c) the justification of the experimental design, (d) randomisation, and (e) the justification of certain inclusion/exclusion criteria.

Justification of the Number of Patients

A statistical justification of the number of patients is provided unless adequate reasons exist as to why this is not possible or appropriate. These reasons should be stated. The justification normally states the following:

* I am happy to acknowledge the input of my statistical colleagues within ICI and in particular that of S. H. Ellis, who had a major influence on the topic of protocol deviations.

© Springer-Verlag Berlin · Heidelberg 1988

1. The relevant primary end point
2. The main treatment comparison of interest
3. The assumed control mean or rate
4. The treatment effect to be detected
5. The estimated underlying variability
6. The values of type-I and type-II errors

Any nonstandard methodology is described in more detail, if necessary in an appendix. Detailed explorations of power curves should also appear in an appendix.

If a trial is designated to detect 'no difference', a minimum difference which it would be important to detect should be used in power calculations.

If plausible assumptions for the relevant control and treated results cannot be made, then the following actions are possible:

1. Base power calculations on a simpler end point, e.g. percentage response rate
2. Use trial to assess required numbers in future work
3. Carry out interim analysis to assess required trial size

In general, the level of α should reflect the prior probability of the hypothesis to be tested. The level of β should reflect the probability of ever replicating the trial, or the importance of getting a definitive result with this trial alone.

It may be necessary to allow for a proportion of patients who will not complete the trial, and if so, this should be stated.

If there are several primary end points, the number of patients should be adequate to satisfy the most stringent requirement.

Trials with inadequate power should be undertaken only if there are plans to combine the results with those from other trials to achieve adequate power, or if it can be shown that the information gained from such a trial will have a clear purpose irrespective of power considerations.

The following is an example of the justification of patient numbers:

Example 1. It is hoped that the addition of treatment X to treatment A will produce a minimum further fall in diastolic blood pressure of 5 mmHg, and this is the minimum difference this trial is aiming to detect. Based on the relevant estimate of variability from an earlier trial (residual within patient sd of 8 mmHg, Bloggs and Bloggs, ICI 065432/0010, data on file), power calculations show that about 20 patients will be required in this crossover trial ($\alpha=0.05$, $\beta=0.1$). The planned size of 24 patients will allow for patients who do not complete the trial.

A simple statement to cover the situation when patient numbers cannot be justified might be as follow:

Example 2. This is the first hospital trial of ICI 123,546 in which ear-lobe distension has been measured as the primary end point. No reliable data exist on which to base estimates of patient numbers, either in the literature or in earlier studies of ICI 123,546. The trial size is therefore based on feasibility, and its adequacy will be assessed at the time of analysis.

Methods of Statistical Analysis

The proposed methods of statistical analysis are outlined, unless no analysis is anticipated. The following topics should be addressed: The primary and secondary end points should be specified unless they are clear from the rest of the protocol. Similarly, the main treatment comparisons to be investigated should be clarified if necessary. The intention to summarise all other data should be stated.

It should be stated that the influence of patients who do not complete the trial will be examined. If possible, the relevant methodology should be specified, e.g. the use of 'intent to treat' analysis.

Any plans to use baseline values, covariates, or factors in analysis of variance to improve precision and/or remove bias should be stated.

Estimation, in addition to significance testing, should receive appropriate mention. Critical *P*-values should not be stated in advance except in the case of early stopping rules. It is better to leave the specific significance tests unstated, unless it is quite obvious and helps the description of methodology.

Any preplanned subgroup analyses should be specified. Any preplanned interim analysis, sequential analysis, or group sequential analysis should be described together with the stopping rules.

If it is anticipated that end points will be combined (by addition or averaging or otherwise) or transformed, then the ways in which they will be combined or transformed should be specified as completely as possible to avoid post hoc selection bias.

The intention to use one-tailed significance tests should be stated and justified.

The personnel responsible for the analysis should be identified. Mention of the statistical software, e.g. the SAS package, is not essential but is occasionally helpful.

The following is a sample statement regarding the methods of statistical analysis proposed:

The primary end points of this two-period crossover trial are post-exercise systolic and diastolic blood pressure. Secondary end points are standing and sitting blood pressure and heart rate. The main treatment comparison of interest is the randomised comparison of treatments A und B. Primary and secondary end points will be subjected to analysis of variance in order to estimate the difference between the effects of A and B and to test its statistical significance. In order to improve precision and to remove bias, the analysis will attempt to allow for differences between patients and between periods, and for any carryover effects of treatment. The measurements made during the run-in and washout periods will also be used to improve precision where possible. Any potential biasing influence of withdrawals and protocol deviants will be explored and minimised. Information on patient characteristics, adverse effects and compliance will be summarised. The analysis will be carried out by the statistical staff of ICI Pharmaceuticals Division.

Justification of the Design

Design justification should appear whenever the rationale for, and detail of, the design would not be clear to a reviewing experienced statistician. For example: (a) crossover designs, in a field of medicine where reasonable doubt may exist about their validity; (b) complex or unbalanced crossover designs; (c) group sequential designs; (d) Zelen (randomised consent) designs.

Randomisation

Specific details are required whenever there are points which would need to be clarified to an experienced reviewing statistician.

Examples are the use of stratification and the use of 'blocking'.

Inclusion/Exclusion Criteria

Occasionally, issues arise which need to be addressed by the statistician in the protocol. For example, statistical comment should accompany the intention to allow retrospective exclusion of patients after entry to the trial on the grounds of a baseline measurement, which requires several days to assay.

Protocol Deviations

The term 'protocol deviations' is taken here to include any foreseen or unforeseen departures from the ideal experimental procedures. Thus, it includes withdrawals, for example. Patients may deviate from the protocol in two main ways: (a) by violation of the entry criteria, or (b) by deviation from the protocol after entry.

Some deviations are envisaged in the protocol and appropriate actions are specified. For example, further follow-up of the patients who are withdrawn may be required and specific methods of statistical analysis may be planned. Other unanticipated deviations are discovered during the conduct of the trial or after its completion. One aim underlies all attempts to compensate for the effects of departures from the protocol, namely the avoidance or minimisation of bias in the treatment comparisons of interest.

Violations of the Entry Criteria

Entry criteria serve two broad purposes. First, they attempt to maximise the treatment effects of interest (generally efficacy) by selection of a group of patients who are expected to benefit. These are usually the inclusion criteria. Second, they attempt to exclude a subgroup of these patients who may be potentially harmed by entry to the trial. These are usually the exclusion criteria.

It is clearly important for all those involved with the trial to try to minimise the number of ineligible patients who enter the trial. This can be done by the use of eligibility checklists, and by drawing the investigators' attention to patients entered in error. During protocol design, attempts should be made to relax the entry criteria as far as possible. Treatment effects often persist in a far wider population than is originally supposed, and patients are generally in short supply.

The post hoc detection of violators of the entry criteria is possible only if the relevant entry data are collected, preferably in machine-readable form.

When patients actively taking part in the trial are found to have violated the entry criteria, the appropriate immediate action depends upon the type of criterion involved. If it is one concerned with efficacy, then the patient is likely to be dropped eventually from the analysis, and hence continued follow-up is necessary only if there are cogent safety considerations. On the other hand, if such a patient violated a safety criterion, then he may well eventually contribute useful efficacy data to the analysis. In this case the preferred action is continued participation and follow-up, but, again, safety considerations must come first.

As indicated above, the analysis of efficacy should generally include violators of safety criteria who successfully complete the trial and should exclude violators of efficacy criteria. The analysis of safety should include all patients.

If the reason for detecting a violator of the entry criteria is related to the treatment the patient is receiving (e.g. an operative procedure may uncover underlying medical conditions), then such a patient should be retained in the analysis whatever the type of criterion violated. Otherwise, bias may be introduced by selective removal of patients from one arm of the trial only.

Retrospective exclusion of patients is sometimes proposed when a rather long assay procedure (for example) is required to determine an essential baseline characteristic. The time lag may be so long that the patient has to start randomised treatment before the result is known. Such retrospective exclusion is permissible, provided that the result and its interpretation cannot conceivably be influenced by the allocated treatment.

Deviations After Entry

Patients may deviate from the protocol in a large number of ways, of which the following are the most common:

1. Withdrawal by the clinician
2. Withdrawal by the patient (dropout)
3. Poor tablet compliance
4. Poor visit compliance
5. Wrong treatment given
6. Missing/unreliable data

The first aim should be to avoid or foresee as many of these problems as possible, and to plan appropriate actions which should follow such deviations. Clear explanations and written instructions to the patient obviously help. Early detection of deviations may help the investigator to avoid them with later patients. Follow-up of withdrawn patients, for example, may be possible only if it is planned ahead of time in the protocol.

Withdrawn patients pose the most common problem. Withdrawal should be avoided whenever possible - temporary cessation of treatment is generally to be preferred to complete withdrawal. When patients are withdrawn it is important to ascertain the reasons, so that they can be classified as treatment failures (side effects, lack of efficacy), random reasons, or even treatment successes (cure). This should be pursued when the patient drops out. Continued follow-up after withdrawal, as per protocol, is nearly always helpful and may be essential in the case of adverse reactions.

The most widely known method of analysis which satisfactorily allows for withdrawals is the so-called intention-to-treat analysis. This is appropriate whenever it is possible to define an end point for each patient on a single scale, irrespective of withdrawal which is directly related to the hypothesis under test. Mortality studies to investigate treatment *policies* are ideal in this respect. The use of extreme values (Gould's method) to represent treatment successes or failures also exemplifies this approach. Such methods estimate without bias the effect of the treatment policy but usually underestimate the magnitude of the treatment effect in compliant patients. Hence, it is usually worth exploring the 'on-treatment' effect in addition, in order to demonstrate that the effect is enhanced in accordance with common sense.

An *explanatory* analysis will generally be more appropriate to the earlier phases of drug development. This is concerned with explaining and exploring the scientific phenomena underlying the treatment effect. Hence, it will focus on patients who comply and will risk potential upward bias in the magnitude of the treatment effect.

A 'last-value' analysis is often helpful.

Overall, the aim of analysis should be to show that any conclusions drawn are robust to different plausible assumptions concerning the withdrawals. This will often involve alternative analyses.

Poor tablet compliance can be reduced by eliminating patients who show poor compliance during a run-in prerandomisation period. If it is intended to divide patients into different compliance categories during the analysis, it is always better if those categories are defined in the protocol. Attempts to associate efficacy with the degree of compliance are sometimes satisfactory. In general, tablet counts should be regarded with a healthy scepticism as they are subject to so many unknown influences. Blood levels are more acceptable, but great care should be taken to avoid the mixing up of samples.

Poor visit compliance is commonly handled by defining 'visit windows' within which the visit is acceptable, and hence the data analysable. Such windows are best defined in the protocol.

If the wrong treatment is administered to a patient, then the appropriate policy depends upon the reason for that treatment being given. If it was purely random then the patient may be analysed as treated. If it was deliberate (e.g. the patient was thought to need that treatment) then the patient should be excluded from the analysis.

This policy should not be followed if the trial is clearly intended to examine treatment policy via an 'intention-to-treat' philosophy. Under these circumstances, patients should be analysed as randomised, regardless of the treatment administered.

The *replacement* of withdrawn patients is not good practice. This means that patients, once entered, should feature in the analysis as fully as their data allow. If the dropout rate is giving cause for concern, then further patients should be added by extending the random scheme.

Crossover Trials

Crossover trials pose some special problems. For instance, if a patient withdraws with an adverse reaction during the second period of a two-period crossover trial, then a 'within-patient' comparison of the treatment is not available from that patient. In addition, if he or she withdraws due to an adverse effect, it may be impossible to determine which treatment was responsible. For these reasons, crossover trials should be avoided if a substantial withdrawal rate is anticipated.

During the conduct of a crossover trial, patients who withdraw from an early treatment period should always be reinstated on their later treatment period(s) where possible. This minimises potential biases and maximises the available information.

The concept of 'intention to treat' cannot be applied to a crossover trial.

The analysis of a multiperiod crossover trial should make use of all available data from withdrawn patients, because useful information relating to treatment comparisons is available in the completed treatment periods. If only one treatment period is available, then no harm is done by leaving that patient in the analysis, and this is the current policy.

The Design of Cancer Prevention Trials

D. P. Byar

Biometry Branch, Division of Cancer Prevention and Control, National Cancer Institute, Blair Building, Room 5A05, 9000 Rockville Pike, Bethesda, MD 20892-4200, USA

The idea of using randomized clinical trials to study cancer prevention is relatively new. In fact, to my knowledge, only a few such trials have been completed and only a few dozen such trials are currently underway in the entire world. This situation contrasts sharply with that for cardiovascular disease, where large-scale randomized intervention trials have been used as a method of study for several decades. In this article I want to show how the design of cancer prevention trials depends on our general concept of carcinogenesis and then describe some real trials which are underway or in the planning stages in order to illustrate some special design considerations that arise in these trials. Finally, I will summarize what seem to me to be some of the major differences between treatment and prevention trials.

Carcinogenesis and Types of Prevention Trials

Our current concept of the process of carcinogenesis has been described as "an over-simplified schematic of a poorly understood process" (Bertram et al. 1987). Nevertheless, it is now pretty well known from experimental research that the process of carcinogenesis is divided into at least two stages which have been called "initiation" and "promotion" (Fig. 1). These terms come largely from animal experiments where cancer is deliberately produced in rodents by using chemicals or other insults. It has been observed that the order in which one applies such carcinogens is important. Certain agents appear to initiate cancer, while those designated as promoters are effective only after cancer has been initiated with some other agent. Some agents may act as both initiators and promoters. The importance of these observations is that they demonstrate that the process of carcinogenesis has at least two steps. It is then assumed that some of these initiated and promoted cells develop into precancerous lesions. There are many names for such lesions, depending on the sites where they arise. Examples include leukoplakia in the mouth, dysplasia in the esophagus, cervical dysplasia, polyps in the colon, and superficial recurrent papillomas in the urinary bladder. The characteristic feature is that there is an anatomical abnormality which may be diagnosed by direct inspection, endoscopic examination, or microscopic study.

Recent Results in Cancer Research, Vol. 111
© Springer-Verlag Berlin · Heidelberg 1988

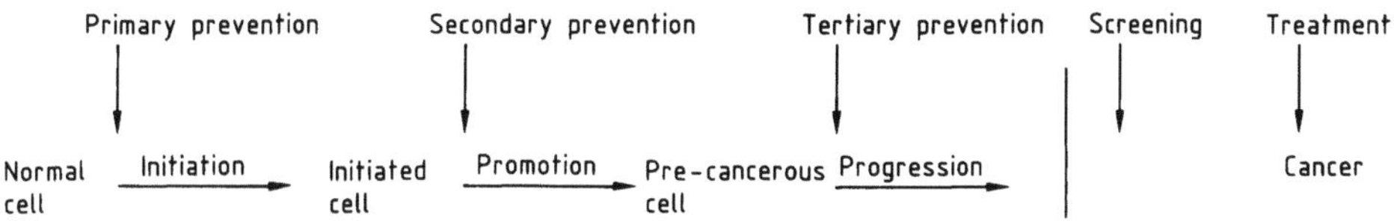

Fig. 1. Stages in the process of carcinogenesis at which various preventive measures are presumed to act and where screening and treatment occur

The vertical line in Fig. 1 designates the point at which most pathologists would no longer designate lesions as precancerous but would actually diagnose cancer. Screening and treatment trials, of course, are concerned with that portion of the horizontal line representing the carcinogenic process after a definite diagnosis of cancer has been made. Conceptually, then, prevention trials can take place anywhere along the line before that point. One difficulty is that we do not know how long the line is for any particular cancer, but we suspect that it must be at least decades in length for certain cancers because we know, for example, that the age at menarche is a risk factor for breast cancer and that subjects may smoke for 20–30 years before developing lung cancer. Bertram et al. (1987) proposed dividing cancer prevention trials into three categories - primary, secondary, and tertiary - depending on where in the carcinogenic process the preventive measure is supposed to intervene. For example, a trial designed to encourage teenagers to avoid taking up tobacco smoking would be called a primary prevention trial. On the other hand, a trial designed to encourage smokers to quit or a trial of dietary modification may be termed a secondary prevention trial if it is assumed that the carcinogenic process has already begun and we are attempting to interrupt it by decreasing cancer promotion. The subjects in primary and secondary prevention trials do not have detectable lesions although they may be chosen to be at high risk for developing cancer. After precancerous lesions are present we may then speak of tertiary prevention trials whose goal is to alter these lesions either by making them regress or disappear, or by preventing their development into cancer. Screening trials have sometimes been called secondary prevention trials, but this usage is confusing and should be avoided. The design of tertiary prevention trials is similar to that of treatment trials and will not be dealt with in this article because an abundant literature deals with such designs. Instead, I will discuss a few special design features that may be considered for primary and secondary prevention trials.

Factorial Designs

A complete factorial design refers to an experiment where two or more factors are under study at two or more levels each, and all combinations of treatments and levels are represented in the design. The simplest example is the 2^2 or 2×2 factorial design, in which each of two factors may be either present or absent, so that we have four treatment groups: one receiving neither factor, one each receiving a single factor, and, finally, a group receiving both factors. Such a design in effect allows us to answer two questions for the price of one. All the data are used to

Table 1. Results and analysis of a 2×2 factorial trial with N subjects in each cell

		B	
		No	Yes
A	No	$\overline{X}$	$\overline{X}_B$
	Yes	$\overline{X}_A$	$\overline{X}_{AB}$

Main Effect of A $= \dfrac{(\overline{X}_{AB}-\overline{X}_B)+(\overline{X}_A-\overline{X})}{2}$

Main Effect of B $= \dfrac{(\overline{X}_{AB}-\overline{X}_A)+(\overline{X}_B-\overline{X})}{2}$

Interaction of A with B $= (\overline{X}_{AB}-\overline{X}_B)-(\overline{X}_A-\overline{X})$

Interaction of B with A $= (\overline{X}_{AB}-\overline{X}_A)-(\overline{X}_B-\overline{X})$

answer each of the questions: does factor A work, and does factor B work? In addition, information is available on their joint action, which could not have been obtained by two separate studies. To illustrate these ideas, suppose that we have studied N patients in a simple 2 × 2 factorial trial and that the responses for each of these four groups can be summarized as means, designated as $\overline{X}$ in Table 1. Below the table are the simple formulae used to compute the main effects of A and B and their interaction. For example, we have two estimates of the effect of A, $\overline{X}_A$-$\overline{X}$ and $\overline{X}_{AB}$-$\overline{X}_B$, so we simply average these two measures to estimate what is called the main effect of A. A similar procedure is followed for estimating the main effect of B. Factors A with B are said to interact on this linear scale if the effect of factor A is different in the presence and absence of factor B. We thus compute the difference in the estimate of the effect of factor A in the presence or absence of factor B. If this difference is zero we conclude that there is no interaction. An interaction of A with B means precisely the same thing as an interaction of B with A. Note that the two formulae are algebraically identical.

These ideas generalize easily to more than two factors. For example, the design for a complete balanced 2^3 or 2 × 2 × 2 factorial design is illustrated in Table 2. Below the layout for the eight treatment groups, I have given the estimates for the main effects of A, the AB interaction, and the ABC interaction. Again, the important thing to note is that all the data are used for all the estimates, but that some of the algebraic signs of the means for the various treatment groups change. The only other thing that changes as we estimate higher orders of interactions is the number of independent estimates provided by the design, and this is reflected by the fractions in front of the estimates for the main effect of A and the AB interaction. Because there are four separate estimates in the 2^3 design for the main effect of A, we divide by four in order to average these; there are two estimates of the AB interaction (in the presence and absence of C), so we divide by two; and there is only a single estimate of the ABC or highest-order interaction. The practical consequence is that we have more statistical power to estimate the main effects than the two-way interactions, and more power for the two-way interactions than for the three-

Table 2. Results and analysis of a 2^3 or $2 \times 2 \times 2$ complete, balanced factorial design

A	B	C	Results
−	−	−	$\overline{X}$
−	−	+	$\overline{X}_C$
−	+	−	$\overline{X}_B$
−	+	+	$\overline{X}_{BC}$
+	−	−	$\overline{X}_A$
+	−	+	$\overline{X}_{AC}$
+	+	−	$\overline{X}_{AB}$
+	+	+	$\overline{X}_{ABC}$

Main effect of A: $\frac{1}{4}(\overline{X}_{ABC}-\overline{X}_{BC})+\frac{1}{4}(\overline{X}_{AC}-\overline{X}_{C})+\frac{1}{4}(\overline{X}_{AB}-\overline{X}_{B})+\frac{1}{4}(\overline{X}_{A}-\overline{X})$

AB interaction: $\frac{1}{2}[(\overline{X}_{ABC}-\overline{X}_{BC})-(\overline{X}_{AC}-\overline{X}_{C})]+\frac{1}{2}[(\overline{X}_{AB}-\overline{X}_{B})-(\overline{X}_{A}-\overline{X})]$

ABC interaction: $[(\overline{X}_{ABC}-\overline{X}_{BC})-(\overline{X}_{AC}-\overline{X}_{C})]-[(\overline{X}_{AB}-\overline{X}_{B})-(\overline{X}_{A}-\overline{X})]$

way interaction. In fact, the ratios of the variances for these three orders of effect are 1:4:16.

As the number of two-level factors (e.g., present and absent) increases, the number of treatment groups increases accordingly as the powers of two. For example, for studying four factors a 2^4 factorial design would have 16 treatment groups. We might find that 16 is too many treatment groups to manage easily in a human intervention study, so a fractional factorial design could be used, in which only a fraction of the total number of treatment groups is studied. For example, in a half-fractional 2^4 design, one studies only eight groups rather than 16. The technique for deciding which cells to study is quite simple. For a half-fractional design one first identifies what is referred to as the "defining interaction." The estimate for this interaction, like that for all the other effects in the full factorial design, will have eight pluses and eight minuses attached to the means of the 16 treatment groups. One simply chooses those treatment groups corresponding either to the pluses or to the minuses to form the half-fractional factorial design. For example, if one chooses the highest-order interaction, that is, the four-way interaction between factors A, B, C and D as the defining interaction, then in a half-fractional factorial design one could study the treatment group receiving none of the factors, the six groups receiving two factors at a time, and the group receiving all four factors. Alternatively, one could choose the complementary set, that is, the four groups receiving only one factor plus the four groups receiving three factors at a time. These two designs are shown schematically in Table 3. The choice between the two designs will generally depend on nonstatistical considerations. For example, design 2 might be preferred if it were deemed unethical to have one group receiving no treatment.

Also shown in Table 3 are the estimates of the main effect of A and of the AB interaction for the two designs. The estimates (except for the constants) can be obtained from the equivalent estimates for the full, balanced 2^4 design by simply deleting the means corresponding to treatment groups not studied in the fractional

Table 3. Two one-half fractional factorial designs for studying four factors

Defining interaction: ABCD	
Design 1	Design 2
Ø	A
AB	B
AC	C
AD	D
BC	ABC
BD	ABD
CD	ACD
ABCD	BCD

Design 1

Main effect of A: $\frac{1}{4}$ [(ABCD + AB) + (AC + AD) − (BC + BD) − (CD + Ø)]

AB interaction: $\frac{1}{2}$ [(ABCD + AB) − (AC + AD) − (BC + BD) + (CD + Ø)]

Design 2

Main effect of A: $\frac{1}{4}$ [(ABC + ABD) + (ACD + A) − (BCD + B) − (C + D)]

AB interaction: $\frac{1}{2}$ [(ABC + ABD) − (ACD + A) − (BCD + B) + (C + D)]

designs. Note that the estimate of the main effect of A simply contrasts the four treatment groups containing factor A with the four lacking factor A. Such fractional factorial designs are used only when the number of separate treatment groups required by a complete factorial design becomes unmanageable. In agricultural and industrial applications very large numbers of factors may be studied together using only a small fraction of the total number of possible factor combinations, but I know of no medical applications for such designs.

The disadvantage of fractional factorial designs is that each of the possible estimates refers to two or more effects. For example, in the half-fractional 2^4 design just discussed, with ABCD as the defining interaction, the estimate of the main effect of A cannot be distinguished from that for the BCD interaction, and thus one says that A is *aliased* with BCD. This means that when we choose to estimate the main effect of A we are assuming that the BCD interaction equals zero, and vice versa. In this design the main effects are not aliased with the two-factor interactions, but the two-factor interactions are aliased with each other in pairs, AB with CD, AC with BD, and AD with BC. However, this is not as bad as it seems. A large effect for A or BCD is much more likely to represent an effect of A than a three-factor interaction of B, C and D. Likewise, if the main effects of both A and B are relatively small, then a large effect for the AB-CD pair is assumed more likely to represent a CD interaction, provided C and D have appreciable effects.

In Table 4 I have listed some of the main design features of a secondary intervention study currently in progress in Linxian, a county in North Central China

Table 4. Design features of a nutrition intervention trial in Linxian, People's Republic of China

Goal:	To reduce mortality from esophageal cancer			
Design:	$\frac{1}{2}$ fractional 2^4 factorial			
Factors:	A	B	C	D
	Retinol β-carotene Zinc	Riboflavin Niacin	Vitamin C Molybdenum	Vitamin E Selenium
Sample size:	25 000			

(Blot and Li 1985). In some communes of this county about one fourth of the population dies of esophageal cancer. The reason for this unusually high incidence of esophageal cancer is unknown, but it is known that the citizens of this region are deficient in a number of micronutrients and vitamins. Accordingly, a one-half fractional 2^4 factorial design was chosen to study the possible effects of some of these agents in decreasing the incidence of esophageal cancer in a trial involving 25 000 adults. As noted in Table 4, the four factors are themselves the presence or absence of combinations of two or three vitamins and trace elements. For example, the presence of factor A means that a subject receives retinol, β-carotene, and zinc, while when factor A is absent the subject receives none of the three. Factorial designs require that all the factors can be given in various combinations without alteration in dosage. This requirement is generally not met in cancer treatment trials, with the exception of simple 2×2 factorial designs comparing chemotherapy with and without radiotherapy, for example. But factorial designs are well adapted to prevention studies where the factors under study have little or no toxicity and thus may easily be given together without reducing dosage.

Factorial designs should be considered whenever one is genuinely interested in studying two or more factors that can actually be given together. This is most likely to be the case when it is known that their mechanisms of action are different, when they are known not to interfere with each other, and when their combined toxicity, if any, is acceptable. These designs are most powerful when large interactions among the factors under study are not expected, but if interactions are of special interest, then factorial designs provide a systematic way of studying them, although because of the increased variance of interaction estimates, larger sample sizes may be needed if one wishes to have adequate power for studying interactions. Byar and Piantadosi (1985) discuss these ideas in more detail.

Cluster Randomization

Cluster randomization refers to randomizing groups of individuals rather than the individuals themselves. I want to illustrate this kind of design with a trial currently in the planning stages at the National Cancer Institute (Table 5). The trial is called the Community Intervention Trial for Smoking Cessation, or COMMIT for short.

Table 5. Design features of the Community Intervention Trial

1. Aimed at heavy smokers
2. Community-based: total population of 50000–170000 per community
3. Design
   A. Randomize 11 community pairs
   B. End point for each community is the quit rate in a random sample of 500 heavy smokers
4. Phase I: Planning and protocol writing (9 months)
   Phase II: Implementation (48 months)
   Phase III: Analysis and reporting (18 months)
5. Intervention channels
   A. Media
   B. Health care settings
   C. Worksites
   D. Hotlines
   E. Networks
   F. Youth and schools
   G. General community

This is a secondary prevention trial designed to encourage heavy smokers (25 or more cigarettes per day) to give up smoking. It is known that heavy smokers experience great difficulty in giving up smoking when the usual methods focused on individuals are used. Cluster randomization was chosen, based upon the hypothesis that heavy smokers will find it easier to stop smoking when cessation assistance is made widely available in an environment where smoking is made less socially acceptable. In this situation intervention must be assigned to social units larger than the individual. This intervention hypothesis led to a decision to study pairs of communities with populations of 50000–170000, with one community of each pair assigned randomly to intervention and the other to serve as a control community. The pairs are formed by matching communities from the same state on economic and demographic variables.

The end point for each community will be the quit rate in a random sample of 500 heavy smokers recruited by a random digit-dialing telephone survey. The random sample in each community will be followed up as a cohort during the 4 years of implementation of the trial, and self-reported smoking cessation will be confirmed by salivary cotinine determinations. Although the sample size calculations presented below are based on using the quit rates in these cohorts as a principal end point, cross-sectional smoking prevalence surveys will also be conducted at the beginning and end of the study, as well as smaller surveys annually during the intervening years. The cross-sectional surveys will provide different information from that obtained from the cohort. In particular, cross-sectional surveys will allow estimation of the number of light, moderate, and heavy smokers in various age and sex categories, provide information about ex-smokers returning to smoking, and show the effects of migration into and out of the communities.

The proposed intervention channels to be used in the intervention cities will include media, health care settings, work sites, smoking cessation hotlines, networks, programs for youths in schools, and changes in local policies related to smoking. The basic idea is that a small field staff working with the trial investigators who are experienced in smoking cessation methodology will act as a catalyst in each of the intervention cities to mobilize community resources for an integrated and comprehensive smoking cessation program.

I would now like to turn to the statistical design developed largely by Mitchell Gail and myself which led to the selection of 11 pairs of communities. The fundamental test statistic will be the average difference in quit rate in the cohorts of 500 heavy smokers across the pairs of communities. In particular, if we designate the estimated proportion of heavy smokers quitting in the intervention cohorts by $p_{i\mathrm{I}}$ and that in the control cohorts by $p_{i\mathrm{C}}$, then the average difference for m pairs of communities is given by

$$\overline{\mathrm{D}} = \frac{\sum_{i=1}^{m} \mathrm{D}_i}{m} = \frac{\sum_{i=1}^{m} (\hat{p}_{i\mathrm{I}}-\hat{p}_{i\mathrm{C}})}{m}. \tag{1}$$

Although we are planning to test the null hypothesis of no intervention effect by comparing $\overline{\mathrm{D}}$ with its permutational distribution ($2^{11}=2048$ possibilities), this procedure is well approximated by the following paired t-test, which yields simple sample size estimates. An estimate of the variance of the m community differences is given by

$$\mathrm{S}_{\mathrm{D}}^2 = \frac{\sum_{i=1}^{m} (\mathrm{D}_i-\overline{\mathrm{D}})^2}{m-1}. \tag{2}$$

Thus, the paired t-test is given by

$$\mathrm{T} = \overline{\mathrm{D}}/(\mathrm{S}_{\mathrm{D}}/\sqrt{m}). \tag{3}$$

The number of pairs of communities needed to obtain a prespecified statistical power may be computed from the usual formula for approximately normal test statistics, namely

$$m^* = \frac{(\mathrm{Z}_\alpha+\mathrm{Z}_\beta)^2\, \sigma_{\mathrm{D}}^2}{\Delta^2} \tag{4}$$

where the Z_α and Z_β are the normal deviates corresponding to the size and power of the statistical test respectively, Δ is equal to the expected value of $\overline{\mathrm{D}}$, and σ_{D}^2 is the variance of the differences. Since the number of degrees of freedom is small, we adjust the value of m^* using the approximation presented by Snedecor and Cochran (1967) to obtain the final number of required communities m by the following equation

$$m = \frac{m^*(\mathrm{INT}(m^*)+2)}{\mathrm{INT}(m^*)} \tag{5}$$

where INT( ) represents rounding to the next higher integer.

The only difficult part of this sample size calculation is in obtaining an estimate for σ_{D}^2 before doing the experiment. Using standard results from cluster sampling

(Donner et al. 1981), the variance of the differences in each community pair is seen to have four terms, two due to binomial variation within each community, and two representing the extra binomial variation between the communities in a pair. Letting $\bar{p}_I$ represent the average quit rate in the intervention communities and $\bar{p}_C$ represent the average quit rate in the control communities, then

$$\sigma_D^2 = \frac{\bar{p}_I(1-\bar{p}_I)}{n} + \frac{\bar{p}_C(1-\bar{p}_C)}{n} + \sigma_{p_I}^2 + \sigma_{p_C}^2 \tag{6}$$

where n is the number of subjects in the cohort to be followed in each of the communities. Once one specifies the expected quit rate in the control and intervention communities ($\bar{p}_C$ and $\bar{p}_I$) and n, it is easy to compute the first two terms of Eq. 6, but the hart part is obtaining estimates for the last two terms, $\sigma_{p_I}^2$ and $\sigma_{p_C}^2$.

In order to plan this trial we obtained unpublished data from the Multiple Risk Factor Intervention Study (MRFIT), in which individual subjects at high risk for coronary heart disease were randomized to usual care or special intervention in 22 different clinics. Some of the smoking cessation results of the MRFIT study are described by Neaton et al. (1981). The data we used are shown in Table 6, where variance estimates are given at the bottom of the columns. The average number of subjects per group in each treatment in each clinic was 155. In this study the average difference in quit rates between usual care and special intervention was 16.1%. We chose to design the COMMIT trial with a one-tailed 5% probability for type-I error and an average difference of 10% in the quit rates. We used the MRFIT data to compute both the required number of communities assuming matching as good as randomization of individuals and the number required assuming completely ineffective matching for various sizes of cohorts. Matching as good as randomizing individuals would be approximated by using the variance given in the fourth column of Table 6, because these differences arose following randomization of individuals within each clinic. Here we are thinking of each clinic as representing a community pair in our trial. On the other hand, completely ineffective matching would correspond to taking a usual care group at random from the second column in Table 6 and pairing it with a randomly selected group from the third column. The estimated variance of the difference would then be the sum of variances given at the bottom of columns 2 and 3 in Table 6. For the actual protocol, the values $\bar{p}_I = 0.25$ and $\bar{p}_C = 0.15$ were used in Eq. 6, instead of the values observed in MRFIT, but this change has little effect on required numbers of community pairs.

The results of our sample size calculations are shown in Table 7. It may be surprising to note that only two communities would be required if we had matching as good as randomizing individuals, $n = 500$, for 80% power. However, this is not surprising if one considers that individual randomization assures no systematic differences between communities, and the binomial variability is small for samples of size 500. The calculations in the lower part of the table show that very little is gained by increasing the size of the cohorts from 500 to 1000, so we selected eight community pairs corresponding to a power of 90% for $n = 500$ as our design of choice. In fact, we are currently planning to study 11 pairs in order to have some extra insurance in case unforeseen events might require dropping some pairs of cities from the study, or in case the variation between matched communities greatly exceeds that observed between clinics in the MRFIT study.

Table 6. Proportions quitting in 22 MRFIT clinics (thiocyanate adjusted at 6th annual visit)

Clinic	Usual care ($\hat{p}_{iC}$)	Special intervention ($\hat{p}_{iI}$)	Difference
1	0.318	0.514	0.196
2	0.350	0.505	0.155
3	0.322	0.444	0.122
4	0.396	0.568	0.172
5	0.222	0.498	0.276
6	0.364	0.462	0.098
7	0.304	0.436	0.132
8	0.301	0.343	0.042
9	0.394	0.504	0.110
10	0.221	0.364	0.143
11	0.279	0.433	0.154
12	0.250	0.451	0.201
13	0.260	0.419	0.159
14	0.261	0.500	0.239
15	0.252	0.399	0.147
16	0.384	0.583	0.199
17	0.296	0.477	0.181
18	0.200	0.398	0.198
19	0.290	0.556	0.266
20	0.216	0.322	0.106
21	0.426	0.496	0.070
22	0.226	0.401	0.175
mean	0.29691	0.45786	0.16095
$s^2=\sum\frac{(X_i-X)^2}{m-1}$	$43.588\cdot10^{-4}$	$49.398\cdot10^{-4}$	$34.141\cdot10^{-4}$

Table 7. Required number of pairs of communities, m, for $\alpha=0.05$ (one-tail) and $\Delta=10\%$

	Power	
Matching as good as randomizing individuals	*0.8*	*0.9*
$n=155$ $\sigma_D^2=34.14\cdot10^{-4}$	4	5
$n=500$ $\sigma_D^2=10.584\cdot10^{-4}$	2	3
Completely ineffective matching		
$n=155$ $\sigma_D^2=92.99\cdot10^{-4}$	8	10
$n=500$ $\sigma_D^2=72.64\cdot10^{-4}$	7	8
$n=1000$ $\sigma_D^2=68.07\cdot10^{-4}$	6	8

Although the COMMIT trial discussed in the previous section is a secondary prevention study, smoking cessation rather than cancer incidence is the end point. This end point was chosen because the relationship between tobacco smoking and lung cancer is regarded as firmly established by most scientists, based on data from a great many studies of various sorts, and because the benefits of smoking cessation are generally accepted. In addition, it was not judged feasible to conduct a trial of sufficient size and duration to demonstrate directly that smoking cessation reduced the incidence of lung cancer.

Sample Size Calculations for a Trial Designed to Affect Cancer Incidence

In this section I want to describe the sample size calculations worked out by Steve Self and Ross Prentice for a proposed trial of the effect of dietary modification on the incidence of breast cancer. International correlations between both incidence and mortality of breast cancer across various countries versus estimates of the amount of fat consumed suggest a strong linear relationship. It is well known that ecological correlations can be misleading, but they are useful for suggesting hypotheses to be tested by other methods. Case-control and cohort studies have not provided a consistent picture concerning the possible relationship between dietary fat and breast cancer, but a considerable body of animal experimental data suggests that mammary cancer can be reduced by limiting dietary fat. Accordingly, a large-scale secondary prevention study called the Womens Health Trial (WHT) has been proposed to examine this question. Some of the principal features of this proposed trial are shown in Table 8. The current design calls for 32000 women aged 45-69 at increased risk of breast cancer to be randomized in a ratio of 2:3 to intervention and control. Unequal randomization was chosen because of the greater cost of intervention versus control. The women will be taught to eat a low fat diet containing about 20% of calories as fat. The usual American diet contains about 40% of calories as fat. After a 3-year recruitment period, women in the study will be followed up for an average of 8.5 years.

The basic equation used for sample size calculation for this trial is again the simple normal approximation, except that the quantity of interest is the log odds ratio between intervention and control groups rather than a difference in proportions as in the preceding example. In particular, the normal approximation is

$$N_{\text{total}} = \frac{(Z_\alpha + Z_\beta)^2 Q}{(\ln R)^2} \tag{7}$$

where

$$R = \frac{p_i/(1-p_i)}{p_c/(1-p_c)} \tag{8}$$

and

$$Q = \frac{1}{f\, p_i(1-p_i)} + \frac{1}{(1-f)\, p_c(1-p_c)} \tag{9}$$

Here p_i is the probability of developing breast cancer for intervention women, p_c is the probability of developing breast cancer for control women, and f is the fraction randomized to intervention. This would be a very simple quantity to compute if we knew what values of p_i and p_c to use in the calculation. Like the variance of D_i in the preceding section, the difficult part is to obtain sensible values for p_i and p_c.

Table 8. Design features of the Women's Health Trial

Subjects	- 32000 women aged 45-69 at increased risk of breast cancer
Design	- ~ 20 clinics randomizing 1600 women on average - 12800 intervention versus 19200 controls
Hypothesis	- A low-fat diet (20% of cals) will lead to a 16% reduction in the incidence of breast cancer by the end of the trial.
Duration	- 10 years - 3 years recruitment 8.5 years average follow-up

The first step is to model the cancer incidence rates allowing for the effects of known risk factors as well as for the postulated effect of dietary fat. Accordingly, the investigators proposed the following model for the age-specific incidence rate for breast cancer:

$$\lambda(t, t_e, \underset{\sim}{Z}) = \lambda_o(t)\exp(\underset{\sim}{\beta}'\underset{\sim}{Z})[1+0.0025\int_{0}^{t-t_e}(\mathrm{F}(u)-40)du] \qquad (10)$$

where $\lambda()$ = age-specific incidence rate for breast cancer
t = current age
t_e = age at entry to the study
$\underset{\sim}{Z}$ = a vector of risk factors
$\lambda_o(t)$ = baseline age-specific incidence rate for breast cancer in the absence of risk factors
$\underset{\sim}{\beta}$ = a vector of regression coefficients representing the relative risks associated with the risk factor $\underset{\sim}{Z}$
$\mathrm{F}(u)$ = average percent fat in the diet at time u

The last factor in square brackets represents the effect of dietary fat as estimated from the international correlations described above. This equation refers to the age-specific incidence rate for an individual woman. We may then use this quantity to compute the probability of developing breast cancer during the trial for an individual woman followed up for d years using the following formula:

$$\int_{t_e}^{t_e+d} \lambda_i(t, t_e, Z)\exp\{-\int_{t_e}^{t}(\lambda(s, t_e, \underset{\sim}{Z})+\psi(s))ds\}dt \qquad (11)$$

where $\psi(s)$ is the age-specific mortality for competing causes of death and the other symbols are defined as for Eq. 10.

Note that Eq. 11 is in the form of a competing risk probability. The first term in the product inside the integral represents the instantaneous probability of developing breast cancer given the patients age and risk factor configuration and duration of time on study, while the second term represents the probability of having not previously been diagnosed with breast cancer or dying of some other cause. In cancer prevention trials of long duration it is important to take competing risks of death from other causes into account explicitly. Ordinarily, such considerations are neglected in planning sample sizes for treatment trials because the patients under study already have cancer, and in many instances the probability of dying of other causes over a short period of time may be neglected. In the Women's Health Trial, we expect overall about 1000 incident breast cancer cases, but we also expect about 750–1000 deaths from other causes.

Other assumptions required for computing sample size concern compliance with the low-fat diet in the intervention group and failure to modify the usual diet in the control group. The sample size of 32000 is based on the assumption that the control group will drop over 8.5 years from 40% of calories as fat to about 38%. The intervention group is assumed to drop promptly to an average of 20% of calories as fat in the first 6 months and then rebound to 23% by the end of the first year, followed by a gradual increase to 26% by the end of the trial. These compliance assumptions provide us with values of $F(u)$ for Eq. 10. Of course, these compliance assumptions are arbitrary and if compliance in either or both groups is less than assumed, statistical power will be diminished. Fortunately, we have data from a pilot study which shows that the reported percent calories as fat in the intervention group fell to 20% by 14 weeks and has remained close to that value for 2 years.

The risk factors currently required for entry into this trial are any one or more of the following: a family history of breast cancer in a first-degree relative, two or more biopsies for benign breast disease, nulliparity or first live birth at age 25 or older, or biopsy evidence of atypical hyperplasia or fibroadenoma with age at diagnosis 45 or greater. In addition, estimated fat intake must exceed 38% of calories. When planning this trial, detailed cost models were developed in order to explore other sets of risk factors in order to see whether or not a more efficient design could be developed. Essentially, the problem is whether it is better to study a smaller group of high-risk women who are difficult to find and require screening very large numbers of potential candidates, or whether in the most extreme case the only risk factor should be age, so that a much larger proportion of the women screened for entering the trial could in fact be admitted. We noted, for example, that if age were the only entry criteria (age 45–69) then 56000 women would be required to obtained the same statistical power as the design requiring 32000 women, but only something like one fourth as many women would need to be screened in order to obtain this number. However, the cost model showed that such an approach would in fact be more expensive since the cost of teaching the women to eat the low-fat diet substantially exceeds the cost of screening. Nevertheless, this was a very useful exercise, and similar exercises should be conducted by anyone contemplating a large-scale primary or secondary cancer prevention trial.

Case-Cohort Monitoring

Another special feature of the Womens Health Trial is the plan to use the case-cohort approach for monitoring compliance to the study diets as well as for exploratory analysis after the trial is completed. The case-cohort approach has recently been described by Prentice (1986) and differs in important ways from the so-called synthetic retrospective approach, first described by Mantel (1973), in several important ways. Essentially, the case-cohort approach involves identifying at the beginning of the study a random subcohort of subjects. Covariates are measured only in this subcohort and in all subjects who become cases during the study. It is assumed that censoring and failure times are known for all cohort members. In the Women's Health Trial the subcohort will consist of a 10% sample of all study subjects, and the important covariates will be the results of blood tests and analyses of the dietary records. Blood samples and dietary records will be obtained from all study subjects, but only those for the subcohort and for all cases who develop during the study will be analyzed. The reason for this is to save money. In a cancer prevention study where the number of end points, i.e., new cancer cases, is low, most of the control information is redundant. It has been estimated that the use of the case-cohort approach in this study will save something like $30 million.

The synthetic retrospective or case-control approach mentioned above consists of selecting controls for all the cases that develop during the trial after the trial is completed. This approach was also developed to save money and time, but there are several important differences. First, the case-cohort approach can be used to monitor the study while it is being conducted. Second, it is more efficient than the synthetic case-control approach because the controls are used more than once in the pseudo-likelihood analysis required for this method. In addition, new controls need not be selected for each cause of death or other end point one wishes to analyze - the same subcohort serves as a control group for all end points. The price one pays for using this method is a more complicated analysis. The reader is referred to the article by Prentice (1986) for details.

Principal Differences Between Cancer Prevention and Treatment Trials

Primary and secondary cancer prevention trials differ from treatment trials in several important ways (Table 9). First, the ideas to be tested generally originate from epidemiology and from animal experiments. This means that the statisticians involved in such trials need to learn a lot about epidemiologic methodology, because they will have to play an important role in interpreting any data suggesting

Table 9. Major differences between cancer treatment and prevention trials

1. *Origin of ideas* - Epidemiology	
2. *Kinds of intervention* -	Vitamins and micronutrients Life-style changes Screening
3. *Substantive expertise* -	Nutrition Social psychology Health promotion
4. *Size* - Because most subjects in a prevention trial do not develop the disease	
5. *Duration* - Compliance and competing risks become important	
6. *Cost* - Very great	
7. *Need for pilot studies* - Because of size, duration, and cost	

that a trial is justified. When case-control and cohort studies present conflicting or unconvincing evidence, randomized cancer prevention trials may be regarded as experimental epidemiology, providing the most reliable method for testing important hypotheses about cancer etiology.

A second important difference is the kinds of interventions under study. Instead of surgery, chemotherapy, and radiotherapy, one is more likely to study life-style changes such as smoking cessation or dietary alteration, or the administration of putative cancer preventive agents such as vitamins and micronutrients. This requires becoming familiar with new areas of scientific knowledge and with substantive experts who use a very different vocabulary. For example, these kinds of interventions require working with nutritionists, social psychologists, and experts in the area of health promotion.

Because most subjects in a primary or secondary prevention trial will not develop cancer, the size of such trials may be one or two orders of magnitude larger than those required for most treatment trials. For the same reason, the duration of the trial is likely to be much longer, and therefore special attention has to be paid to compliance and to the problem of competing risks. The requirement for much larger and longer trials means that costs also will be very much greater, so very careful planning and justification for the hypothesis to be tested will certainly be required. Generally, because of these considerations, appropriate pilot studies designed to evaluate the ability to recruit subjects and the willingness of the subjects to comply with the interventions will be required. Despite the enormous difficulties and the commitment of time, energy, and money required to untertake primary and secondary prevention studies, the possible payoff seems worth the price, both from the point of view of increasing our understanding of the process of carcinogenesis and how it may be modified, as well as in terms of the potential human suffering to be avoided if prevention trials are successful.

References

Bertram JS, Kolonel LN, Meyskens FL (1987) Rationale and strategies for chemoprevention of cancer in humans. Cancer Res 47: 3012-3031

Blot WJ, Li JY (1985) Some considerations in the design of a nutrition intervention trial in Linxian, People's Republic of China.

Fourth symposium on epidemiology and cancer registries in the Pacific basin. Natl Cancer Inst Monogr 69: 29-34 (NIH publ no 85-2768)

Byar DP, Piantadosi S (1985) Factorial designs for randomized clinical trials. Cancer Treat Rep 69: 1055-1063

Donner A, Birkett N, Buck C (1981) Randomization by cluster: sample size requirements and analysis. Am J Epidemiol 114: 906-914

Mantel N (1973) Synthetic retrospective studies and related topics. Biometrics 29: 479-486

Neaton JD, Broste S, Cohen L, Fishman EL, Kjelsberg MO, Schoenberger J (1981) The multiple risk factor intervention trial (MRFIT). VII. A comparison of risk factor changes between the two study groups. Prev Med 10: 519-543

Prentice RL (1986) A case-cohort design for epidemiologic cohort studies and disease prevention trials. Biometrika 73: 1-11

Snedecor GW, Cochran WG (1967) Statistical methods. Iowa State University Press, Ames, Iowa, pp 113-114

*Strategies for Subgroup Analysis in Clinical Trials**

H. E. Rockette and R. J. Caplan

Department of Biostatistics, Graduate School of Public Health, University of Pittsburgh, Pittsburgh, PA 15261, USA

Introduction

Standard methods of assigning *p* values to quantify the probability of falsely rejecting a null hypothesis are often misinterpreted when multiple comparisons are made. The *p* value of a test statistic is usually applicable to an individual comparison which is assumed to have been selected a priori, and the probability of falsely rejecting at least one of several comparisons (often called the experimentwise error rate) may be much higher than the individual (or comparisonwise) *p* value. In a clinical trial multiple comparisons occur when analyses are repeated at several points in time, when pairwise comparisons are made among more than two treatment groups, when there is more than one end point being tested, or when the same hypothesis is tested on different subgroups of patients.

The major focus of this paper will be to discuss problems arising from subgroup analysis in clinical trials. Specifically we plan to: (a) demonstrate the magnitude of the experimentwise error rate that may occur in subset analyses of a large randomized clinical trial, (b) discuss some methods of controlling the experimentwise error, and (c) discuss some general problems in deciding upon strategies for subset analysis.

Although the increase in the experimentwise error rate when one does subgroup analysis is well recognized (Pocock 1984), the magnitude of the increase depends on many factors including the sample size within the subgroups, the correlations among the variables used to define patient subgroups, and the number of subgroup comparisons. An upper bound on the experimentwise error rate could be obtained by applying Bonferroni's inequality but this may be overly conservative given the dependence that often exists among variables used to define patient subgroups. Some indication of the magnitude of the problem can be made using computer simulation. Since our objective is to obtain a reasonable estimate of the magnitude of the experimentwise error rate that might occur in the analyses of

* The research was partially supported by the National Cancer Institute, U10CA 12027, and American Cancer Society Grant RC13.

© Springer-Verlag Berlin · Heidelberg 1988

currently conducted clinical trials, we have employed statistical procedures in common use and have selected values of the parameters necessary for simulation from a recently conducted randomized clinical trial of rectal cancer. A similar approach has been used to ascertain the magnitude of the experimentwise error rate of a commonly employed strategy of analyzing occupational epidemiological data (Rockette and Arena 1987).

Methods

Parameters for the simulation were taken from two treatment arms of a randomized trial of patients with operable rectal cancer (Fisher et al. to be published). A total of 351 patients were randomly assigned to one of the two treatment arms. The average time of follow-up was 54 months and there were 192 events. Age ($\leq$ 64 years, >64 years), sex and Dukes Class (B or C) were the three dichotomous stratification variables. The number of patients and the average death rate in the control arm for the substrata defined by these stratification variables are given in Table 1. Time until death for each patient was assumed to obey an exponential distribution and was generated using IMSL (1980). For each patient in the control group the parameter of the exponential distribution used to generate time until death was selected from Table 1 to be consistent with that patient's stratification variables. The simulated time until death for patients was compared to their time in the study. If the generated time until death was greater than the time in the study the patient was considered to be a censored observation. Simulated data for patients in the treatment group was generated by reducing the hazard function by a specified percentage from the rates given in Table 1. Five hundred simulations were conducted when there was no treatment effect (0% reduction in hazard) and 100 simulations were conducted for cases where there was a treatment effect (20%, 40%, and 50% reduction in hazard).

In analyzing this data set we have employed some general strategies which are often employed in the analysis of subgroups. The treatment effect is tested by employing a proportional hazards model for a given group of patients and testing whether the coefficient of the treatment variable is statistically significant ($p=0.05$). Interaction for an individual stratification variable was considered sig-

Table 1. Average death rates by stratum

Age (years)	Sex	Dukes class	Treatment A (control)	Treatment B (treatment)	Monthly failure rate
$\leq$64	Male	B	25	24	0.019
$\leq$64	Male	C	46	49	0.041
>64	Male	B	19	18	0.012
>64	Male	C	22	24	0.019
$\leq$64	Female	B	12	13	0.007
$\leq$64	Female	C	30	25	0.024
>64	Female	B	8	12	0.013
>64	Female	C	11	13	0.018

nificant if the coefficient of that interaction term was significant. A global test for interaction incorporated all interaction terms for the various strata in the model and compared this full model to the likelihood with no interaction terms in the model. Critical regions of the global test for interaction were obtained using the χ^2 statistic as the asymptotic distribution of the likelihood ratio test.

Potential Errors in Subgroup Analysis

When conducting subgroup analysis there are several types of errors that can be made when the comparison of two treatment arms within a subgroup finds them to be significantly different. One may falsely identify a treatment effect in a subgroup when no treatment effect exists for any subgroup of patients. This false acceptance of an ineffective treatment is the most recognized aspect of the multiple comparisons problem. However, there may be a homogeneous benefit from treatment but the investigator falsely attributes the benefit to a specific subgroup of patients. Thus the investigator falsely identifies a heterogeneous effect of treatment when the effect is homogeneous (Pocock 1984; Byar 1985). A third type of error may occur if there is an effect of treatment in some or all of the patient subgroups and the investigator fails to distinguish a crossover interaction from differences in treatment effect that have the same direction but different magnitudes. A test of crossover interaction has recently been proposed by Gail and Simon (1985).

Results

Table 2 summarizes the probability of falsely declaring a significant treatment effect at each of the two levels of the three stratification variables. The probability that at least one of the subsets is declared to be statistically significant is 0.22. Since we only have three strata and are only making six subset comparisons, the effect is much less dramatic than it would be if there were more stratification variables or if subsets were formed using combinations of stratification variables. The comparisonwise error rate of 0.053 is the average of the type I error for each of the individual subgroups and its deviation from 0.05 includes simulation error.

Table 2. Percentage of false rejections in the presence of no treatment effect (500 simulations)

Subgroup	Percentage rejections
Young ($\leq$64)	5.8
Old ($>$64)	6.8
Male	5.2
Female	4.2
Dukes B	4.2
Dukes C	5.8
Comparisonwise error	5.3
Experimentwise error	21.6

A review of the published literature indicates there is no uniformly applied strategy for identifying heterogeneity of patient response. The statistician would most naturally investigate a heterogeneous response to treatment by formally testing for interaction within the context of a mathematical model. However, clinicians will often look only at the p values for various levels of a variable and conclude heterogeneity if within some levels there is a statistically significant effect and within other levels no such effect exists. Although such conclusions depend on a p value, the lack of any formal test for interaction has prompted us to call such an approach "clinical interaction."

Table 3. Percentage of false declarations of "clinical interaction" when none exists

Factor	Reduction in hazard			
	0%	20%	40%	50%
Age	12.2	32.0	54.0	25.0
Sex	8.6	38.0	50.0	28.0
Dukes class	9.6	31.0	55.0	27.0
Comparisonwise error	10.1	33.7	53.0	26.7
Experimentwise error	21.2	48.0	76.0	43.0

Table 3 summarizes the percentage of rejections of the test for "clinical interaction" for selected homogeneous reductions in the hazard function for all patients on treatment B. For example, if there is a true benefit resulting in a 20% reduction in the hazard function for patients receiving treatment B, for 32% of the simulations one age level will show a statistically significant difference at $p = 0.05$ and at the other age level there will be failure to reject. The probability of this occurring is a function of the relative sample sizes of the two levels of the stratum and thus differs for the three stratification variables. In the presence of no treatment effect the experimentwise error rate of 0.21 is similar to the value given in Table 2; in at least one of the six subsets the null hypothesis is rejected. However, the error rate of falsely declaring patient heterogeneity if there is a moderate but homogeneous treatment effect is much higher. If treatment B has a true reduction in hazard of 40% for all patients such a strategy results in a false declaration of patient heterogeneity in 76% of the simulations. The decrease in error rate for a 50% reduction in the hazard occurs because as the treatment effect becomes larger the null hypothesis is more likely to be rejected at both levels of the stratification variables.

The elevated type I error could be controlled using a formal test for interaction. The requirement might be made that if some levels of a variable show a significant treatment effect and not others, then heterogeneity be accepted only if the test for interaction is significant (strategy S1). If the investigator desires to control the experimentwise error rate resulting from testing multiple stratification variables then the implications of a test for clinical interaction might be accepted only if the global test for interaction rejects (strategy S2). Table 4 demonstrates that the effect of superimposing tests for interaction post hoc onto exploratory data analysis of subsets by pairwise tests does control the excess false rejection rate. How-

Table 4. Percentage of false declarations of interaction when none exists for various strategies

Factor	Reduction in hazard					
	0%		20%		50%	
	S1	S2	S1	S2	S1	S2
Age	4.4	1.4	6.0	4.0	2.0	0.0
Sex	1.8	1.2	4.0	4.0	3.0	2.0
Dukes class	2.2	1.0	3.0	4.0	3.0	1.0
Comparisonwise error	2.8	1.2	4.3	4.0	2.7	1.0
Experimentwise error	8.4	3.0	13.0	4.0	8.0	3.0

S1, *S2*, strategies 1 and 2.

ever, such a strategy is not recommended. The test is not only unnecessarily conservative but the true alpha error is dependent on the magnitude of the relative treatment effect in the two arms. Both of these problems can be avoided by using only tests of interactions to determine heterogeneity and ignoring p values associated with individual subsets. To control adequately for the number of comparisons it is recommended that the strategy of employing the global test for interaction be used.

The failure to properly distinguish a crossover interaction from a noncrossover interaction may have important ethical ramifications. Utilizing the test proposed by Gail and Simon (1985) our simulations confirm their assertion that the test is of relatively low power in detecting a crossover difference. This is in part due to the extremely conservative nature of the test for a variety of frequently occurring situations. In 300 simulations where there was a homogeneous treatment effect ranging from 20% to 50% there were no rejections at the $p = 0.05$ level.

Since the existence of a detrimental effect of treatment has many ramifications other than those associated with misleading type I errors, we will not discuss it in detail in this paper. However, it should be noted that in dealing with crossover interactions a conservative decision for the statistician (i.e., protection from falsely identifying patient heterogeneity) may not be conservative relative to the medical management of the patient.

Conclusions

As regards specific results, we can make the following conclusions:

1. Subset analysis should be done very cautiously because of the multiple comparison problem. With an increasing number of strata or the use of combinations of variables to define subsets the magnitude of the type I error increases.
2. A less recognized aspect of subgroup analysis is that if there is a homogeneous treatment effect a response may be identified in only some subgroups of patients. If the concept of "clinical interaction" is used to identify subsets, then even with a small number of subsets a moderate homogeneous treatment effect can produce a large number of false assertions of patient heterogeneity.

3. The concept of "clinical interaction" should not be employed even if attempts are made to adjust for the elevated type I error; instead formal tests for interaction should be used. The reporting of p values associated with specific subsets should not be used to highlight subsets visualized as having the greatest response.
4. The global test for interaction should be used to place the experimentwise error rate in perspective. This requires specification of the number of variables investigated in the subgroup analysis.

The following general comments concern strategies of dealing with subgroup analysis:

1. Statistical analysis is only one aspect of the decision-making process to determine efficacy of treatment; the biological reasonableness of the result as well as the ethics that may enter into new trials based on the results of old trials must be brought into the decision.
2. It is important to distinguish between strategies to stop a trial, strategies used in the analysis of a trial, and strategies to be employed in reporting the results of a trial. Certainly the reporting of the experimentwise error rate and a description of the strategy employed in the analysis is crucial for the reader to place conclusions based on subgroup analysis in proper perspective. However, decisions as to whether results based on subgroups should not be reported or if reported not included in the abstract is more a philosophical than statistical issue.
3. It is unlikely that uniform methods capable of controlling all aspects of the multiple comparison problem will ever be employed in large scale research projects. We have ourselves ignored multiple ways of classifying a variable in a model (continuous, categorical), multiple endpoints (survival and disease-free survival), and the impact of multiple tests over time on our subsetting strategies. Nevertheless, published clinical trials could be better interpreted by the reader if investigators better formalized their strategies of subgroup analysis and included some indication of the experimentwise error rate. Furthermore, when ethical considerations do not preclude its use replication remains the most convincing argument for accepting the results of secondary hypothesis testing.

References

Byar D (1985) Assessing apparent treatment-covariate interactions in randomized clinical trials. Stat Med 4: 255–263

Fisher B, Wolmark N, Rockette H, Redmond C, Deutsch M, Wickerham L, Fisher E, Caplan R, Lerner H, Gordon P, Feldman M, Cruz A, Legault-Poisson S (to be published) Postoperative adjuvant chemotherapy or radiation therapy for rectal cancer: results from NSABP protocol R-01

Gail M, Simon R (1985) Testing for qualitative interactions between treatment effects and patient subsets. Biometrics 41: 361–372

IMSL (1980) IMSL reference manual. IMSL, Houston

Pocock SJ (1984) Clinical trials: a practical approach. Wiley, New York

Rockette HE, Arena VC (1987) An evaluation of the proportionate mortality index in the presence of multiple comparisons. Stat Med 6: 71–77

Statistical Tools for Subset Analysis in Clinical Trials

R. Simon

National Cancer Institute, Landow Building, Room 4B06, Bethesda, MD 20892, USA

Introduction

The topic of subset analysis is complex, yet it has evoked simplistic solutions and strong feelings as a results of these simplistic solutions. There are some clinical investigators who ransack their data to find a subset of patients in which their new therapy looks effective. They report the findings in apparent ignorance of the problems of multiple comparisons, and their statistically significant finding looks good to the mass of statistically unsophisticated readers. Many of us react strongly to this, and the phrase "subset analysis" itself acquires a connotation of deception and sophistry. We hear individuals say that it is all right to look at subset results, but don't believe them. We hear that subset analyses can only generate hypotheses to be tested in other clinical trials. Does this mean that one must entirely ignore subset results regardless of how strong they are? Is it practical to design future studies and treat future patients on this basis? Does this also hold for clinical trials of cardiovascular disease or cancer prevention which may involve enormous numbers of patients and cost tens of millions of dollars? Is this sensible statistically?

Unfortunately, the heat generated by controversies about subset analysis polarizes us and inhibits us from discussing the problem intelligently. There are no easy solutions to the problem; perhaps there are no solutions at all. But there are tools we can use and steps we can take to help understand how and whether treatment effectiveness varies among subsets of patients. This objective is particularly important when we are dealing with expensive or toxic new treatments. With a cheap nontoxic treatment, if the average effect is positive then one need not be too concerned about subset effects. It may seem unlikely that the treatment will actually harm some patients, and distinguishing degrees of benefit is not a priority. But for expensive or toxic treatments the situation is very different. Not to substantially benefit from such a treatment may mean to be harmed in other ways even if survival itself is not reduced.

Most of our clinical trials are not large enough to support reliable subset analysis unless the treatment effects are large. We are all, I believe, familiar with the multiple comparison problem for subset analysis. If an experimental treatment is completely equivalent to a control treatment in K disjoint subsets of patients, then

Recent Results in Cancer Research, Vol. 111
© Springer-Verlag Berlin · Heidelberg 1988

the probability that at least one treatment versus control comparison will be significant at the α level by chance alone is

$$1-(1-\alpha)^n. \quad (1)$$

For $\alpha = 0.05$ and $n = 10$ the probability in Eq. 1 is 0.40. Hence, the probability of obtaining a "statistically significant" difference between treatments in one or more subsets is substantial by chance alone.

The multiple comparison problem noted above is exacerbated by the lack of statistical power for comparing treatments within subsets. Suppose, for example, that there are two subsets with equal numbers of patients. Let d_1 and d_2 be the observed treatment differences in the two subsets, and assume that the true treatment differences in the subsets are identical. Let *Ser* denote the standard error for the average treatment difference and let $Ser_i = Ser\sqrt{2}$ denote the standard error for the treatment difference within each subset $i = 1,2$. If the average treatment difference is just statistically significant at the 0.05 level

$$\frac{(d_1 + d_2)/2}{Ser} = 2$$

then at least one of the treatment differences within subsets does not even approach statistical significance:

$$P\left[\min_{i=1,2}\left|\frac{d_i}{Ser_i}\right| < 1\right] = 0.56 \quad (2)$$

Note that d_i/Ser_i is the "z value" for testing treatment difference within subset i. Equation 2 indicates that even when the relative treatment effect is constant across subsets, if the average treatment difference is not overwhelming then lack of statistical significance within subsets means nothing.

The obstacles to making reliable inferences about subset effects are thus considerable. Nevertheless, it is still appropriate to address subset questions provided we have the scientific integrity and statistical sophistication to interpret and report the results sensibly, often admitting ambiguity and uncertainty. In the next section I will review some statistical tools that are available for conducting subset analyses.

Tools for Subset Analysis

In many cases, the tools available for subset analyses may not provide clear-cut answers about subset effects. They help to avoid misleading conclusions, however, and help to quantify the support for the existence of substantial subset effects.

Specifying Major Subset Hypotheses in the Protocol

In any extensive set of data one will often be able to find spurious exciting patterns if one looks hard enough. This gives rise to the statistical maxim: "If you torture a set of data enough it will confess to anything." One way of reducing the magnitude of this "curse of dimensionality" is to specify in advance one or a very few subset hypotheses of major interest. This should be done more often in cancer clinical trials. Although the Neyman-Pearson theory of hypothesis tests is not the model of all scientific inquiry that some think it is, it is correct to ascribe more credence to confirmation of a prespecified hypothesis than to a hypothesis generated by the data themselves. If the major subset hypotheses are specified in advance, then the magnitude of the multiple comparison problem is known and can be adjusted for if one wishes. Otherwise, one is relegated to trying to determine retrospectively how many subsets were examined and how many would have been examined if the "interesting" results had not been observed when they were. The Bayesian, like the frequentist, is influenced by the prior credence he or she places on a hypothesis. For the Bayesian this requires specification of a model and prior distributions for subset effects at the start of the study. For the frequentist this requires specification of one or a few major subset hypotheses. Of course, specifying in advance a few major subset hypotheses does not in itself provide enough patients to enable treatment differences within subsets to be detected with sufficient statistical power. If the subset hypotheses are really of a priori importance, however, then they should influence the sample size of the clinical trial.

Writing a Protocol for the Subset Analysis

If more than a very few prespecified subset hypotheses are to be evaluated, it is useful to write a protocol for how the analysis will be conducted. This protocol should ideally be part of the study protocol to assure that the plan has not been influenced by the data. The purpose of the subset analysis protocol is to provide a reliable assessment of the size of the multiple comparison problem involved, so that proper analytic adjustments can be made and so that this information can be communicated in reports of the clinical trial. The multiple comparison problem is often horrendously large. For example, 146 subset comparisons were made in the Beta-Blocker Heart Attack Trial (Furberg and Byington 1983). When one starts looking at subsets defined by combination of variables, the size of the multiple comparison problem increases rapidly. This is compounded by the analysis of multiple end points. A protocol for analysis should also specify a hierarchy of importance for the hypotheses to be evaluated and perhaps prior beliefs for these hypotheses. Analysis of numerous subsets without a structured approach generally precludes being able to quantify the level of credence to be placed in results.

Confidence Intervals for Treatment Effects

The most prevalent approach to subset analysis is the performance of statistical significance tests for treatment effects within subsets. This is almost guaranteed to give misleading results. The lack of statistical power for detecting treatment effects within subsets is not apparent when a significance test is performed or reported. Because of the lack of power, the absence of a statistically significant difference in a subset is not strong evidence that the treatments are equivalent for the subset patients. The error of claiming subset-specific effects based on the fallacy of finding a significant effect in one subset and not finding it in another is common, however.

The use of confidence intervals instead of significance tests enables one to avoid the significant/nonsignificant fallacy. Reporting a confidence interval for treatment effect within a subset shows immediately whether the subset results are "negative" or "indeterminate" (Simon 1986). Although confidence intervals do not avoid the multiple comparison problem, their use would substantially improve the interpretation of subset analyses.

Interaction Tests

A treatment by subset interaction means that the treatment effect (i.e., the difference in effectiveness between the two treatments) varies among subsets of patients. One way of controlling the multiple comparison problem is by requiring that a statistically significant global interaction be demonstrated as a requirement for comparing treatments within individual subsets. This is the approach traditionally used in the analysis of variance. Global interaction means that the test should simultaneously evaluate all the treatment by subset interactions of potential interest. Performing separate interaction tests for each subset effect of potential interest carries with it its own multiple comparison problem. Of course, if the global interaction test is statistically significant, then one needs to isolate what subset effect is responsible.

Suppose that there are K disjoint subsets of interest and that d_k is an estimate of the treatment difference in the k'th subset. If d_k is normally distributed with variance σ_k^2, then the hypothesis of no treatment by subset interaction can be tested by calculating

$$\sum_{k=1}^{K} w_k(d_k - \bar{d})^2 \tag{3}$$

where

$$1/w_k = \sigma_k^2$$

and $\bar{d}$ is the weighted average of the d_k

$$\bar{d} = \frac{\sum_{k=1}^{K} w_k \, d_k}{\sum_{k=1}^{K} w_k}$$

If there is no interaction, then (3) has a chi-square distribution with K-1 degrees of freedom.

Frequently, the subsets of interest are not disjoint. For example, the sex subsets are not disjoint from the stage subsets. In general, interaction tests can be performed using likelihood ratio tests. For example, we may have a logit model

$$logit\, p_i = \alpha \, t_i + \beta \, x_i \tag{4}$$

where t_i is a binary (0 or 1) indicator of which treatment is assigned to the i'th patient, x_i is a vector of binary covariates for the i'th patient, α is a regression coefficient for the main effect of treatment, and β is a vector of regression coefficients for the covariate effects. We can add all possible first-order treatment by covariate subset effects to Eq. 4 and obtain

$$logit\, p_i = \alpha\, t_i + \beta\, x_i + \gamma\, x_i\, t_i \tag{5}$$

Under the hypothesis of no treatment by subset interactions minus 2 times the logarithm of the ratio of maximized likelihoods for Eq. 5 relative to Eq. 4 is asymptotically chi-square distributed with degrees of freedom equal to the number of interactions in Eq. 5. Interaction tests are described in more detail by Simon (1982).

Because most clinical trials are not planned to be sufficiently large for reliable subset analysis, the power of interaction tests will be low. In fact, the power may be hopelessly low unless one specifies a very few major subset hypotheses and plans the subset analysis as suggested above. A priori, the presence of important true interactions is unknown whereas the spurious appearance of large differences in treatment effects among subsets is highly likely. Consequently, it seems appropriate to require quantitative documentation, via interaction tests, that apparent subset differences are unlikely to be the result of chance fluctuations. Occasionally, subset hypotheses are considered important enough that sufficient patients have been accrued to separate subsets for independent analysis with sufficient statistical power. In such cases a significant interaction test should not be viewed as a prerequisite for separate analysis of the subsets. The separate subsets should probably be viewed as separate studies, each of which has better statistical power than the interaction test itself.

Qualitative Interactions

Peto (1982) has distinguished ordinary interactions from qualitative or cross-over interactions. Let $(\delta_k\ k=1, \ldots, K)$ denote the true treatment differences within K disjoint subsets. An ordinary treatment by subset interaction means that not all of the δ_k are equal. A qualitative interaction means that some of the δ_k are positive and others are negative. A qualitative interaction means that one treatment is superior to the other for some subset but is inferior for some other subset. Peto has argued that only qualitative interactions are important, since some variability in the magnitude of treatment effects will almost always exist among subsets defined by important prognostic factors. Since the definition of interaction is model dependent, it is also possible that nonqualitative interactions could be eliminated by a monotone scale transformation. Since there is usually no self-evidently appropriate scale of response measurement, nonqualitative interactions may not be important clinically.

Gail and Simon (1985) developed a statistical significance test for qualitative interactions. Let $(d_k\ k=1, \ldots, K)$ be independent, normally distributed estimators of $(\delta_k\ k=1, \ldots, K)$ and let d_k have variance σ_k^2. The test statistic is $Q = \min(Q^-, Q^+)$ where

$$Q^{+} = \sum_{d_k > 0} (d_k^2/\sigma_k^2)$$

and

$$Q^{-} = \sum_{d_k < 0} (d_k^2/\sigma_k^2).$$

Gail and Simon have tabulated critical values of c for rejecting the hypothesis of no qualitative interaction when $Q > c$. The critical value is a function of the size of the test α and of the number of subsets K.

When dealing with toxic or expensive treatments one cannot dismiss the importance of treatment by subset interactions of the form $\delta_k > \delta'$ for some subsets and $\delta_k < \delta'$ for other subsets, where δ' is some positive value which represents the minimal improvement which would lead one to select a new toxic experimental treatment over a less toxic standard treatment. For example, intensive adjuvant chemotherapy may substantially prolong survival for one subset of patients but have little or no positive impact on another subset. This may be a very important non-qualitative interaction. The Gail and Simon test is, however, applicable in this situation. One simply applies the test described to the translated estimates $(d_i - \delta')$. One can thereby test the hypothesis that a "clinically significant" treatment difference exists uniformly across subsets.

Sample Splitting

It is part of the conventional wisdom that subset analyses primarily generate hypotheses to be tested in other studies. We have already pointed out how a very few major subset hypotheses can be specified in advance to be tested in a study. It is also possible to generate and "independently" test subset hypotheses in the same study. For purposes of subset analysis one could split the data into two portions. In one portion one can screen the subset results and formulate a very few subset hypotheses to be tested in the second portion of the data. In general, this procedure is inefficient compared with analyzing the entire set of data as a whole and applying a multiple correction adjustment to account for the number of subsets examined (Thomas et al. 1985). The sample-splitting approach does permit one to use judgement and prior information in selecting the subset hypotheses for test. It also has an intuitive appeal and can be applied by persons without a detailed knowledge of statistics. Subset analyses for large studies are sometimes conducted by professional statisticians in an unstructured manner. If the process were adequately structured, then multiple comparison corrections could be applied. Otherwise, sample splitting may be useful. In either case, however, the power for detecting subset-specific differences will be small unless the initial dimension of the problem is not large and the subset differences are substantial.

Empirical Bayesian Methods

If one places sufficient structure on the subset problem, then additional tools become available. Continuing the notation used above, let the observed treatment differences within K disjoint subsets be denoted (d_k) and assume that these quantities are independently normally distributed with means (δ_k) and variances (σ_k^2). We shall assume that the variances (σ_k^2) are known. The empirical Bayesian approach structures the problem by treating the (δ_k) as random variables with a specified distributional form. For example, assume that for k = 1,. . .,K

$$\delta_k \sim NID\,(\mu,\, \sigma_0^2). \tag{6}$$

One is assuming here that the subset effects are distributed as independent random variables from the same normal distribution. The parameters μ and σ_0^2 of this distribution are easily estimated from the data (Efron and Morris 1973)

$$\hat{\mu} = \frac{\sum w_k\, d_k}{\sum w_k} \tag{7}$$

where $w_k = 1/\sigma_k^2$. All summations here are over the range k = 1,. . .,K. $\hat{\sigma}_0^2$ is the value A, which is the solution to

$$A = \frac{\sum (d_k^2 - \sigma_k^2)\; I_k(A)}{\sum I_k(A)} \tag{8}$$

where

$$I_k(A) = \frac{1}{2\,(A + \sigma_k^2)^2}.$$

The posterior density of δ_k is normal with mean $\lambda_k = \pi\hat{\mu} + (1-\pi)\; d_k$ where $\pi = w_0/(w_0 + w_k)$. The variance of the posterior density of δ_k is $\gamma^2 = (w_0 + w_k)^{-1}$.

The posterior mean of the unknown treatment effect within subset k is a weighted average of the overall average treatment effect μ estimated by Eq. 7 and the observed difference d_k within subset k. In calculating this weighted average, the weights are determined by the size of the variance of d_k around δ_k relative to the size of σ_0^2 estimated by the value of A that satisfies Eq. 8. The posterior mean of δ_k is thus a "shrinkage estimator"; the estimate is shrunk from d_k toward the overall mean μ. If the data indicate that there are large differences between subsets in relative treatment efficacy, then there is little shrinkage and each subset difference is taken at face value. If, on the other hand, the data indicate that there is little inter-subset difference in relative efficacy, then inferences for treatments within subset are based primarily on overall effects, since the posterior means are dominated by the $\hat{\mu}$ terms.

Inference about relative treatment efficacy within a subset is quite simply based on the posterior density of δ_k for that subset. For example, the posterior probability that the true treatment difference is at least as large as δ' is

$$p_{post}(\delta_k \geq \delta') = \Phi\left[\frac{\lambda_k - \delta'}{\gamma_k}\right] \tag{9}$$

where Φ is the standard cumulative normal distribution function.

Table 1. Effect of propranolol on postinfarction patients with mechanical or electrical complaints

Abnormality	d_k	σ_k	d_k/σ_k	λ_k	γ_k	λ_k/γ_k	$\Pr(\delta_k > 0)$
None	0.4	1.1	0.36	0.92	0.94	0.98	0.16
Electrical	5.7	1.8	3.17	4.01	1.3	3.16	0.0008
Mechanical	6.4	3.3	1.94	3.26	1.6	2.06	0.020
Both	4.2	3.4	1.23	2.73	1.6	1.72	0.043

Table 1 shows an example of the empirical Bayesian approach. The first two columns show the difference in mortality for four subsets of postinfarction patients randomized to receive either propranolol or placebo as part of the Beta-Blocker Heart Attack Trial (BHAT) (Furberg et al. 1983). The patients are classified into subsets based upon the presence or absence of findings indicative of electrical (rhythm) and/or mechanical (pump) complications early during hospitalization. A positive difference in mortality in the second column of Table 1 favors propranolol over placebo. The third column shows the approximate standard errors of the differences in column two. Using Eqs. 7 and 8 above, one obtains $\hat{\mu} = 2.315$ and $\hat{\sigma}_0^2 = 3.2616$. The fourth column shows d_k/σ_k. The remaining columns show the posterior mean and variance of the δ_k and the posterior probabilities that $\delta_k \geq 0$. In comparing d_k with λ_k one sees that all treatment effects have been "shrunk" toward the mean of 2.315. This causes a decrease of effect for the last three subsets and an increase for the first. The change is particularly strong for the third subset; its extreme value of 6.4 is shrunk to 3.26 because its standard error σ_k is large relative to $\hat{\sigma}_0$. Comparing the σ_k column with the γ_k column, one sees that precision of estimation has been substantially enhanced in the posterior analysis. Comparing column 4 with column 7, one sees the size of the effects per standard error compared for the prior and posterior analysis. For subsets two and three, the shrinkage of effect is approximately compensated by the improvement in precision. For the first subset the prior precision was already good and the main effect of the analysis is a slight increase in the estimate of treatment effect. For the fourth subset there is a moderate shrinkage but a large improvement in precision. Consequently, the inference that propranolol is superior to placebo for the fourth subset is strengthened by the posterior analysis. Confidence limits for δ_k are easily calculated from the normal distribution with mean λ_k and variance γ_k^2.

The empirical Bayesian analysis is appealing. This appeal is achieved by assuming that the subset-specific treatment effects δ_k can be regarded as random variables from a distribution with a finite number of parameters and known form. The assumption in Eq. 6 gave results particularly easy to use, but any other "mixture" assumption would provide the same conceptual solution to the problem. There does not appear to be any particular reason to believe that Eq. 6 should be correct. With many subsets one could test the assumption. Figure 1 of Furberg and Byington (1983) shows d_k values for 146 subsets in the BHAT trial. The effects do appear to be normally distributed. The larger differences are associated with larger standard errors, and an empirical Bayesian analysis as described above would have been useful. More complex analyses can be achieved by replacing Eq. 6 with a mixture assumption that provides more flexibility for the relationships among the δ_k. Thomas et al. (1985) use a mixture of two normals and Laird (1978) uses a nonparametric maximum likelihood estimate of the mixture distribution. The empirical Bayesian approach provides an interesting tool for looking at subset effects. The results will be dependent upon the mixture assumption and hence should be evaluated in conjunction with other tools.

Bayesian Methods

It was observed above that the results of an empirical Bayesian analysis are somewhat subjective due to the selection of a mixture distribution. If some subjectivity is acceptable for dealing with a very difficult problem, one might ask, "Why not perform a pure Bayesian analysis?" In fact, the empirical Bayesian analysis described above is very similar to a Bayesian analysis with noninformative priors on μ and σ_0^2. Such a formulation, however, is somewhat restrictive with regard to the degree of correlation among the δ_k. Bayesian formulations of the subset problem have been described by Cornfield (1976) and by Donner (1982) but also under restrictive assumptions and without a full analysis.

I would like to present a Bayesian model here which is also restrictive but which is simple and potentially useful for interpreting some subset results. Assume that the patients in the study are partitioned into two subsets, say male and female. If δ_1 and δ_2 are the treatment differences within the two subsets, let $\theta = \delta_1 - \delta_2$ represent the difference of the two subset-specific treatment effects. If there is no treatment by subset interaction then $\theta = 0$. Let $\hat{\theta}$ denote an estimate of θ calculated from the data and assume that $\hat{\theta}$ is normally distributed with mean θ and variance σ^2, as would be the case asymptotically for maximum likelihood estimators. We shall also adopt a prior for θ

$$\theta \sim N(0, \tau^2) \tag{10}$$

Such a symmetrical prior might be appropriate in situations where we do not have biological hypotheses about how relative treatment efficacy might vary among subsets.

Under these assumptions, one can show that the posterior distribution of θ is normal wih mean

$$\lambda_{post} = \hat{\theta}(1 + \sigma^2/\tau^2)^{-1} \tag{11}$$

and variance

$$\gamma^2 = (\sigma^{-2} + \tau^{-2})^{-1}. \tag{12}$$

The posterior mean depends on the observed $\hat{\theta}$ but the posterior variance does not. Let θ' denote a degree of difference between the subset-specific treatment differences that is considered of minimal clinical significance. Then a measure of whether there is a clinically significant treatment by subset interaction is given by

$$p_{post}(\theta \geq \theta') = \Phi\left[\frac{\lambda_{post} - \theta'}{\gamma}\right]. \tag{13}$$

We will consider an example for the situation where treatment effectiveness is measured by 5-year survival proportion. Let $\theta' = 0.10$, so that a 10% difference in relative treatment efficacy is the smallest treatment by subset interaction of clinical significance. Of course, the clinical significance of an interaction of a given size depends somewhat on the magnitude of the overall treatment difference. But for overall differences of about 5%–20% an interaction of 10% is important. Assume that a priori differences of θ' and $-\theta'$ are considered equally likely and each is associated with a probability of one in ten. This means that a clinically significant interaction in one direction or the other is given an a priori probability of one in five. A reasonable a priori probability for an overall treatment difference of clinical significance might be one in two, so a value of one in five for an interaction for a subset of no special interest certainly does not seem too low. The analysis described here can be repeated for various partitioning variables. Using the one-in-five assumption, we obtain for the value of the prior standard deviation $\tau = \theta'/1.28$, because 1.28 is the 90th percentile of the standard normal distribution. Thus, $\tau = 0.078125$.

We shall also assume that the standard error of the overall treatment difference is 0.031. This value provides a statistical power of about 0.90 for detecting an overall treatment difference of 0.10 using a two-sided significance test of size 0.05. These assumptions seem reasonable for some large clinical trials that are not planned with sufficient sample size for within-subset treatment comparisons. Under these assumptions, σ equals 0.031 times the square root of 2, since σ is the standard error of the interaction estimate. Hence, $\sigma = 0.04384$.

From Eqs. 11 and 12 we obtain that the posterior mean of θ is 0.7605 $\hat{\theta}$ and the posterior standard deviation is 0.0382, where $\hat{\theta}$ is the observed interaction effect, the observed difference in subset-specific treatment differences. Finally, assume that the observed interaction effect is three times its standard error, $\hat{\theta} = 3\sigma = 0.1315$. This corresponds to a situation with an apparently highly significant interaction. Then Eq. 11 gives 0.10 for the posterior mean and Eq. 13 gives 0.50 for the posterior probability that this interaction exceeds the level of minimal clinical significance. The posterior probability of 0.50 clearly does not represent compelling evidence for the interaction. It is about the size that one would use to justify a confirmatory trial. The value of 0.50 is based upon the numerous assumptions made, but it does seem to represent an assessment of the credence that might be placed on a subset finding for one common scenario. The model deserves further study because of its simplicity and the naturalness by which the prior may be specified.

Bayesian methods are infrequently used for the analysis of clinical trials. Subset analysis, however, is one area where they should be more adequately explored.

Discussion

Many of the most important and most expensive clinical trials in cancer, cardiovascular disease, and other areas result in conclusions based on subset analyses. In some of these cases it is surprising that the methodology used is almost guaranteed to give misleading results. Some of the problems of subset analysis are inherent in trying to answer too many questions with too few patients. Good methodology is not a substitute for more patients, but more patients are not a substitute for good methodology.

It is unwise to base scientific conclusions on data from a single study. Most subset findings can be reliably evaluated only in light of confirmation or refutation by similar studies. Few would disagree with this philosophically, but some investigators do not report their results with this in mind. It is not enough to say "these results require confirmation." The medical community would be better served if the authors contacted organizers of similar studies that had been completed to determine whether the claimed subset effects were also found in those trials. Whereas statistically significant effects for subsets will be too much to expect for each similar study, it is important to know the extent to which results of similar studies are consistent with the claimed effect. In view of the importance placed by authors on subset findings, it does not seem inappropriate to require that they attempt to assess this by contacting original sources where necessary, the degree to which their findings are consistent with those of other studies. This assessment would require judgement, because two studies are seldom exactly alike.

Utilizing the best statistical methodology for the design and analysis of subsets is particularly important when there are no confirmatory trials available. This may be the case for very expensive prevention trials and for some therapeutic trials. Subset findings for such studies may create serious dilemmas in prescribing treatments for future individuals and in the planning of future trials. The resolution of these dilemmas requires consideration of losses for incorrect actions as well as assessment of the existence and magnitude of subset effects. The ethical difficulties in deciding whether to design a follow-up trial based on believing or ignoring a subset effect can be substantial. Targeting separate follow-up trials to separate subsets can also result in too few patients per trial to answer any further question. Hence, such targeting based on an unconfirmed result is hazardous; it must be based on the best statistical practice in the design and analysis of the original study.

For most clinical trials it will not seem practical or appropriate to plan the sample size large enough to support definitive subset analyses. Most subset findings identified by naive analysis of such trials will not be confirmed by other trials. This will be largely because the findings are spurious, but it may also be due in part to the limited size of the "confirmatory" trials. If there are serious subset questions suggested by such a set of trials, a meta-analysis based on primary data is required. There are some clinical situations, however, where sufficient sample size for separate analysis of major subsets seems clearly needed; for example, evaluation of hormonal treatment for patients with estrogen receptor-positive or -negative primary breast cancer. In such circumstances, planning sample size sufficient only for a pooled analysis does not seem justified.

I have not attempted to provide a complete compendium of tools for subset analysis. There are other general tools not covered. One method which should at least be mentioned is the use of regression models to attempt to "adjust away" subset effects based on imbalances for other variables. There may also be special aspects of particular clinical trials which can be taken advantage of in the analysis. For example, some clinical trials have two experimental treatments and one control therapy. If the two treatments are very dissimilar but the same type of interaction occurs for both relative to the control, one must question whether the control results are a fluke. Biological rationale for the interactions and consistency of results with regard to different end points must also be considered.

John Tukey said: "It is right for each physician to want to know about the behavior to be expected from the intervention or therapy applied to his individual patient ... it is not right, however, for a physician to expect to know this." Subset analyses can, however, discover specificities of fundamental importance. Approaching subset analyses in a structured manner utilizing the best statistical tools available is necessary if we are to reduce the proliferation of misleading results while analyzing and reporting our studies thoroughly and responsibly.

References

Cornfield J (1976) Recent methodological contributions to clinical trials. Am J Epidemiol 104: 408-421

Donner A (1982) A Bayesian approach to the interpretation of subgroup results in clinical trials. J Chronic Dis 35: 429-435

Efron B, Morris C (1973) Stein's estimation rule and its competitors - an empirical Bayes approach. J Am Stat Assoc 68: 117-130

Furberg CD, Byington RP (1983) What do subgroup analyses reveal about differential response to beta-blocker therapy? Circulation 67 (suppl I): I98-I101

Furberg CD, Hawkins CM, Lichstein E (1983) Effect of propranolol in postinfarction patients with mechanical or electrical complications. Circulation 69: 761-765

Gail M, Simon R (1985) Testing for qualitative interactions between treatment effects and patient subsets. Biometrics 41: 361-372

Laird NM (1978) Nonparametric maximum likelihood estimation of a mixing distribution. J Am Statist Assn 73: 805-811

Peto R (1982) Statistical aspects of cancer trials. In: Halnan KE (ed) Treatment of cancer. Chapman and Hall, London, pp 867-871

Simon R (1982) Patient subsets and variation in therapeutic efficacy. Br J Clin Pharmacol 14: 473-482

Simon R (1986) Confidence intervals for reporting results of clinical trials. Ann Intern Med 105: 429-435

Thomas DC, Siemiatycki J, Dewar R, Robins J, Goldberg M, Armstrong BG (1985) The problem of multiple inference in studies designed to generate hypotheses. Am J Epidemiol 122: 1080-1095

*Competing Risks, Interactions and Crossing Hazards**

R. Kay

Department of Probability and Statistics, University of Sheffield,
Sheffield S3 7RH, Great Britain

Introduction

Byar (1985a) has analysed some data from a randomised clinical trial comparing treatment for patients with prostate cancer in stages 3 and 4. A full listing of the data is given in Byar (1985b). Treatment consisted of different doses of diethylstilbestrol (DES): 0 (placebo), 0.2 mg, 1 mg and 5 mg daily. Byar identified important treatment and covariate interactions in an exponential regression model for survival time, and by carefully considering the nature of the disease and treatment concluded that the beneficial effects of DES with regard to cancer death were compensated by increased risk of cardiovascular death for the high DES doses. He proceeded to outline methods for choosing optimal treatment for patients based on covariate information.

Including such interactions is a rather indirect way of investigating the effects of treatment on the risk of death from different causes. I will show, in addition, that the data are not well described by such a model.

This approach also does not fully appreciate the competing-risks nature of survival. Using methods which allow the risks of cardiovascular death and cancer death to be assessed separately, a more direct and more easily interpretable method of analysis is possible. The purpose of this paper is to use such methods in the analysis of these data. Choice of optimal treatment is also considered under this alternative approach and important differences in principle between this and the methods proposed by Byar (1985a) are discussed. Considerations throughout are based on the more general proportional-hazards model rather than on the exponential special case.

* This article is based partially on Kay R. (1986) Treatment effects in competing-risks analysis of prostate cancer data. Biometrics 42: 203-211. With permission from The Biometric Society.

Recent Results in Cancer Research, Vol. 111
© Springer-Verlag Berlin · Heidelberg 1988

The Data

The data set consists of 506 patients randomly allocated to one of four treatment regimes; placebo, 0.2 mg, 1.0 mg and 5.0 mg DES daily. For the purposes of analysis, 0 (placebo) and 0.2 mg were designated as low-dose DES and 1.0 mg and 5.0 mg as high-dose and the treatment indicator was put equal to 0 or 1 for low and high dose respectively. There were additionally seven covariates of interest: age (0, <75 years; 1, 75-80 years; 2, >80 years), weight index (wt.-ht.+200; 0, ⩾100; 1, 80-99; 2, <80), performance rating (0, normal; 1, limitation of activity), history of cardiovascular disease (0, no; 1, yes), serum haemoglobin (0, ⩾ 12 g/100 ml; 1, 9-12 g/100 ml; 2, <9 g/100 ml), size of primary lesion (0, < 30 cm^2; 1, ⩾30 cm^2) and Gleason stage/grade category (0, ⩽10; 1, >10). These will be denoted, as in Byar (1985 b), respectively by AG, WT, PF, HX, HG, SZ and SG. There were 483 patients with complete information on all relevant variables and the analysis was conducted on this subset. Of these, 344 died, with 149 classified as cancer deaths and 139 suffering cardiovascular death. The remaining 56 died of other causes. Survival time was recorded in months.

The Proportional-Hazards Model for Competing Risks

Byar (1985 a) used the exponential special case of the proportional-hazards model (Cox 1972) to analyse these data. The latter model is most easily described using the hazard function $\lambda(t)$ (the instantaneous rate at which patients are dying through time) with

$$\lambda(t) = \lambda_o(t) \exp(\beta_1 x_1 + \beta_2 x_2 + \cdots + \beta_p x_p) \tag{1}$$

where $x_1, x_2, \ldots, x_p$ are the explanatory variables (treatment indications and covariates). An extension according to Kalbfleisch and Prentice (1980) considers separate hazard functions for the different causes of death, so that $\lambda(t)$ is made up of a series of J hazard functions (corresponding to the J causes of death) with

$$\lambda(t) = \lambda_1(t) + \ldots + \lambda_J(t).$$

Here $\lambda_1(t)$ is the hazard function for death from cause 1, $\lambda_2(t)$ from cause 2 and so on. These authors then allow each cause-specific hazard to depend on the explanatory variables in a unique way, i.e.

$$\lambda_j(t) = \lambda_{oj}(t) \exp(\beta_{j1} x_1 + \ldots + \beta_{jp} x_p) \tag{2}$$

Parameter estimation uses the method of partial likelihood and details of this are given in Kalbfleisch and Prentice (1980). Briefly, the $\underset{\sim}{\beta}_j$'s are estimated separately for each cause, with deaths from remaining causes treated as censored observations. Details of the fit of Eq. 2 to the prostate cancer data are discussed in the next section. Standard errors of parameter estimators are obtained through estimated second derivatives of the log partial likelihood, and significance tests are based on comparing parameter estimates with standard errors.

Data Analysis

Table 1 gives details of model-fitting to the prostate cancer data. Equation 1 is used to investigate overall survival while Eq. 2 investigates the effects of the explanatory variables on the causes separately. For overall survival the treatment effect is not quite significant, with treatment group 1 (high-dose DES) doing better. All covariates have significant coefficients, with higher values in each case giving poorer survival. The effects of the variables, however, are explained more appropriately through the cause-specific analysis. Indeed, as I will show later, both the form of Eq. 1 fitted here and that including treatment x covariate interactions as considered by Byar (1985a) show significant lack of fit. Treatment group 1 (high-dose DES) does better as regards risk of cancer death (estimated relative risk $e^{-0.55}=0.57$) yet worse as regards cardiovascular death (estimated relative risk $e^{0.35}=1.42$). Older patients are at higher risk of cardiovascular death, as are those with a history of cardiovascular disease. Haemoglobin, tumour size and stage/grade significantly affect risk of cancer death, with higher values being associated with higher risk. 'Other causes' included deaths from respiratory disease, other specified or unspecified noncancer causes and unknown causes. Older patients and those with a higher weight index were at higher risk of dying from these, as were patients in treatment group 1. The weight-index effect puts patients who are lighter relative to their height, and therefore probably weaker, at higher risk. The treatment effect here is possibly caused by patients whose cancers have not been checked by treatment (group 0) but who have died from a noncancer/noncardiovascular cause.

As regards choice of optimal treatment, with which Byar (1985a) was particularly concerned, this is also easily accomplished within the competing-risks framework. For a patient with covariate values $x_2,\ldots x_p$ the hazard for cause j can be estimated by replacing the β's with their estimated values to give $\hat{\lambda}_j(t)$ for x_1 (the

Table 1. Parameter estimates for overall survival (Eq. 1) and cause-specific hazards (Eq. 2); standard errors are given in *parentheses*

Coefficient	Eq. 1	Eq. 2 cause specific: Cardiovascular disease	Eq. 2 cause specific: Cancer	Eq. 2 cause specific: Other causes
Treatment	−0.18 (0.11)	0.35 (0.17)*	−0.55 (0.17)*	−0.58 (0.28)*
AG	0.29 (0.09)*	0.34 (0.13)*	0.01 (0.14)	0.77 (0.20)*
WT	0.20 (0.09)*	0.04 (0.15)	0.19 (0.13)	0.53 (0.21)*
PF	0.40 (0.16)*	0.47 (0.26)	0.25 (0.24)	0.54 (0.41)
HX	0.44 (0.11)*	1.14 (0.18)*	−0.09 (0.17)	0.02 (0.27)
HG	0.29 (0.12)*	0.02 (0.20)	0.47 (0.17)*	0.36 (0.29)
SZ	0.67 (0.15)*	−0.22 (0.35)	1.15 (0.19)*	0.72 (0.41)
SG	0.40 (0.11)*	−0.02 (0.17)	1.34 (0.20)*	−0.45 (0.28)
log-ligelihood		−763.00	−771.17	−297.74

Asterisks denote individual significance at approximately the 5% level at least, corresponding to $\dfrac{\beta}{\text{s.e.}(\beta)} > 2$.

binary treatment indicator) equal to 0 and 1. Here, also, the underlying hazard has been replaced by an estimated function. Details are given in Kay (1986). This, in turn, leads to an estimated overall hazard function $\hat{\lambda}(t) = \hat{\lambda}_1(t) + \ldots + \hat{\lambda}_J(t)$ and estimated predicted survival function S(t) for the two treatment possibilities. If S(t) for $x_1 = 0$ is consistently higher than S(t) when $x_1 = 1$, then treatment 0 is preferred and vice versa. If these functions cross, however, clinical considerations are needed in the choice of preferred treatment.

Choice of Optimal Treatment

The type of model considered by Byar (1985a) includes a common underlying hazard $\lambda_o(t)$ for all patients, and therefore, since $\lambda(t)$ when $x_1 = 0$ is then either uniformly smaller or uniformly larger than $\lambda(t)$ when $x_1 = 1$, optimal treatment can be defined unambiguously. Equation 2, however, contains fewer constraints than Eq. 1. In terms of resulting survival obtained from the sum of the cause-specific hazard rates and for Eq. 2, it may be that overall survivor functions for the two treatments cross. Crossing survivor functions of the kind described here are not unexpected, and indeed, Eq. 1, which does not allow them, might therefore be considered unrealistic. This creates problems, however, as regards choice of optimal treatment, since under Eq. 2 there may not be a uniformly superior treatment. For a particular patient, one treatment regime may be preferred for short-term survival while a second treatment predicts better long-term survival. Note that in this case, Eq. 1, which constrains the treatment effect to be consistent, averages out the effect to produce predicted survivor functions which display a uniform but spurious treatment difference. In terms of the clinical decision on optimal treatment, crossing survival curves require some subjective judgement to choose an appropriate treatment regime for that patient. For the prostate cancer data these considerations do not usually apply, as optimal treatment can be defined unambiguously in almost all cases. For example, Figs. 1 and 2 show the predicted survival curves for patients with covariate combinations HG = SZ = SG = 1, remaining covariates = 0 and HX = 1 and remaining covariates = 0 respectively. In both cases one treatment gives consistently better survival. In the former case low-dose DES is preferred, while in the latter case the reverse is true. Crossing survival curves do, however, occur for some patients. Figure 3 displays these curves for a patient with AG = 2, HX = SG = 1, and remaining covariates = 0. Short-term survival to about 15 months is more likely for high-dose DES, with better long-term survival prospects under low-dose DES. It should be pointed out, however, that these differences are small and the two treatment regimes in this case produce very similar predicted survival patterns. Nevertheless, this example illustrates that, in principle, crossing survival curves can result.

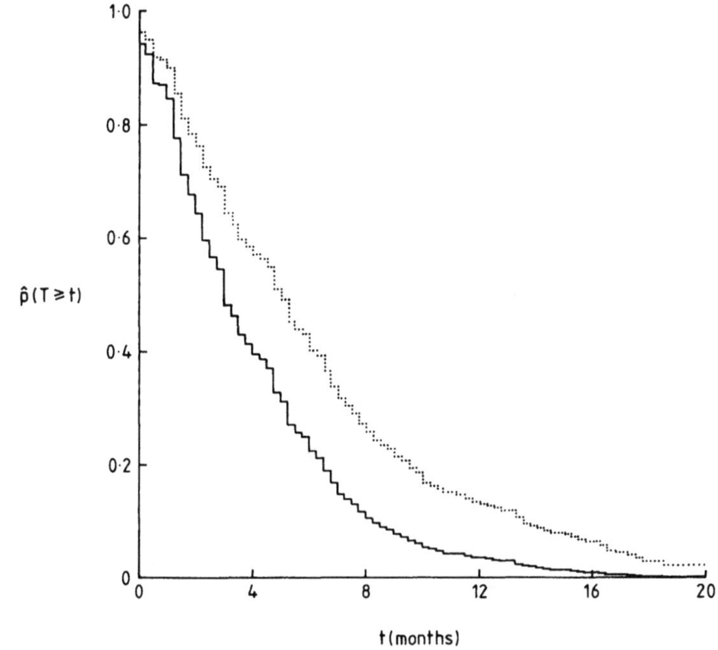

Fig. 1. Estimated survival curves for treatment groups and a patient with AG = WT = PF = HX = 0, HG = SZ = SG = 1. —,low-dose DES; · · · · ·,high-dose DES

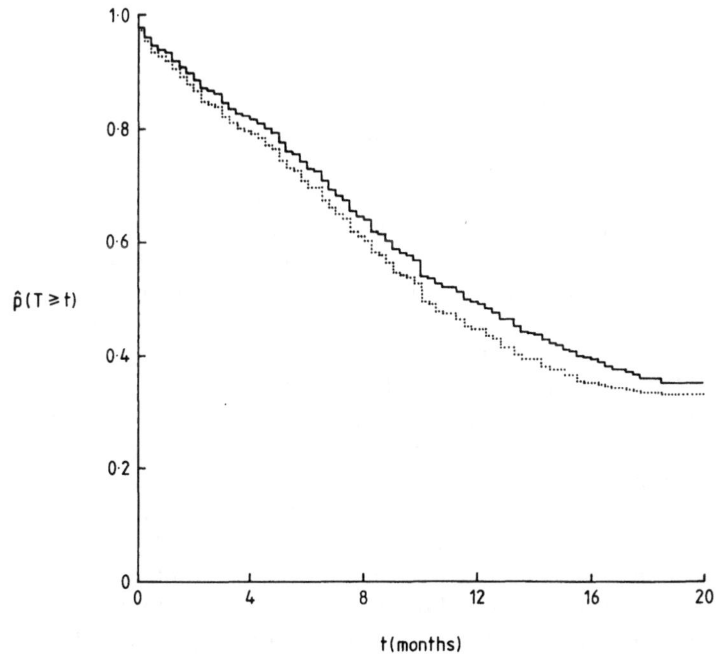

Fig. 2. Estimated survival curves for treatment groups and a patient with AG = WT = PF = HG = SZ = SG = 0, HX = 1. —,low-dose DES; · · · · ·,high-dose DES

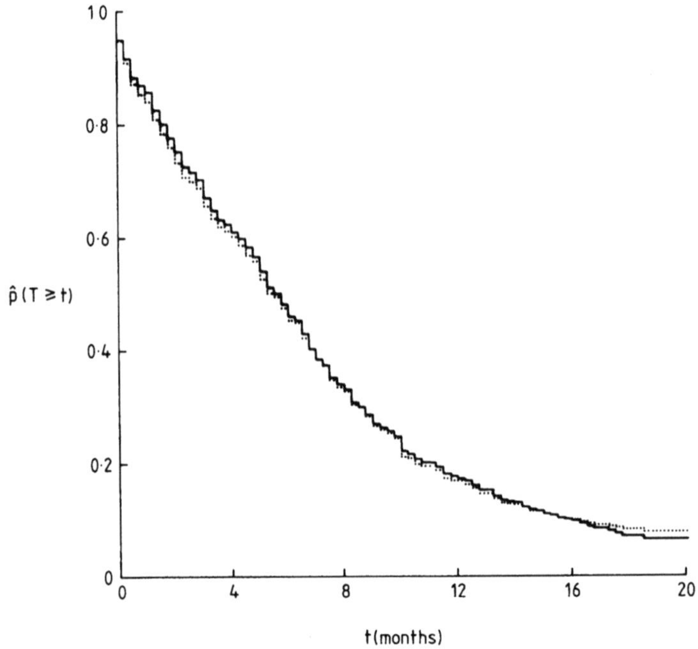

Fig. 3. Estimated survival curves for treatment groups and a patient with WT = PF = HG = SZ = 0, AG = 2, HX = SG = 1. —, low-dose DES; ·····, high-dose DES

Model Checking

Equation 2 assumes that the explanatory variables affect each cause-specific hazard in a multiplicative way that is the same for all t. This assumption, which can in certain situations be invalid, needs to be checked. This may be done for each cause j by dividing the time axis into r disjoint intervals and allowing the coefficient $\underset{\sim}{\beta}_j$ in Eq. 2 to be different for the different intervals. Estimation of the different $\underset{\sim}{\beta}_j$ values is straightforward, and a test of constant $\underset{\sim}{\beta}_j$ is based on a likelihood ratio test procedure. Details are given in Kay (1986).

For Eq. 1 these methods are simpler with a single subdivision of the time scale and go through in an obvious way.

For the prostate cancer data three intervals were chosen for both cardiovascular death and cancer death. The cut points for each cause were chosen to ensure approximately equal numbers of deaths from that cause in each of the intervals. For cardiovascular death the intervals used were (0, 12], (12, 31], and (31, ∞), and a likelihood ratio test for constant coefficients for this cause gives a χ^2_{16} statistic of 13.30, which is not significant. In particular, the three estimated coefficients of the treatment variable are, with standard errors in brackets, 0.46(0.30), 0.34(0.29) and 0.31(0.30) respectively. For cancer deaths the intervals were (0, 14], (14, 31], (31, ∞), and the χ^2_{16} statistic is 21.94, again nonsignificant. The estimated coefficients of treatment and standard errors are −0.30(0.28), −0.83(0.30), −0.75(0.29). These results suggest that the assumption of proportionality for Eq. 2 for these two causes is not violated. Similar results were noted for the remaining death category 'other causes'.

In contrast, the overall survival Eq. 1 does not fit the data well. Using a model with the three-interval subdivision (0, 13], (13, 32], (33, ∞] gives a χ^2_{16} statistic of 28.23, which is significant at the 5% level. The coefficients of the treatment indicator with standard errors were 0.09(0.19), −0.40(0.19), −0.31(0.20). The differential effect of treatment is consistent with our interpretation of the effects of treatment on the risks of cancer and cardiovascular death. Most cardiovascular deaths occur relatively quickly after start of treatment and then cancer deaths predominate. The treatment effect in favour of high-dose DES is therefore seen only later in time. The effects of additional covariates were also seen to vary with time in this model.

The proportional-hazards model is unable to model such nonconstant effects, although nonproportional hazards could be obtained from this model by introducing interaction terms of covariates and treatment with time. This alternative, however, presents considerable computational problems and also involves some subjectivity in the choice of modelling schemes for the time dependency. The form of the proportional-hazards model fitted by Byar (1985a), which included the interactions of treatment with AG and SG covariates also displays significant lack of fit ($\chi^2_{20}=31.63$, $P<0.05$) using the same three interval subdivision of the time scale as above for Eq. 1.

Discussion

The method of analysis presented here does not make any assumptions regarding the dependence of competing causes of death. Modelling and inferences are undertaken with in the competing-risks framework, and questions regarding risks following removal of one or more possible causes of death are not addressed. The fitted model merely describes which risks pertain for the patients in the course of the trial and how these risks are related to treatment and covariates. Further discussion on more general issues relating to this is provided in Kalbfleisch and Prentice (1980, Chap. 7).

Byar (1985a) was concerned mainly with two aspects of these data: firstly, which covariates were important with regard to death from the various causes, and secondly, how should treatment be chosen for a particular individual to provide the best chance of survival? The competing-risks analysis gives more direct answers to both these questions. In addition, these methods contain less 'modelling' than was used by Byar. In particular, for any patient overall survival curves for the two treatments are allowed to cross in the competing-risks model while this is not the case in Byar's work. That this should be allowed is intuitively clear.

Acknowledgements. The prostate cancer data were initially made available by David Byar through the Multivariate Study Group of the Royal Statistical Society, and I would like to express my thanks to David Byar and Agnes Herzberg for making this possible. Dave Robson wrote the computer programs to produce the figures.

Byar DP (1985a) Assessing apparent treatment-covariate interactions in randomised clinical trials. Stat Med 4: 255-263
Byar DP (1985b) Prognostic variables for survival in a randomised comparison of treatments for prostatic cancer. In: Andrews DF, Herzberg AM (eds) Data. Springer, Berlin Heidelberg New York (Series in statistics)
Cox DR (1972) Regression models and life tables. Stat Soc B 34: 187-220
Kalbfleisch JD, Prentice RL (1980) The statistical analysis of failure time data. Wiley, New York pp 167, 170
Kay R (1986) Treatment effects in competing-risks analysis of prostate cancer data. Biometrics 42: 203-211

*Significance Testing in the Comparison of Survival Curves from Clinical Trials of Cancer Treatment**

J. L. Haybittle**

MRC Cancer Trials Office, Medical Research Council Centre, Hills Road, Cambridge CB2 2QH, Great Britain

The log-rank test (Peto and Peto 1972) is now widely used for comparing survival data from randomised clinical trials of cancer treatment that require prolonged follow-up. The test is optimal when the death rate in one group consistently exceeds that in the other group by a given proportion, the so-called proportional hazards situation. Alternative tests that are sometimes used are Gehan's generalisation of the Wilcoxon rank sum test (Gehan 1965) and its subsequent modifications by Peto and Peto (1972) and by Prentice (1978). Of these, the latter is to be preferred with censored data (Prentice and Marek 1979), and, as shown by Lee et al. (1975) in a simulation experiment comparing survival curves modelled on Weibull distributions, it may perform better in a nonproportional hazards situation. Similarly, Fleming et al. (1980) have demonstrated the loss of power of the log-rank compared with that of the Wilcoxon test in comparing survival curves where the greatest differences occur at early follow-up times, and Harrington and Fleming (1982) have shown a similar loss when the hazard ratio is a maximum at time zero and decreases smoothly towards unity as follow-up increases. The reason for the difference between the performance of the two tests is that the calculation of the Wilcoxon statistic weights the differences between observed and expected events according to the estimated survival at the time of the event, whereas the log-rank calculation gives equal weights at all event times (Tarone and Ware 1977). Thus, the Wilcoxon test gives more weight to differences which appear early in follow-up.

It may be questioned whether the proportional-hazards model is the most appropriate one for many trials of cancer therapy, since the control arm may often contain a subset of long-term survivors or 'cured' patients, and the new therapy being tested is unlikely to effect any improvement of survival in this subset. For example, Nissen-Meyer (1979) has postulated that the effect of adjuvant therapy

---

* This article is reprinted with permission from Pergamon Journals Ltd., from Haybittle JL (1986) Eur J Cancer Clin Oncol 22: 1279–1283.

** I am indebted to Mr. Laurence Freedman for his helpful discussions during the course of this work, and to Professor N. M. Bleehen for allowing me to use the facilities of the MRC Cancer Trials Office, Cambridge.

© Springer-Verlag Berlin · Heidelberg 1988

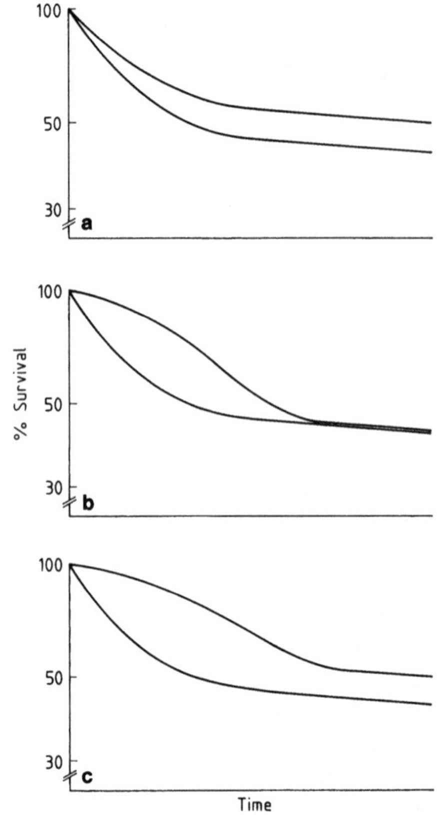

Fig. 1 a–c. Possible outcomes of trials of cancer treatment. **a** Increase in proportion of long-term survivors (type A effect); **b** increased survival time in proportion of short-term survivors (type B effect); **c** combination of both A and B effects

following surgery for primary breast cancer might be either to increase the percentage of long-term survivors, or to delay tumour growth in the remainder while not turning them into long-term survivors, or a combination of both these effects. In none of these situations would the outcome be a reduction of the hazard rate by a constant proportion throughout the duration of follow-up. This is illustrated in Fig. 1, where the three possible outcomes are plotted on log-linear graphs and the ratio of the slopes of the curves at any particular time gives the hazard ratio at that time. Figure 1a shows the effect of an increase in the percentage of long-term survivors (type-A effect). As the patients with a poor prognosis become a progressively smaller fraction of those still at risk, the death rates in the two groups become the same, i.e. that of the long-term survivors. The hazard ratio (Fig. 2) decreases with time towards unity.

In Fig. 1b the percentage of long-term survivors is the same in both groups, but the effect of adjuvant therapy has been to give some increased survival time to the poor-prognosis patients (type-B effect). Now the slope of the upper curve is initially less than that of the lower curve, but later the situation reverses as the delayed

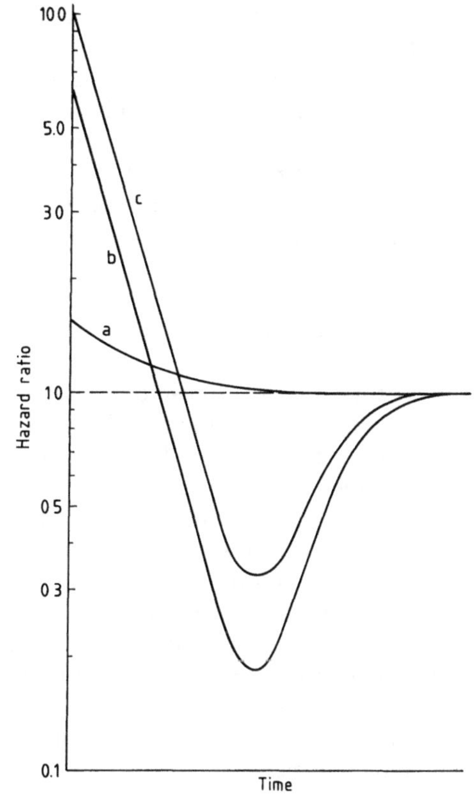

Fig. 2. Plots of hazard ratio (control arm/new treatment arm) for survival curves in Fig. 1

deaths in the poor-prognosis group occur, and eventually the slopes are identical. Thus, the hazard ratio (Fig. 2) decreases with time to a minimum value which is less than unity and then increases towards unity. The combination of both effects is illustrated in Fig. 1c, where the resulting hazard ratio plot (Fig. 2) is similar to that for Fig. 1b.

A further consequence of outcomes such as those in Fig. 1 is that the power of a test may be reduced rather than increased with further follow-up, even though more events will be recorded. This has been discussed by Peto et al. (1977), who suggest that the follow-up period may subdivided and the log-rank test applied separately in each period, so that the significance of early differences can be assessed. They warn, however, that the point of subdivision should not be chosen *after* examination of the two survival curves, but should be based on some consideration of the overall survival curve of all patients together to find when the overall death rate changes.

In spite of this recommendation, very few published clinical trials have been analysed in this way, and a common report following analysis without subdivision has been that an earlier reported significant difference has been reduced or has disappeared after further follow-up. For example, the results of the trial of adjuvant polyA-polyU in breast cancer after a maximum of 5 years' follow-up (Lacour et al. 1980) showed a significant difference ($P < 0.03$) in relapse-free survival time of node-positive patients; after 8 years' follow-up this difference was nonsignificant (Lacour et al. 1984). A report of a UICC meeting on the management of early breast cancer (Canellos et al. 1982) stated that 'reporting data on the results of adjuvant therapy too early can result in premature acceptance of benefits which subsequently may disappear.' If the benefit was extension of survival in a poor-prognosis fraction of patients, a subsequent nonsignificant result by the log-rank test carried out without subdivision of the time scale does not necessarily mean that this benefit was illusory, but only that the way the test was used was inappropriate.

Simulation experiment

The continued uncritical use of the log-rank test in spite of its known loss of power when hazards are not proportional may be due partly to lack of appreciation of the magnitude of this loss. In the examples simulated by Fleming et al. (1980) the power of the log-rank was found to be less than 50% that of the Wilcoxon test in models showing early differences in the survival curves.

Table 1 gives the results of a simulation experiment specifically designed to reproduce the situations shown in Fig. 1. Two hundred patients were entered into each arm of a trial at a uniform rate over a period of 4 years. Analysis of each trial was made at 4 years after the first patient was entered, i.e. at completion of entry, and also after a further follow-up of 4 years. Four hundred trials were simulated for each set of conditions.

The model for the survival curve of the control arm was taken to be a two-exponential one, namely:

$$S(t) = c \cdot \exp(-\lambda_1 t) + (1-c) \cdot \exp(-\lambda_2 t)$$
$$(t > 0,\ 0 < c < 1)$$

Table 1. Results of simulation experiments

Row no.	Control arm c	New treatment arm			Type of effect	% of trials[a] judged significant[b] (power of test)			
		c	$(1-c)$ fraction Increase in:			At 4 years		At 8 years	
			Mean survival (years)	Half-life (years)		Log-rank	Wil-coxon	Log-rank	Wil-coxon
1	0.6	0.8	0	0	A	70	68	87	88
2	0.3	0.5	0	0	A	57	53	86	80
3	0.6	0.6	1.5	0	B	88	95	31	56
4	0.3	0.3	1.0	0	B	98	100	55	94
5	0.6	0.7	1.0	0	A+B	84	89	63	79
6	0.6	0.6	0	1.5	B	51	53	39	50
7	0.3	0.3	0	1.5	B	90	90	92	96

[a] Out of a total of 400 trials for each row.
[b] Using $\chi^2 \geqslant 3.841$, $P \leqslant 0.05$ as the criterion for significance.

where S(t) is the surviving fraction at time t, λ_1 and λ_2 are constants with $\lambda_2 >> \lambda_1$, and c is the fraction of patients having the smaller mortality, i.e. the potentially long-term survivors. With $c = 0.6$ and λ_1 and λ_2 corresponding to half-lives of 20 and 1.5 years respectively, the model is a reasonably good representation of relapse-free survival up to 8 years as published by Lacour et al. (1984) for their control group of node-positive breast cancer patients.

To simulate the effect of the new treatment in the second arm, c could be increased by a specific amount and/or the survival times of patients with the higher mortality (λ_2) could be increased. Two methods of achieving this latter change were used. In one the survival times were increased by the simple addition of an amount derived from a normal distribution of increments with a specified mean, μ, and standard deviation, σ. σ was taken to be $\mu/3$ and the distribution was truncated at -3σ so that none of the survival times in the new treatment arm were actually decreased. In the second method, λ_2 was decreased, i.e. the half-life for the poor-prognosis group was increased.

All simulations were carried out with λ_1 and λ_2 in the control arm corresponding to half-lives of 20 and 1.5 years respectively. λ_1 was always kept corresponding to a half-life of 20 years in the new treatment arm. Four simulations were made with $c = 0.6$ in the control arm; three were made with $c = 0.3$.

Rows 1 and 2 of Table 1 show that when the effect of the new treatment was solely to increase the proportion of long-term survivors (type-A effect; Fig. 1a), both tests behaved very similarly, although there is some indication of a small power advantage for the log-rank test in row 2 when the proportion of long-term survivors is smaller.

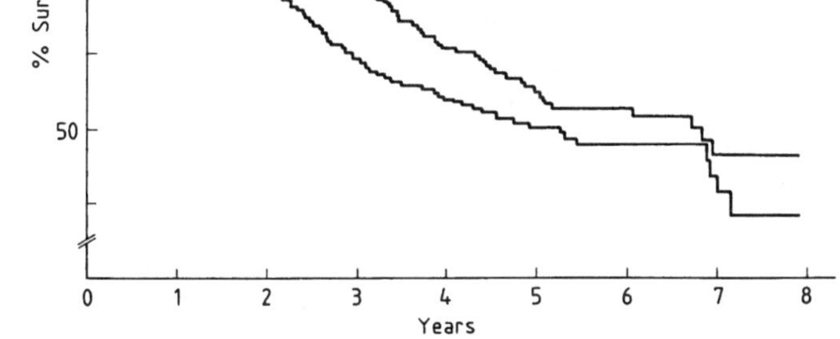

Fig. 3. Simulated trial result at 8 years after entry of first patient; 200 patients per arm entered over 4 years. Control group assumed to have 60% long-term survivors dying exponentially with a half-life of 20 years and 40% short-term survivors dying exponentially with a half-life of 1.5 years. New treatment arm *(upper curve)* similar to control, except that survival times of short-term survivors increased additively by amounts drawn randomly from a normal distribution of increments of mean 1.5 years and standard deviation 0.5 years

When the effect of the new treatment was solely to increase survival in an additive manner in the poor-prognosis patients (type-B effect), then the picture was very different (rows 3 and 4). The tests had similar power at 4 years, but both lost power with further follow-up due to the curves coming together from about 5 years onwards. However, the loss of power was much less marked with the Wilcoxon than with the log-rank test. At 8 years in each simulation the power of the log-rank was less than 60% that of the Wilcoxon. Figure 3 is an example of one simulated trial where both tests gave significant results at 4 years but only the Wilcoxon test still showed a significant difference at 8 years.

Row 5 shows the results when both increase of c and additively increased survival of poor-prognosis patients were simulated. Again, the loss of power at 8 years with the Wilcoxon is less marked than the loss with the log-rank test.

Rows 6 and 7 give the results when the type-B effect was simulated by doubling the half-life in the poor-prognosis group. In this subgroup the hazards then maintain a constant ratio, but, because of the unaffected good-prognosis fraction, the overall picture is still one of nonproportional hazards. The results in row 6 when $c = 0.6$ are qualitatively similar to those in row 3, in that power decreases with further follow-up, though less markedly, and the Wilcoxon test has a higher power than the log-rank at the later follow-up point. When c is smaller (row 7) the overall situation is nearer to that of proportional hazards, and both tests behave similarly with some increase of power at later follow-up.

Discussion

The results demonstrate that the loss of power of the log-rank in comparison with that of the Wilcoxon test can be considerable in some situations where the ratio of the hazard rates does not remain constant. The loss is most marked when the new treatment has a type-B effect only, i.e. prolongs survival of a subset of patients with a poor prognosis but does not increase the number of long-term survivors. This could well be the effect to be expected of a number of new cancer treatments and, unless the follow-up period is to be subdivided for analysis (with the disadvantages that may arise from an arbitrary choice of division points), the Wilcoxon test is more suitable than the log-rank for use in such trials.

The choice of test to be used should be governed by the hypothesis to be tested, and clinicians initiating trials should give some thought to the way in which the hoped-for benefit of a new treatment is likely to be expressed. Statisticians can then be guided accordingly in the choice of the test to be used. In any case, when the result of a trial is analysed, an examination should be made of the way in which the hazard ratio varies with follow-up time. The log-rank test should not be used for an overall comparison of curves such as those shown in Fig. 3.

References

Canellos GP, Hellman S, Veronesi U (1982) The management of early breast cancer. N Engl J Med 306: 1430-1432

Fleming TR, O'Fallon JR, O'Brien PC, Harrington DP (1980) Modified Kolmogorov-Smirnov test procedures with application to arbitrarily right-censored data. Biometrics 36: 607-625

Gehan EA (1965) A generalized Wilcoxon test for comparing arbitrarily singly censored samples. Biometrika 52: 203-217

Harrington DP, Fleming TR (1982) A class of rank test procedures for censored survival data. Biometrika 69: 553-566

Lacour J, Lacour F, Spira A, Michelson M, Petit J-Y, Delage G, Sarrazin D, Contesso G, Viguier J (1980) Adjuvant treatment with polyadenylic-polyuridylic acid (PolyA.PolyU) in operable breast cancer. Lancet ii: 161-164

Lacour J, Lacour F, Spira A, Michelson M, Petit J-Y, Delage G, Sarrazin D, Contesso G, Viguier J (1984) Adjuvant treatment with polyadenylic-polyuridylic acid in operable breast cancer: updated results of a randomized trial. Br Med J 288: 589-592

Lee ET, Desu MM, Gehan EA (1975) A Monte Carlo study of the power of some two-sample tests. Biometrika 62: 425-432

Nissen-Meyer R (1979) Adjuvant cytostatic and endocrine therapy: increased cure rate or delayed manifest disease. Comm Res Breast Dis 1: 95-109

Peto R, Peto J (1972) Asymptotically efficient rank invariant test procedures. J R Stat Soc A 135: 185-198

Peto R, Pike MC, Armitage P, Breslow NE, Cox DR, Howard SV, Mantel N, McPherson K, Peto J, Smith PG (1977) Design and analysis of randomized clinical trials requiring prolonged observation of each patient. II. Analysis and examples. Br J Cancer 35: 1-39

Prentice RL (1978) Linear rank tests with right-censored data. Biometrika 65: 167-179

Prentice RL, Marek P (1979) A qualitative discrepancy between censored-data rank tests. Biometrics 35: 861-867

Tarone RE, Ware J (1977) On distribution-free tests for equality of survival distributions. Biometrika 64: 156-160

Estimating the Magnitude of Benefits from Adjuvant Therapy

I. C. Henderson

Dana-Farber Cancer Institute, Harvard University, 44 Binney Street, Boston, MA 02115, USA

The physician at the bedside considering the appropriateness of a treatment for a particular patient should ask at least five questions:

1. Does the therapy have any benefit?
2. What is the nature of the benefit? Does it improve patient survival? Quality of life?
3. What is the magnitude of the benefit?
4. Does the benefit outweigh the cost?
5. Are the available data applicable to this particular patient? Were the patients included in the clinical trial enough like this patient to conclude that benefits observed in the trial apply in this clinical situation as well?

Most of these questions have been or will be considered at other times in this symposium. I will focus only on question 3: What is the magnitude of the benefit? I believe that most physicians take the absolute difference in disease-free survival or absolute survival at one point in time - usually the last point on a Kaplan-Meier plot - as an estimate of the magnitude of the benefit. Unfortunately, this is the least certain point, or the estimate with the widest confidence intervals along the entire plot. As a result, others use the level of statistical significance as a reflection of the size of benefit of the therapy. This is equally dangerous, since a very small benefit may result in a very high level of statistical significance in a large trial or in an overview. (In fact, "inflation" of statistical significance is an important source of the misinterpretation and misapplication of overview results.) A third approach to estimating the magnitude of benefit is to calculate the ratio reduction in mortality or the ratio reduction in some other undesirable end point. This approach may distort the magnitude of the effect by ignoring a large percentage of the population. For example, if eight of 100 patients in the control group and six of 100 patients in the treated group die during a period of observation, this 2% change in mortality may be expressed as a 25% reduction in mortality over the observational period. The expression of an effect as a ratio reduction in mortality may ignore the lack of effect or even negative effects of treatment on patients unlikely to die without treatment but likely to experience the toxicities of treatment.

Recent Results in Cancer Research, Vol. 111
© Springer-Verlag Berlin · Heidelberg 1988

Ideally, any measure chosen to express the magnitude of treatment effect should fulfill two criteria:

1. It should reflect the biologic effects or the mechanism of treatment benefit for the treatment under consideration.
2. The effects of treatment and the costs of treatment should be expressed in the same units of measurement.

The importance of considering the mechanism of treatment benefit can be illustrated using two modalities of treatment for patients with early breast cancer. The traditional treatments, mastectomy and radiotherapy, are given in anticipation that the entire tumor can be removed prior to its metastasis to a distant organ. When this happens the patient will be "cured," with restoration of her life expectancy prior to the diagnosis of breast cancer. There is no evidence that life will be prolonged among patients whose disease has metastasized prior to the initiation of treatment. There is no concept of a "partial response" to mastectomy or local/regional radiotherapy. The effect is "all or none." In this context it is probably reasonable to accept the differences in survival of two treatment groups on a life-table plot as an estimate of the percentage of patients whose tumor will be totally eradicated as a result of treatment.

Although the goal of adjuvant systemic therapy may be total eradication of all foci of micrometastases, it is likely that tumor reduction at most sites will be incomplete. In addition, the degree of tumor reduction is likely to vary greatly from one patient to the next (and even from one site to another). We know this is true for patients with metastatic breast cancer, a condition which permits measurement of tumor reduction. The response to endocrine therapy or cytotoxic chemotherapy in patients with measurable lesions will vary from apparent stabilization of growth in some patients to total eradication of disease for a variable period of time in others. A similar spectrum of response is likely to occur with micrometastases. This is shown schematically in Fig. 1. The ordinate represents the total body tumor cell burden; the abscissa represents time elapsed from diagnosis of the cancer and initiation of treatment. Patients whose tumor is untreated or is intrinsically resistant to treatment will have continuous tumor growth, shown here as logarithmic growth (curve A), ignoring for illustrative purposes probable growth plateaus which may occur during the periods of clinically evident metastatic disease. These patients will die at point I. Patients whose disease is cured by systemic chemotherapy are likely to have a pattern of disease reduction similar to that shown by curve B. Each course of chemotherapy will result in a sharp reduction in tumor burden followed by a small regrowth of tumor before administration of the next course of therapy. If the disease is very sensitive and does not become resistant to therapy during the course of treatment, the total body tumor burden will fall to a point which can be then eliminated by the body's own immune response. A more likely response to chemotherapy is shown by curve C. Patients may initially have a response to chemotherapy somewhat less than that illustrated by curve B and may eventually develop resistance to the therapy. Tumor regrowth in these patients is likely to be at the same rate as the original tumor, and the patient's death will occur at point II, when the tumor burden has once again become lethal. The response to endocrine therapy, which appears to be more cytostatic than cytocidal,

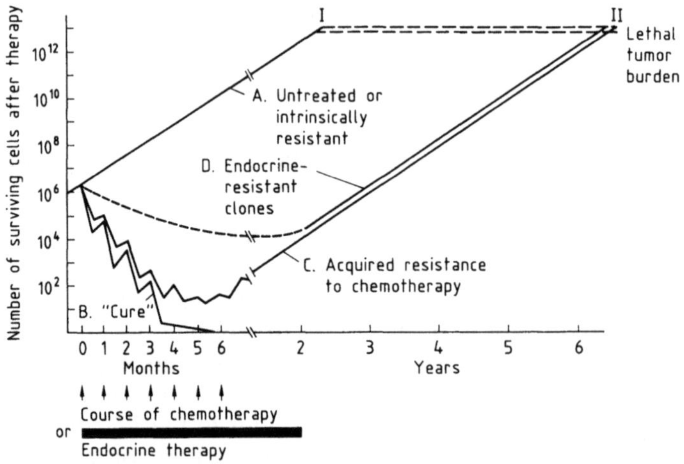

Fig. 1. Potential effects of adjuvant therapy on breast cancer micrometastases and interrelationship with patient survival. (From Henderson 1987)

may result in a less complete reduction of tumor cell burden, but the time interval before tumor regrowth and patient death may be as prolonged as that in the patient with a partial response to chemotherapy. In an individual patient the interval between point I and point II represents the difference in the time at which the patient would have died without treatment and the time when she dies with treatment. This interval reflects a benefit which is less than total, but this may be considered by patient or physician as sufficient to justify the cost of treatment. The duration of this interval is likely to vary considerably among patients. It should be assumed that many or most patients will have some prolongation of life as a result of treatment.

These effects of adjuvant systemic therapy contrast to the "all-or-none" effects of local treatment. While it is appropriate to describe the benefits of local therapy as a percentage of the population affected, the benefits of adjuvant therapy should be expressed as an average effect on each and every treated patient.

Practically, this means that the effects of therapy should be measured along the abscissa - the time axis of a life-table plot - rather than the ordinate. Conceptually, the easiest way to illustrate this is by calculating the difference in median survival for the control and treated groups. This is illustrated in Fig. 2. The data shown here are from the original Milan trial in which patients were randomized to receive either 1 year of Cyclophosphamide Methotrexate 5-Fluorouracil (CMF) or mastectomy without systemic therapy of any type (Bonadonna et al. 1985). All patients entered into this trial had histologically involved nodes, and patients were stratified into premenopausal and postmenopausal groups. Figure 2 is an actuarial plot of the survival of the premenopausal women through the first 10 years of follow-up. As illustrated in Fig. 2a, the difference in the survival of the treated and control populations at the 10th year is 14.2%. Although over half of the control patients had died, only about 40% of the treated patients were dead by the 10th year, and a true difference in "medians" can not be determined at the present time.

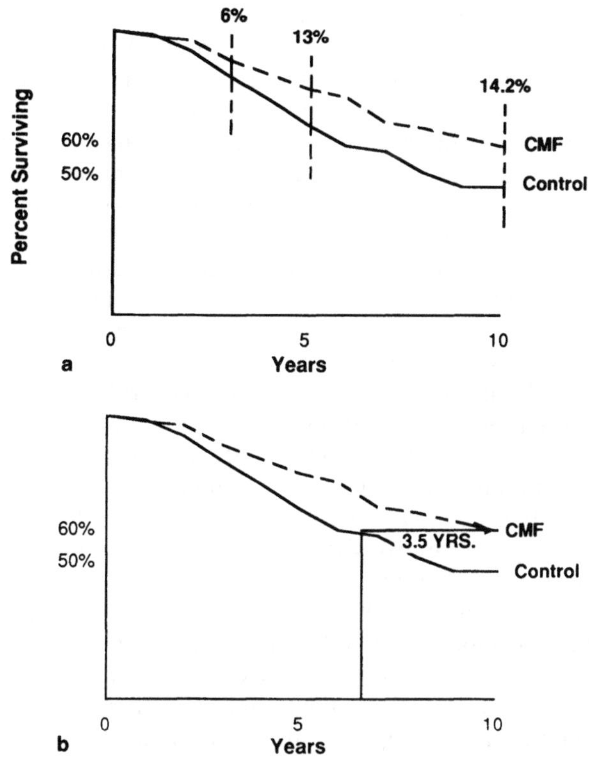

Fig. 2a, b. Overall survival for premenopausal women randomized to receive either adjuvant CMF or no treatment control. **a** is a representation of the data with emphasis on the vertical distance between the two life-table plots. **b** utilizes the same data with emphasis on the horizontal difference between the curves at the 60th percentile. (Modified from Bonadonna et al. 1985)

However, a horizontal drawn at the 60th percent level permits a calculation of the time separation of these two curves at a point close to the median. It is plausible that the effects seen when both populations have reached a median survival will be similar. As illustrated here, this difference is now 3.5 years. If this were indeed a difference in medians, it would suggest that 50% of the patients had lived an additional 3.5 years *or more* as a result of treatment. The other 50% of the patients had a benefit of less than 3.5 years (or possibly lived for a shorter period of time than they would have without treatment).

Another method for estimating the prolongation of survival is a determination of the difference in means. This could be achieved by measuring the area under the treatment curve and the area under the control curve and then subtracting the two areas.

There are obvious limitations to these two methods. First, both require very long follow-up. A difference in medians is not valid until the minimum follow-up of all patients entered into the trial equals the median follow-up of the group of patients with the best survival. For the data illustrated in Fig. 2, a valid difference in medians may not be possible for another 5-10 years. A difference in means cannot be determined until all the patients are dead. This will likely be several decades into the future. Second, a difference in medians is calculated at one point in time. Unless the curves are parallel throughout all or most of the follow-up, this single point may not accurately reflect the average effect of treatment. It is possible that some patients treated with systemic therapy will be "cured." A few patients with very prolonged survival as a result of therapy would distort a difference in means and overestimate the average effect for the majority of patients with a more modest prolongation of survival. It would be desirable to have an estimate of the confidence intervals around these averages, whether a difference in medians or a difference in means, and this is particularly important if the possibility of a detrimental effect is very large.

Although estimates of the average prolongation of survival are conceptually preferrable to calculations of rate differences at a single time point, average prolongation of survival is more difficult to determine. Probably the best approach to this problem is the use of mathematical models with assumptions which can be clearly stated and varied. This at least permits the physician to ascertain if these assumptions are consistent with his understanding of the disease and the usual effects of the therapies.

The additional advantage of expressing a survival benefit as years or months of prolongation of life is that this number can be more readily compared with years or months of quality of life lost due to toxicity. In general, the toxicities of therapies occur while the patient is receiving therapy, are readily apparent to patient and physician, and apply to all treated patients. Toxicities are inherently subjective, and it is difficult to apply objective numerical values to them. However, expressing survival benefits as months or years gained allows the physician or patient to personally subtract the numbers of months or years he/she feels have been lost due to toxicity. In the example of adjuvant CMF for premenopausal women just described, the physician and the patient might compare an average survival benefit of 3-4 years with a toxic cost of 1 year (i.e., the duration of CMF therapy in the Milan study). Some patients will choose to ignore the cost and will consider any prolongation of survival an improvement and an increased chance of being alive at a particular date as worth almost any cost short of death itself. In situations where the average prolongation of survival is equal to or shorter than the time during which the patient experienced the toxicities of therapy, many patients would elect no treatment no matter how statistically significant the survival benefit or how large the increased certainty of survival at a defined future date.

References

Bonadonna G, Valagussa P, Rossi A, Tancini G, Brambilla C, Zambetti M, Veronesi U (1985) Ten-year experience with CMF-based adjuvant chemotherapy in resectable breast cancer. Breast Cancer Res Treat 5: 95-115

Henderson IC (1987) Adjuvant systemic therapy of early breast cancer. In: Harris JR, Hellman S, Henderson IC et al (eds) Breast diseases. Lippincott, Philadelphia, pp 324-353

*Treatment by Protocol: Assessment of Gains and Losses**

H. Scheurlen**

Institut für Medizinische Biometrie und Informatik der Universität,
Im Neuenheimer Feld 325, 6900 Heidelberg, FRG

The Protocol

Treatment as a mutilating and hazardous intervention - an injury in legal terms - requires an explanation. With a perception of the biology of a given disease in mind, based on available evidence accumulated so far, one first of all has to weigh costs, risks, and benefits of all feasible interventions. Diagnostic procedures prior to remedial interventions and subsequent differential treatments should be specified in advance. Finally, an attempt should be made to account for the outcome of an intervention. In a broad sense, it is this three-point statement - background information, strategy for actions, strategy for analyzing results - that constitutes a protocol. Any intervention by protocol may be called a therapy.

Protocols may differ considerably in form and quality according to the following properties:

1. They may be explicit if explained by a written text or just implicit if not.
2. They may be flexible over time if changed whenever new evidence comes into fashion or fixed if physicians are less credulous.
3. They may differentiate between subgroups and thereby be rather complicated, or they may be simple.
4. They may be either completely determinate with respect to the measures to be taken against a particular disease or indeterminate to some extent.
5. They may or may not require informed consent.

In a determinate protocol every subgroup of patients can be assigned to one and only one treatment: the treatment of choice. Any other assignment can be considered malpractice or at least an exceptional treatment in the context of the protocol. However, sometimes a clear-cut treatment of choice may not exist and it may be unclear to which of two or more procedures preference should be given. If this

* To Professor Herbert Immich on his 70th birthday.

** I would like to thank John Haybittle, Richard Kay, and Martin Schumacher for their helpful suggestions.

© Springer-Verlag Berlin · Heidelberg 1988

happens, the protocol may provide a random procedure as a means of decision-making.

Seeking consent implies that a patient has the say, and that in an indeterminate protocol a patient also will have to be informed about uncertainty and possibly about random allocation. In a formal randomized clinical multicenter trial one would expect the proportions of patients randomized not to vary too much from hospital to hospital, and the preferences of the nonconsenting patients should not be too differently distributed. In those breast cancer trials of which I am in charge, this is far from what actually happens, indicating that the patient's consent may depend to a considerable degree on the doctor's understanding of uncertainty.

As concerns the outcomes of interventions, a few remarks should be made on the reliability of treatment comparisons to be guaranteed by the protocol. Within a protocol considering treatments to be completely determinate, any conclusions drawn from a comparison between the predominant treatment of choice and an exceptional treatment can only be invalid, as only unfavorable circumstances can have prevented a patient from being treated "lege artis." Not surprisingly, the treatment of choice most often appears to be superior to any other treatment, even after adjustment for prognostic factors. In a comparison between protocols patients should be grouped by prognostic factors without exclusions, irrespective of the treatment actually given and in particular of the treatment being considered a protocol deviation or not. The only valuable treatment comparison may be that of randomized patients in an 'indeterminate' protocol with the patients grouped according to the treatment intended by random allocation.

Patients not giving consent are looked upon as being inappropriate for an unbiased estimation of treatment effects and are therefore as a rule not considered for comparisons. However, we think that all patients who fulfill the clinical entry criteria should indeed be entered into a formal comprehensive cohort study (Scheurlen et al. 1984). In a protocol providing randomization one has to look at the self-selection mechanisms using clinical and sociodemographic variables as predictors and at the patient's consent to randomization as the (binary) outcome variable. The most important question concerns the range of validity: Are we allowed to generalize a conclusion drawn from the subgroup of properly randomized patients to the total population of the clinically eligible patients? This topic is dealt with later in this volume in a paper by Schumacher and Davis.

On Treatment Effects

It has been tacitly assumed so far that an account of the outcomes of interventions can be given only by comparing differently treated groups of patients using some measurement, e.g., survival time, presumably to be related to success or failure of treatments. What we call a treatment effect is essentially a summary statistic of those outcomes expressing the deviation from what we would expect if the treatment alternatives were equally effective, e.g., the difference between two proportions of patients surviving t years, the difference between the total of observed deaths and the total of the extents of exposure to risk of death at each time of an observed death, the risk or odds ratio, or the reduction in mortality.

These figures, however, tell us little about a patient's gain or loss through therapy when taking his or her natural history into account. They are meaningful mainly in cases where all patients react nearly the same way to therapy, regardless of their natural history. To see what happens to an individual patient one should be able to observe a pair of survival times: t_T - the patient's survival time if treated or if given an additional treatment (target variable), and t_0 - the patient's survival time if not treated or if not given the additional treatment (natural history). As obviously we cannot both treat a patient and not treat him or her at the same time, a model with the patient serving as his or her own control in a none vs. some or an add or drop comparison can be only speculative in survival analysis of a potentially progressive disease, e.g., primary operable breast cancer, with the patients not exhibiting signs and symptoms of disease residuals after primary surgery and with adjuvant therapy either to be given or not.

In a graphical presentation of this speculative deep model a point (t_0, t_T) above the break-even line $t_T = t_0$ indicates a beneficial treatment effect and a point below the line an adverse effect, with gain or loss to be expressed by the vertical distance $t_T - t_0$ of a point from the line. When we are considering a cohort of patients, a regression line $\hat{t}_T = f(t_0)$ may be fitted to the swarm of points with the points either tightly clustered or widely scattered around the line, where $\hat{t}_T$ is an estimate of the mean survival time following treatment given a specified value of the natural history t_0. Those points of a control group in a two-or-more sample comparison should all come to lie on the break-even line. In a hypothetical example, as displayed in Fig. 1, it is assumed (a) that therapy on average is harmful to patients who have a very bad prognosis, (b) that those patients with a moderately bad prognosis will profit most by therapy, (c) that gain decreases gradually as prognosis improves, and (d) that very-good prognosis patients do not profit at all or even lose.

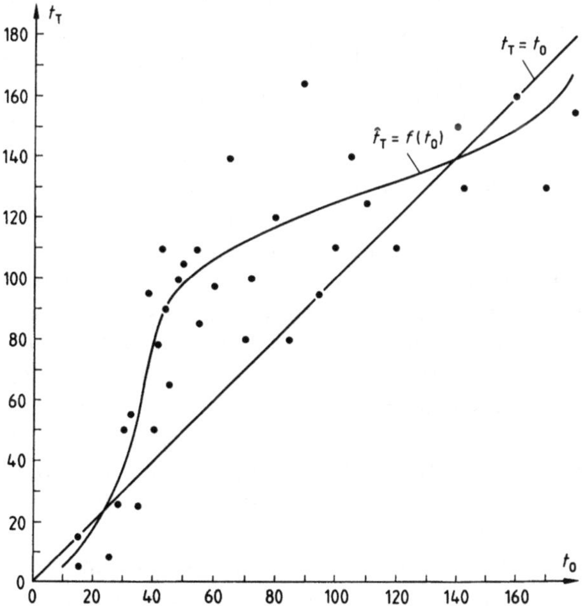

Fig. 1. Deep model: paired observations (hypothetical) and regression line of survival times following treatment (t_T) or natural history (t_0)

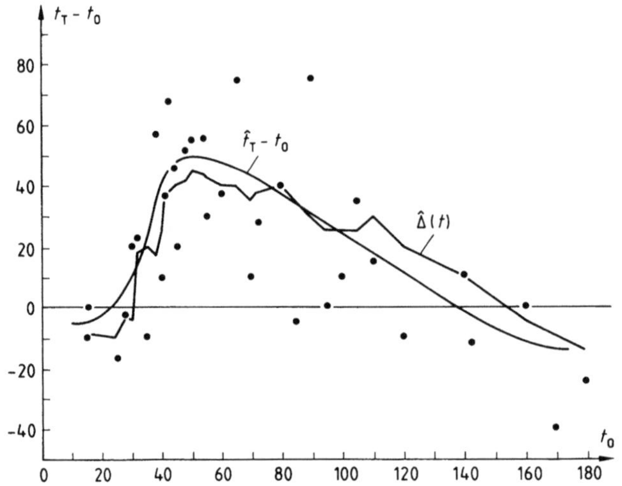

Fig. 2. Deep model: paired observations, gain and shift functions

Let us now consider some special cases of a functional relationship between the target variable t_T and natural history t_0. A straight line parallel to the break-even line will be obtained if gains and losses are uniformly distributed over the range of natural histories with no interaction between natural history and treatment. All other possible lines, either straight or not, imply some kind of an interaction. It is quantitative if the regression line runs totally above (or below) the break-even line, or qualitative if it runs somewhere across the break-even line. The main effect of a treatment may be expressed in terms of the average of distances $t_T - t_0$.

As we want to know how gain or loss $t_T - t_0$ rather than survival time following treatment t_T is related to natural history t_0, let us change the ordinate of the coordinate system accordingly (Fig. 2). The new regression function $\hat{t}_T - t_0 = g(t_0) = f(t_0) - t_0$ relating average gain or loss to natural history may be called gain function. Such an estimate of the average gain $\hat{t}_T - t_0$ given natural history t_0, however, will depend to a considerable degree on the mathematical model assumed for the shape of the gain function. Note that in our hypothetical example the points (t_0, t_T) are adapted somehow to a preassumed "regression line" and the points (t_0,$t_T - t_0$) to a preassumed "gain function," and that these lines can hardly be reproduced by formal regression analysis given the points.

Taking up an idea by Doksum (1974), the gain function $g(t_0)$ may be replaced by the shift function $\hat{\Delta}(t_0)$ without any assumptions to be made on the type of a functional relationship. To arrive at the shift function, let us go back to the points (t_0, t_T), draw the survival curves $\hat{S}_0(t)$ using the t_0 and $\hat{S}_T(t)$ using the t_T of the paired observations (Fig. 3), and take the horizontal distances $\hat{\Delta}(t)$ between any two points on the survival curves at time t and at $t + \hat{\Delta}(t)$ respectively, satisfying the condition $\hat{S}_0(t) = \hat{S}_T(t + \hat{\Delta}(t))$. In our example the estimate $\hat{\Delta}(t_0)$ relating the horizontal shift to natural history comes fairly close to the gain function $g(t_0)$ assumed in advance (Fig. 2).

Eventually, however, we will have to translate the deep model into a surface model, as only the real survival time can be obtained from a patient who has either

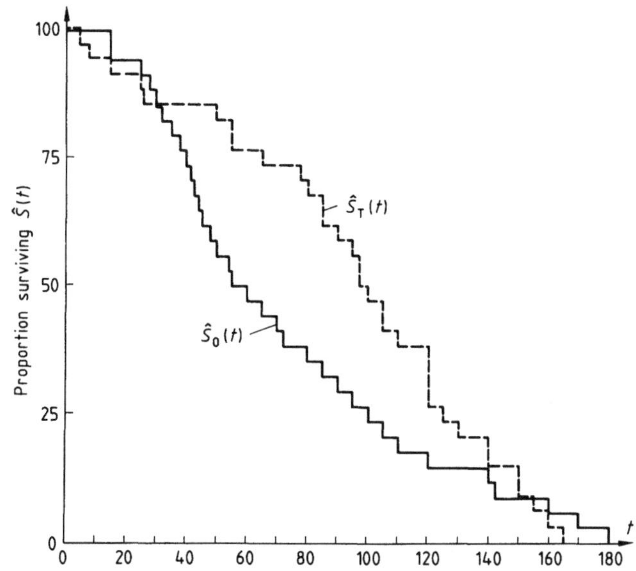

Fig. 3. Deep model: survival curves

been treated or not. Here the question arises whether or not any of the information considered in the deep model may come to the surface when survival curves derived from real survival data are compared.

In the surface model we have the two survival curves of a control and a treatment group and from these a shift function may be obtained, proceeding the same way as we did with the deep model. It is easy to see that the shift function in the surface model provides an unbiased estimate of the shift function in the deep model and thereby also an estimate of the gain function. In fact, to see how average gain may be related to natural history, the remaining difference between the models - paired observations (t_0, t_T) in the deep model, observations of either t_0 or t_T in the surface model - becomes less striking: Just draw one half of the paired observations (t_0, t_T) of the deep model from a box at random and note t_T to form the treatment group in the surface model and t_0 from the remaining points to form the control group, this being a true description of what is going on in a randomized trial (Fig. 4). Thus, in the surface model we have exactly half the observations of the deep model, this being the only difference between the two models when one is considering survival curves (Fig. 5) and shift functions. Note, however, that the shift function in the surface model leaves us ignorant of the random variation of individual gains and losses, or, putting it another way, that we are left with a sort of regression line without knowing to what points the line is fitted.

To see how gain on average depends on natural history is one thing. We need, however, to predict natural history, i.e., survival following no further treatment in the control group, to identify those patients who will presumably benefit from therapy. It is at this point that prognostic factors will have to come into play. Patients in the trial who have benefited on average from therapy should be identified by separating out that region [t_0^*, t_0^{**}] of the control group where the shift $\hat{\Delta}(t)$ appears to be substantial (a) to see how prognostic factors of the patients dying in

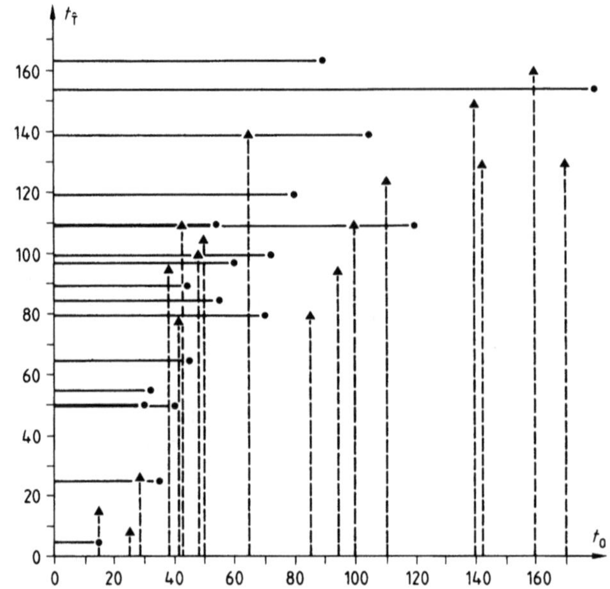

Fig. 4. Random allocation of survival times in the deep model to the treatment and control groups in the surface model

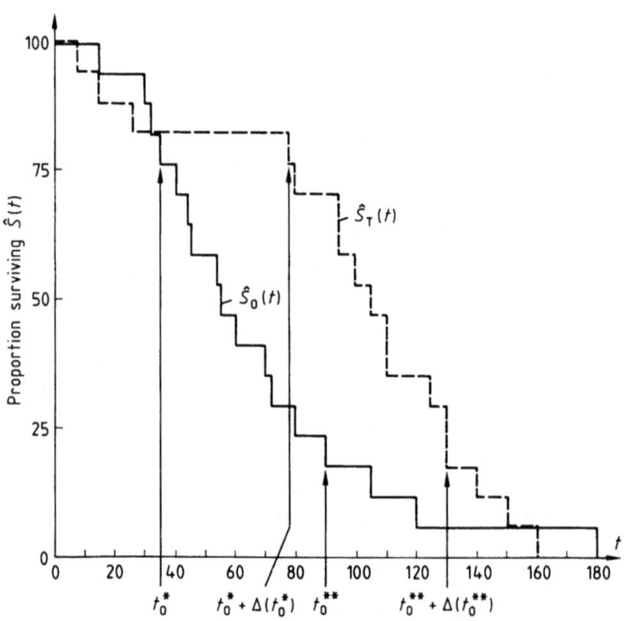

Fig. 5. Surface model: survival curves and region of substantial shift

that interval compare with those of the patients in the treatment group dying in $[t_0^* + \hat{\Delta}(t_0^*), t_0^{**} + \hat{\Delta}(t_0^{**})]$ - there should be no significant difference - and (b) to compare these two groups of patients with those of the control and treatment groups falling outside the regions defined above where $\hat{\Delta}(t)$ is either small or even negative, indicating only little gain or an adverse effect on average (Fig. 5). Therapy is assumed to be effective if the substantially profiting patients prove to be significantly different with respect to prognostic factors from those doing not as well.

Compared with conventional survival analysis, we are now arguing the other way round: Instead of comparing treatments with respect to survival time we compare prognostic factors with respect to a putative benefit of treatment. This allows interactions between treatment and prognostic factors to be assessed directly, as no product terms need be included in a regression model. Furthermore, no proportional-hazards assumption is being made, as the outcomes of treatment are defined in terms of a discrete response variable with two or three categories according to the region of substantial shift and a region to the left and/or to the right of it. This allows the proportional-hazards regression model to be replaced by a logistic regression model.

Of course, the shift function approach has its limitations. It is certainly inappropriate when too many observations are censored and it therefore may fail in an early analysis. It may, however, also fail in an old trial fulfilling the requirements of long-term follow-up if the information about prognostic factors has been transmitted only in fragments or if it has become obsolete. Another problem concerns the separation of a "substantial" shift region which is more or less arbitrary, and some sensitivity analysis should be carried out by repeating a regression procedure under slightly changed conditions, with the bounds of a region of benefit varied over a plausible range to test the stability of conclusions drawn from the procedure.

The question arises whether existing data from a reported trial could be usefully subjected to the shift function approach. As concerns long-term follow-up and completeness of information, trials on adjuvant therapy in primary breast cancer unfortunately meet either the former or the latter requirement at best. For this reason we have to concentrate on those very poor prognosis patients in a trial who do not benefit on average from a treatment that may well be beneficial to other patients who have a better prognosis (i.e., on the region to the left of a substantial shift region). If prognosis and treatment interact in this way, the two survival curves of a treatment and a control group should run closely together at the beginning and diverge after some estimable period of time. In the NATO trial (Baum 1985), such an initial period of questionable benefit from Nolvadex lasts about 2-3 years. Similarly, in the NSABP trial comparing cytotoxic monochemotherapy with no chemotherapy (Protocol B-05; Fisher et al. 1986) a period of 4-5 years, and in a Veterans Administration study on estrogen therapy for prostate cancer (Byar and Green 1980) a period of about 2 years can be separated out. If these patients who experienced poor prognosis and no benefit on average from therapy were to be characterized reliably by their profile of prognostic indicators, a first step toward differential treatment could be taken. Otherwise, individual gains or losses will be almost unpredictable because of a swamping random variation in the deep model.

References

Baum M (1985) Selection for endocrine treatment. Rev Endocr Rel Cancer (Suppl) 16: 33-38

Byar DP, Green SB (1980) The choice of treatment for cancer patients based on covariate information: applications to prostate cancer. Bull Cancer (Paris) 67: 477-490

Doksum K (1974) Empirical probability plots and statistical inferences for nonlinear models in the two-sample case. Ann Stat 2: 267-277

Fisher B, Fisher ER, Redmond C et al. (1986) Ten-year results from the NSABP clinical trial evaluating the use of L-phenylalanine mustard (L-PAM) in the management of primary breast cancer. J Clin Oncol 4: 929-941

Scheurlen H, Olschewski M, Leibbrand D (1984) Zur Methodologie kontrollierter klinischer Studien über die Primärbehandlung des operablen Mammakarzinoms. Strahlentherapie 160: 459-468

On Combining Information: Historical Controls, Overviews, and Comprehensive Cohort Studies

The Use of Data Bases and Historical Controls in Treatment Comparisons

D. P. Byar

Biometry Branch, Division of Cancer Prevention and Control, National Cancer Institute, Blair Building, Room 5A05, 9000 Rockville Pike, Bethesda, MD 20892-4200, USA

I suspect that the main reason I was invited to contribute to this symposium was that the organizers believed it would be important to discuss the topic suggested by the title they assigned to me. They were aware that I have been an outspoken critic of the idea that data bases and historical control groups can be used reliably to compare treatments. Since I have already presented my ideas in writing several times, I will merely summarize them briefly here and refer interested readers to the list of references at the end of the contribution, where my previous papers as well as those of some other authors are listed.

The wide availability of computer technology carries many advantages for medical researchers. However, the relative ease with which data can be put into the computer has led many to believe that the construction of elaborate data bases might somehow replace the need for randomized clinical trials to evaluate the relative merits of various forms of therapy for cancer. Although I believe that carefully constructed computerized data bases may serve many useful purposes, I do not believe that the comparison of treatments is among them. The central reason for my view is that the prognosis of individual patients varies markedly for all forms of cancer, even though many factors are known which explain some portion of this variability. Such prognostic variables include the stage of the cancer at diagnosis, the histological type of the tumor, the general physical condition of the patient, and the patient's age (for some cancers). Despite knowledge about these and other prognostic factors, most of the variability in the course of cancer patients remains unexplained. This means that substantial bias is possible when the outcomes for two groups of patients treated differently are compared. The essential problem is that someone has decided what treatment to give to each patient on some basis or another. In general one may assume that the physician caring for the patient chose the treatment believed most likely to affect favorably the course of the disease. This situation contrasts sharply with that in epidemiology, where the observational method has long been used to evaluate possible risk factors for cancer or the effects of certain exposures. In the epidemiologic setting, individuals do not deliberately choose the substances to which they will be exposed nor do they choose their risk factors in the hope that they can increase the probability of developing cancer! Thus, the kinds of biases which may result from the deliberate

Recent Results in Cancer Research, Vol. 111
© Springer-Verlag Berlin · Heidelberg 1988

assignment of treatment to patients with cancer are much less likely in epidemiologic studies. I and many others have argued that randomized clinical trials are greatly to be preferred for comparing two or more treatments for cancer because they simply represent the application of the experimental method - as opposed to observation - to the field of therapy evaluation.

Even though the randomized clinical trial may be regarded as the "gold standard" for therapy evaluation, most publications concerning cancer treatments are not the reports of randomized clinical trials, but instead consist of reports of single cases, series of patients all treated the same way in a particular center, series of cases with historical controls, analyses of outcomes according to treatment for patients in computerized data bases, and other kinds of observational studies such as the recently proposed case-control approach proposed by Horwitz and Feinstein (1981 a, b). I find it useful to arrange these various kinds of evidence into a hierarchy (Table 1) from the least convincing to the most convincing from a methodological point of view. This hierarchy is discussed by Green and Byar (1984).

Probably, the very individuals who defend the use of historical controls or data bases would actually prefer data from randomized clinical trials if such data were already available. However, there are many objections to randomized clinical trials, including questions of ethics, expense, complexity, size, duration, and the necessity for cooperation of a large group of individuals, many of whom will receive little individual credit. Although all these objections can be overcome, as is evident from the large number of clinical trials conducted in the field of cancer therapy, it is nevertheless not surprising that researchers continue to look for alternatives. Gehan and Freireich (1974) advocate the use of historical controls, particularly when there has been a recent sequence of studies admitting similar kinds of patients and using similar criteria for evaluation of response. Although this approach is undoubtedly preferable to obtaining controls from the literature, it provides only limited protection against bias introduced by changes over time in the nature of the patient population, in diagnostic criteria, or in supportive care. Difficulties with the use of historical controls are presented in more detail in Byar et al. (1976) and in Byar (1979).

Although the term "medical data base" has undoubtedly been used to describe a great variety of sets of information stored in computers, I use the term to refer to

Table 1. Hierarchy of strength of evidence concerning efficacy of treatment, from least convincing to most convincing

1. Anecdotal case reports
2. Case series without controls
3. Series with literature controls
4. Analyses using computer data bases
5. "Case-control" observational studies
6. Series with historical control groups
7. Single randomized clinical trials
8. Confirmed randomized clinical trials

a prospective registry of computerized information concerning patients with one or more diseases. Such data are likely to include baseline information collected when patients are first observed, details about treatment, and follow-up information. Unlike a series of recent historical controls all treated in the same manner, medical data bases are likely to contain information on patients treated in a variety of ways according to the training and beliefs of many different physicians. The purpose of setting up medical data bases is often not specified in advance with any clarity. Even when careful protocols are developed for what information should be stored, the overall purpose may rest on nothing more than the notion that if you store enough data in the computer you can later answer almost any question which happens to occur to you. Of course, one of the most pressing questions facing physicians is how to treat the next patient, and it is natural to inquire about one's previous experience with various treatments before making such a decision. Unfortunately, medical data bases cannot be expected to give reliable answers to such questions because of a number of special problems, including the definition of data items, problems with missing values, actual errors in the data, difficulty in defining time zero in chronic diseases, problems with subset definition, multiple comparisons, and the need for adjustment procedures. These problems are discussed in some detail in Byar (1980, 1981), Fleming (1982), and Mantel (1983).

I believe that medical data banks can be quite useful for describing the kinds of patients treated at a given medical center and for describing the general course of a disease. In addition, medical data bases can assist in diagnosis and can be used to study prognostic factors. However, they should be used only with great caution for comparing treatments. In the case of rare diseases where it is generally not possible to conduct randomized clinical trials, reliance on previous observation may be the best basis for making treatment decisions.

In summary, I agree with the opinion of Rockette et al. (1982) that "when ethical issues do not preclude its use, the appropriate focus should be on how the principle may be best utilized rather than upon what the alternative approaches to the randomized clinical trial might be."

References

Byar DP (1979) The necessity and justification of randomized clinical trials. In: Tagnon HJ, Staquet MJ (eds) Controversies in cancer: design of trials and treatment. Masson, New York, pp 75-82

Byar DP (1980) Why data bases should not replace randomized clinical trials. Biometrics 36: 337-342

Byar DP (1981) Possibilities and limitations of observational studies and evaluation of medical data bases. In: Victor N, Dudeck J, Broszia EP (eds) Therapiestudien. Proceedings of the 26th annual meeting of the German Society of Medical Documentation, Computer Sciences, and Statistics. Springer, Berlin Heidelberg New York, pp 528-537 (Medizinische Informatik und Statistik, vol 33)

Byar DP, Simon RM, Friedewald WT, Schlesselman JJ, DeMets DK, Ellenberg JH, Gail MH, Ware JH (1976) Randomized clinical trials: perspectives on some recent ideas. N Engl J Med 295: 74-80

Fleming TR (1982) Historical controls, data banks and randomized trials in clinical research: a review. Cancer Treat Rep 66: 1101–1105
Gehan EA, Freireich EJ (1974) Non-randomized controls in cancer clinical trials. N Engl J Med 290: 198–203
Green SB, Byar DP (1984) Using observational data from registries to compare treatments: the fallacy of omnimetrics. Stat Med 3: 361–370
Horwitz RI, Feinstein AR (1981 a) The application of therapeutic-trial principles to improve the design of epidemiologic research: a case-control study suggesting that anticoagulants reduce mortality in patients with myocardial infarction. J Chronic Dis 34: 575–583
Horwitz RI, Feinstein AR (1981 b) Improved observational method for studying therapeutic efficacy: suggestive evidence that lidocaine prophylaxis prevents death in acute myocardial infarction. JAMA 246: 2455–2459
Mantel N (1983) Cautions on the use of medical data bases. Stat Med 2: 355–362
Rockette HE, Redmond CK, Fisher B, Participating NSABP Investigators (1982) Impact of randomized clinical trials on therapy of primary breast cancer: the NSABP overview. Controlled Clin Trials 3: 209–225

*Limitations and Advantages of Meta-analysis in Clinical Trials**

H. E. Rockette and C. K. Redmond

Department of Biostatistics, Graduate School of Public Health, University of Pittsburgh, Pittsburgh, PA 15261, USA

Introduction

Meta-analysis has recently been applied to a variety of areas in medical research (Collins and Langman 1985; Himel et al. 1986; Collins et al. 1985; Tran and Weltman 1985). By meta-analysis we mean a quantitative synthesis of data across several different but related studies. This usually entails the application of uniform methods of statistical analyses and/or data presentation. Reasons for performing a meta-analysis include confirmation of a general hypothesis by combining data from related studies, estimation of a general treatment effect by combining data from related studies, generation of hypotheses for further testing, and convincing others of a finding by presenting a systematic summary of all studies related to that finding.

The use of such analysis raises several questions. These include the following: (a) Which studies should be included? (b) What problems arise as a result of the application of classical hypothesis testing to combined studies? (c) How do we estimate an average treatment effect, and what is its interpretation? (d) Are there differences in the approach to hypothesis generation in a single study and in a meta-analysis? (e) How should results from a meta-analysis be presented?

The purpose of this paper is to discuss some of the considerations important in conducting a meta-analysis in medical research. Particular emphasis will be given to those aspects relevant for adjuvant therapy trials.

Criteria for Study Inclusion

One of the first decisions in a combined analysis is whether both randomized and nonrandomized studies should be included. If one combines over a large number of nonrandomized trials one may obtain statistical significance, because each trial has a small systematic bias in the same direction which reaches statistical signifi-

* The research was partially supported by the National Cancer Institute, U10CA 12027, and by American Cancer Society grant RC13.

© Springer-Verlag Berlin · Heidelberg 1988

cance with a large sample size. To eliminate such systematic bias the inclusion of only randomized trials appears justified.

Another issue related to bias is one of published versus nonpublished studies. Several authors have demonstrated that the process leading to publication tends to favor positive studies (Pocock 1984; Begg 1985; Greenwald 1975; Light and Pillemer 1984). Such a systematic bias increases the chance of falsely identifying a treatment effect and has prompted some investigators to suggest that both published and nonpublished studies should be included in an overview analysis.

Any decision regarding study inclusion also requires one to address the vague concept of combining over "similar studies." The definition of "similar" may be debatable. In September, 1985, the Consensus Development Conference sponsored by the NIH concluded that adjuvant chemotherapy and antiestrogen treatment for breast cancer were effective in reducing mortality (NIH 1985). Conclusions from this Consensus Development Conference were influenced by findings obtained from a meta-analysis, conducted by Peto, of all the randomized trials of either chemotherapy or tamoxifen therapy. The analysis justifying chemotherapy included 4000 patients receiving the combination therapy cyclophosphamide, methotrexate, 5-fluorouracil (CMF), 100 patients receiving CMF plus other cytotoxic agents, 3000 patients receiving multiple agents not including CMF, 3000 patients receiving single agents other than CMF, and 3000 patients receiving cytotoxic agents perioperatively. The primary comparison in the presentation by Peto to evaluate the effect of cytotoxic therapy was between the 11000 patients receiving nonperioperative therapy and those patients receiving no prophylactic cytotoxics. Although this decision is one approach, a different investigator might have selected a different subset of studies on which to perform the primary analysis (i.e., all cytotoxic regimens including perioperative therapy or, alternatively, only CMF regimens).

Role of Classical Hypothesis Testing

There are several differences between a meta-analysis and an individual randomized clinical trial which make the application of formal hypothesis testing more difficult. First, the decision as to which studies are "similar" and therefore included is made after individual studies and their results have been published. There is always the possibility that these decisions could be influenced by knowledge of end results and could invalidate the significance level in a formal test of a primary hypothesis.

Second, most individual trials permit multiple analysis of the data during the follow-up period. If these analyses contribute to the decision to stop the trial they influence the significance level. These "stopping rules" are often not stated in published studies, and even if the rules for stopping the individual trials are stated it may be difficult to obtain an overall *P* value associated with the primary hypothesis of a meta-analysis. If the studies permitted repeated analysis of the data and did not adjust the "stopping rule" to reflect the elevated type-I error, then a combined analysis may include a bias in favor of a positive finding.

In combination therapy it is tempting to test the effect of drug A by comparing results in trials where drug A and drug B are given in combination with results from trials where drug A is given alone. For example, in the breast cancer overview for tamoxifen, NSABP Protocol B-09 was used to draw inferences about the effect of adjuvant tamoxifen. This protocol compared tamoxifen plus PF (L-PAM and 5-FU) with PF alone and may not be an indication of the adjuvant effect tamoxifen would have alone. Gelber and Goldhirsch (1986) have discussed this method of determining a treatment effect and refer to it as the "fallacy of the arithmetic construct."

Estimation of an Average Treatment Effect

The index used to measure average treatment effect impacts on the statistical analysis and may affect the interpretation of the data. Many statistical models measure effect using relative risk or relative odds, but risk differences may be more appropriate for public health decisions. One might consider whether there should be a weighting factor for each study reflecting compliance, completeness of follow-up, and other measures of data quality. Unfortunately, if one decides that a weighted index is appropriate it is not clear what the appropriate weighting index should be. Issues related to data quality become more relevant if the meta-analysis fails to demonstrate a treatment effect.

There is strong justification for viewing the average treatment effect in the context of a random effects model. Such a model assumes treatment effects are heterogeneous, that the data from each study estimate a different treatment effect, and that the overall average is an estimate of the average of the treatment effects of all studies. Utilization of a random effects model will tend to place broader confidence intervals on our estimate and probably provides a more realistic estimate of the average treatment effect. Issues related to the use of random effects models in meta-analysis are addressed by DerSimonian and Laird (1986).

Estimates of an average treatment effect may not adequately summarize the time-dependent nature of the treatment effect. Adjuvant trials in cancer have different lengths of therapy and the conditional probability of recurrence may depend on how recently adjuvant therapy has been given. Even when individual studies have the same response pattern over time, differing lengths of follow-up would make the average treatment effect estimated in a meta-analysis inadequate.

Given that an estimate of treatment effect has been obtained, the interpretation of this estimate may still be unclear. The different studies may have related but different treatment regimens, and the results may be difficult to translate into clinical management of the patient. In practice, a positive finding may be interpreted as justifying any of the many regimens which show a benefit when combined. Alternatively, some might select the regimen with the greatest observed benefit even though it may provide less convincing evidence of a benefit than other regimens when evaluated outside the context of a meta-analysis.

The practical benefit of a therapy is more difficult to evaluate in the presence of interactions. The statement is often made that in meta-analysis, even if there are interactions, as long as these are of a quantitative nature there need be no concern since we are looking for consistent differences in the same direction. However, although such consistent differences may result in the assertion that there is a benefit of therapy, the presence of interaction of outcome with patient characteristics limits the ability to quantify the benefit for the general public, where patient characteristics are likely to be different.

Hypothesis Generation

The larger sample size of a meta-analysis makes it tempting to test hypotheses on various subsets of patients when it may not have been feasible for individual studies. The problems of elevated type-I errors in doing subset analysis have been addressed elsewhere (Pocock 1984; Byar 1985; Rockette and Caplan, this volume). In a meta-analysis the problem is further complicated, since the methods that have been suggested to control the type-I error when doing subset analysis cannot be easily applied. For example, in an individual trial one can control the type-I error when doing subset analysis by using global tests for interactions. However, at the time one does a meta-analysis the investigators who conducted the individual studies have already examined multiple, but an often unspecified number of subsets. The method of analyzing subsets may differ for individual studies, and many studies will not even specify the number of subsets that were investigated. Furthermore, the presentation of results in subsequent publications may be influenced by previous published results from related trials and produce unjustified confidence as to the extent of independent confirmation. Thus, if the secondary hypotheses selected for a meta-analyses are influenced by findings from the individual studies they may be the result of more screening for positive findings than is apparent.

Another problem with testing secondary hypotheses is that of indirect comparisons. For example, in the meta-analysis of adjuvant therapy where only randomized trials have been included, one might, after testing the primary hypothesis, decide to compare all high-dose and low-dose treatment arms. If the corresponding high- and low-dose comparisons are selected from different studies they are no longer randomized comparisons.

If one utilizes the data base of the meta-analysis to generate secondary hypotheses based on subsets, then formal tests of interaction should be employed in an appropriate manner. Such models should include terms to allow for study heterogeneity, and it is possible that the most important interactions would include the variable designating study. If the combined data set is sufficiently large one might generate such hypotheses on part of the data set and attempt to confirm it on the remainder of the data.

Presentation of Results

Often, the presentation of a meta-analysis can be as important as the way the meta-analysis is conducted. In presenting results the objectives of the meta-analysis should be clearly stated. Measures of treatment effect from individual studies should be presented with confidence intervals, not only a summary statistic over all studies. Reasons for excluding studies should be clearly stated, and the similarities of studies should be justified.

Role of Meta-analysis

We have reviewed the limitations associated with the interpretation of meta-analyses. Nevertheless, there are several advantages to performing such analyses that are appealing. First, such analyses fill a gap between scientists and policymakers. Scientists typically have done studies but made little effort to evaluate the practical impact of their scientific findings. Meta-analysis is an attempt to more directly synthesize the information provided from a variety of scientific studies. Meta-analysis also provides a systematic method of synthesizing information rather than the arbitrary or informal manner in which synthesis may occur in a literature review or the Discussion section of a publication. Finally, a meta-analysis which attempts to find both published and nonpublished data may present information to the scientific community that is not readily available.

In deciding the role meta-analysis should have, one might first determine the ranking of a meta-analysis with regard to strength of evidence concerning efficacy of treatment. Green and Byar (1980) have proposed a hierarchy of different types of scientific investigations ranging from anecdotal case reports to a confirmed randomized clinical trial. Where should meta-analysis fit in such a hierarchy? One might try to conceptualize a multi-institutional single trial with characteristics of meta-analysis. In the adjuvant therapy setting one would probably find a study where each institution is permitted to use their own drug dosage and length of therapy, so that there is uniformity within an institution but not between institutions. Furthermore, each institution may have their own data management, their own stopping rules, and their own statistical unit with perhaps a different emphasis on the analysis. Quality control standards, although they could reasonably be assumed to meet some minimal level, would be variable for the different groups. A primary hypothesis would not be defined until after some of the institutions had reached conclusions about their findings. Such a trial would not be viewed with the same degree of belief as a well-controlled randomized clinical trial of the same size. Therefore, one might argue that a meta-analysis in the hierarchy of investigations is like a large single randomized trial that is not done well by current standards.

We have discussed the scientific limitations associated with meta-analysis as well as some of the advantages of these analyses. There are also practical problems that may result if meta-analysis is widely employed and which may have an impact on our scientific approach to problems. Specifically, analyses might encourage small studies since they could always be combined later in a large meta-analysis. Meta-analysis might also interfere with accrual of ongoing studies, since it could be performed on many small ongoing studies and results might be made public prior to the completion of many of the studies. Since many of the criticisms of a meta-analysis relate to combining similar but different studies there could be an attempt to make the studies more similar, which would ultimately affect the diversity of clinical trials.

In summary, meta-analyses provide a useful method to synthesize related research on important issues. The major problems to date probably arise from the failure to adequately appreciate the limitations of such procedures rather than from the way in which they are conducted.

References

Begg CB (1985) A measure to aid in the interpretation of published clinical trials. Stat Med 4: 1-9

Byar D (1985) Assessing apparent treatment-covariate interactions in randomized clinical trials. Stat Med 4: 255-263

Collins R, Langman M (1985) Treatment with histamine-H antagonists in acute upper gastrointestinal hemorrhage. N Engl J Med 313: 659-666

Collins R, Yusuf S, Peto R (1985) Overview of randomized trials of diuretics in pregnancy. B Med J 290: 17-22

DerSimonian R, Laird N (1986) Meta-analysis in clinical trials. Controlled Clin Trials 7: 177-188

Gelber RD, Goldhirsch A (1986) The concept of an overview of cancer clinical trials with special emphasis on early breast cancer. J Clin Oncol 4 (11): 1696-1703

Green S, Byar D (1980) Using observational data from registries to compare treatments: the fallacy of omnimetrics. Stat Med 3: 361-370

Greenwald AG (1975) Consequences of prejudice against the null hypothesis. Psychol Bull 82: 1-20

Himel HN, Liberati AL, Gelber RD, Chalmers TC (1986) Adjuvant chemotherapy for breast cancer: a pooled estimate based on published randomized control trials. JAMA 256: 1148-1159

Light RJ, Pillemer DB (1984) Summing up: the science of reviewing research. Harvard University Press, Cambridge MA

National Institutes of Health (1985) Adjuvant chemotherapy for breast cancer. NIH consensus development conference statement, vol 5, no 12. NIH consensus development conference, September 1985, Bethesda, Maryland

Pocock SJ (1984) Clinical trials: a practical approach. Wiley, New York

Tran ZV, Weltman A (1985) Differential effects of exercise on serum lipid and lipoprotein levels seen with changes in body weight: a meta-analysis. JAMA 254: 919-924

Overview of Adjuvant Radiotherapy for Breast Cancer

J. Cuzick

Imperial Cancer Research Fund, Lincoln's Inn Fields, P.O. Box 123,
London WC2A 3PX, Great Britain

Two papers by Cuzick et al. (1987 a, b) have recently been published in which mortality results from all available mature randomized trials of adjuvant radiotherapy are updated and analyzed collectively. Briefly, these overviews, which were based on individual patient data for over 10000 patients with more than 6000 deaths, showed conclusively that radiotherapy had no appreciable affect on mortality in the first 5-10 years of follow-up, but they suggested rather strongly ($P < 0.001$) that at least some forms of radiotherapy had a deleterious effect on long-term survival as measured by subsequent survival in those patients who survived at least 10 years. This result was based primarily on the earliest generation of trials in which radiotherapy was a randomized option after all patients had received a radical mastectomy, but it was also supported by the King's/CRC trial of simple mastectomy with or without radiotherapy. Overall, the death rate after 10 years among 10-year survivors was estimated to be 35% higher (95% CI, 15%-58%) in those who had been randomized to receive radiotherapy.

These results have prompted further questions which were not addressed in the original study. These are of two types, regarding (a) limitations in the data base and (b) limitations in the analysis. These are briefly addressed below.

Limitations in the Data Base

Because of the large amount of effort necessary to extract data from very old trials, the data collected were kept to a minimum. We were interested in long-term mortality, so that it was essential to record the vital status and date of death of each individual patient. The essential core of data collected on all patients consisted of:

1. Randomized treatment option
2. Age at diagnosis
3. Clinical nodal status

The results of the overview have prompted a number of further questions, including:

© Springer-Verlag Berlin · Heidelberg 1988

1. Which specific cause(s) of mortality are elevated?
2. What is the relation of excess mortality to type of radiotherapy given?
3. What is the laterality of the primary tumour? This will determine doses to other tissues, especially the heart.
4. What was the actual treatment given, not just the allocated treatment?

In order to answer these questions we plan to collect on each individual patient who survived 10 years or more the following additional information:

1. Whether breast cancer was present at death
2. Cause of death, with special attention to the following major groups:
   a) breast cancer
   b) other cancer
   c) cardiac
   d) other vascular
3. Type of radiotherapy given, especially kilovoltage vs megavoltage X-rays
4. Actual radiotherapy given to primary site - dose and fields both at presentation and for relapses in the first 10 years
5. Laterality of original primary tumour
6. Radiotherapy given for contralateral disease

We hope this more detailed overview will help to answer questions about the long-term effects of radiotherapy, which are particularly relevant now because of a shift in primary treatment towards breast conservation with its associated increase in the use of radiotherapy.

Methodologic and Statistical Issues

Two points have arisen regarding the methods of analysis used: (a) the emphasis on subsequent mortality in patients surviving more than 10 years, and (b) the need to accommodate treatment variability in the analysis.

The Subgroup of 10-year Survivors

The majority of deaths in the first 5-10 years are due to occult distant micrometastases which would be unaffected by radiotherapy to the chest wall or axilla. Thus, by focusing on long-term survivors we are avoiding the great mass of deaths which are likely to contribute more to the variance of any treatment difference than to any mean difference. However, the subgroup of 10-year survivors is necessarily a postrandomization selected group and could be biased, if radiotherapy affected survival in the first 10 years in such a way as to unbalance the future survival prospects of those who achieved 10-year survival. For example, if the effect of radiotherapy was only to delay deaths in the 9th year until the 10th year, then the poorer survival after 10 years would be the result of better survival in the first 10 years. However, the survival curves in the first 10 years do not support such a possibility, but because of the far larger number of deaths at early follow-up times such an effect could be masked. This possibility seems sufficiently unlikely on a priori grounds in this particular instance, and most likely it can be discounted.

Treatment Heterogeneity

Although the precise treatment may vary among centres, doctors, or even on an individual patient basis, this fact is usually ignored in clinical trials, except for occasional stratifying by centre. The question arises more naturally when an overview is attempted, since differences in treatment are usually apparent in the separate trial protocols.

The question of a specific treatment difference has already arisen in discussion of the radiotherapy trials. One possible explanation of the differences in long-term survival is a delayed effect of scattered irradiation on heart disease rate. This could be quite different for kilovoltage than for megavoltage treatment. By collecting more information this specific question can be addressed, but there remain other differences in the treatments and it would be unreasonable to suspect that they do not have at least a small effect on survival. A test for heterogeneity between trials can give some idea of the magnitude of this variability, but problems remain in the interpretation of a single summary treatment effect obtained from an overview.

Interpretation will depend to some extent on the degree of heterogeneity as measured, for example, by a χ^2 test. When this is sufficiently large that treatment effects differ by more than their estimated standard error, an attempt should be made to discover which specific treatments were superior, and further trials should be undertaken to confirm this. When differences in treatment effects are small compared with their estimated standard errors, as in the case for the radiotherapy trials, then it is probably more fruitful to think in terms of some average treatment effect and to accept that treatment itself has some measurable variability in addition to that due to the unpredictable nature of the patient's response. This variability can be modeled in various ways, but the most important component will be its variance. Empirical Bayes arguments can then be invoked to estimate the variance and to determine its effect on confidence limits for the mean treatment effect. Generally, the variance and confidence intervals will be increased only if the χ^2 test for heterogeneity exceeds its expected value, and then by an amount related to the magnitude of this difference. Often these considerations have little effect on the resulting estimates, but they are important in principle and need to be considered in each specific overview.

References

Cuzick J, Stewart H, Peto R, Baum B, Fisher B, Host H, Lythgoe JP, Ribeiro G, Scheurlen H, Wallgren A (1987a) Overview of randomized trials of postoperative adjuvant radiotherapy in breast cancer. *Cancer Treat Rep* 71: 15–29

Cuzick J, Stewart H, Peto R, Fisher B, Kaae S, Johansen H, Lythgoe JP, Prescott RJ (1987b) Overview of randomized trials comparing radical mastectomy without radiotherapy against simple mastectomy with radiotherapy in breast cancer. *Cancer Treat Rep* 71: 7–14

Overview of Randomized Trials of Postoperative Adjuvant Radiotherapy in Breast Cancer

J. Cuzick, H. J. Stewart, R. Peto, M. Baum, B. Fisher, H. Host, J. P. Lythgoe, G. Ribeiro, H. Scheurlen, and A. Wallgren*

Imperial Cancer Research Fund, Lincoln's Inn Fields, P. O. Box 123, London WC2A 3PX, Great Britain

Introduction

One of the first major randomized trials in cancer therapy was concerned with the value of postoperative adjuvant radiotherapy for breast cancer. Since then, a large number of trials have addressed this issue, but the impact of this treatment on long-term survival still remains clouded. This is due partly to the long natural history of breast cancer and partly to the changing approach to primary treatment, where a trend toward less surgery and more radiotherapy has taken place. The current interest in procedures aimed at breast conservation (Calle et al. 1978; Hellman et al. 1980; Veronesi et al. 1981; Fisher et al. 1985a) highlights this shift and emphasizes the need for a greater understanding of the role of radiotherapy in primary management.

There is now little doubt that postoperative radiotherapy delays local recurrence (Host and Brennhovd 1977; Wallgreen 1977; Cancer Research Campaign Working Party 1980; Lythgoe and Palmer 1982; Ribeiro 1979). However, this delay has not led to any delay in distant recurrences or to a reduction in mortality, at least over the first 5-10 years of follow-up. Timothy et al. (1979) have argued that local recurrences are best treated as they occur, and that it is overtreatment to irradiate the axilla in all cases, especially since no survival benefits accrue from early treatment. Brady et al. (1977) have pointed out that the need to treat local recurrences can be distressing and awkward, especially if regular follow-up is not stringently adhered to, and that routine adjuvant radiotherapy is to be preferred on this account.

These arguments presuppose that the treatment has little effect on overall survival. The opinion has been voiced by some clinicians (Brady et al. 1977; Watson 1977; Fletcher and Montague 1978) that the sterilizing ability of postoperative radiotherapy has a beneficial effect on survival due to the killing of micrometastases in the local field. On the other hand, Stjernsward (1974, 1977a, b), in a review of published mortality, has suggested that radiotherapy may have a detrimental effect on survival. He hypothesized that this might be due to the destructive effects of radiotherapy on the local immune defenses. Stjernsward's analysis, which has gener-

* We thank Dr. R. Edwards and Ms. I. Stratton for valuable computing assistance.

Recent Results in Cancer Research, Vol. 111
© Springer-Verlag Berlin · Heidelberg 1988

ated much controversy (Levitt and McHugh 1975, 1977, 1978; Stjernsward et al. 1976; Stjernsward and Day 1978), was based on published accounts of trials, and some of the differences in favor of no radiotherapy have been reduced on further follow-up. Published accounts have shown that radiotherapy has little effect on short-term survival, but the possibility remains that there could be important effects on long-term survival.

The purpose of this study was to update and view collectively the effects on long-term survival for all of the randomized trials of postoperative adjuvant radiotherapy. Our criterion for inclusion of a trial was that it must incorporate a randomization between two arms which differed only by the addition of postoperative radiotherapy in one group and that the trial should be sufficiently mature to provide useful information about survival in the period ≥5 years after randomization. The trials fell naturally into two groups; those in which the surgery was some form of radical mastectomy and those in which the surgery was a simple mastectomy with or without node sampling. A related set of trials compared radical mastectomy without radiotherapy against simple mastectomy with radiotherapy. These trials are reviewed in Cuzick et al. (1987).

Trials Under Review

The trials under review are shown in Table 1, along with brief details of the radiotherapy regimens. These regimens vary in many respects, such as energy of the

Table 1. Details of radiotherapy regimens in trials under review[a]

Trial	Year of onset	Type of therapy	Dose (Gy)	No. of fractions	Duration (days)	Biologic dose (rets)
Radical mastectomy ± XRT						
Manchester Q	1949	250 kV	35.0-40.0	15	21	1438-1693
Manchester P	1952	250 kV	32.5-42.5	15	21	1335-1746
Oslo I	1964	200 kV	18.0-36.0	20	28	681-1362
Oslo II	1968	^{60}Co	50.0	20	28	1689
Heidelberg	1969	^{60}Co	54.0	30	42	1905
Stockholm	1971	Nodal, ^{60}Co	45.0	25	35	1406[b]
Simple mastectomy ± XRT						
Manchester Regional	1970	300 kV or	37.0	15	21	1493
		Nodal,	40.0	15	21	1464 (1211[c])
		4 meV	30.0	15	21	
CRC	1970	Ortho or	32.5-46	-	21-42	1335-1483
		meV	35.7-50.6	-	21-42	1306-1453
NSABP-B04	1971	meV	40.0-50	25	35	1224-1530
Edinburgh I	1974	4 meV	42.5	10	28	1661

[a] *XRT*, radiotherapy.
[b] Chest wall, 10-15 meV.
[c] Chest wall, 300 kV.

beam, fields irradiated, duration of treatment, and recommended dose range. All regimens included irradiation to the axilla. Although no conversion can be applied to produce true biologic equivalence, the regimens have been ranked according to their likely biologic effect by applying a relative biologic efficiency correction, using ^{60}Co as the standard beam, and calculating the nominal standard dose value (in rets) for each regimen (Ellis 1965). The range in the ret values thus calculated is wide (681-1905 rets), but with the exception of one trial (representing at most 6% of the irradiated patients), the values are all well above 1200 rets, the minimum value estimated as adequate for local control in several reports in the literature.

Table 2. Method of randomization, patient exclusions, and dates of entry and last follow-up for each trial

Trial	Method of randomization	Exclusions after randomization	Period of entry (years)	Date of last follow-up
Manchester Christie	Even or odd date of birth of patient	None after registration, but impossible to assess allocation	1949-1955	Jan 1982
Oslo	Random number table in central office; unstratified	None; 27 protocol deviations are included in the analysis	1964-1972	Jan 1981
Heidelberg	Random number table 2-8 days postmastectomy by surgeons; patients taken sequentially from operating 800 m books	One perioperative death; 23 protocol deviations are included	1967-1972	Aug 1985
Stockholm	Central telephone (12 strata); randomized blocks in lists before surgery	None	1971-1976	Jan 1983
Manchester Regional (stage I)	Central telephone stratified by center	None	1970-1975	Jan 1981
CRC	Numbered envelopes at each center	Discrepancies noted in 557 patients; all patients analyzed here	1970-1975	June 1985
NSABP-B04	Numbered envelopes at each center; randomized blocks	100 of 1765 (5.7%) patients in entire trial were ineligible and excluded	1971-1974	July 1985
Edinburgh I	Central envelopes by trial secretary (12 strata)	None; ten protocol deviations are included	1974-1979	Mar 1986

Details concerning the method of randomization, exclusion of patients, and dates of entry and last follow-up are shown in Table 2. Further details on each trial are given below.

Radical Mastectomy with or Without Radiotherapy

Historically, this was the first category of trials to be undertaken and individual trials were started between 1949 and 1971. The specific trials included are as follows.

Manchester Christie

This trial randomized 1461 patients between 1949 and 1955 (Ribeiro 1979; Paterson 1962; Paterson and Russell 1959; Easson 1968; Palmer and Ribeiro 1985). All patients were treated surgically by a Halsted radical mastectomy. Two different regimens of kilovoltage radiotherapy were used, initially the so-called quadrate technique and later the peripheral technique; these are labeled as the Q and P series, respectively, in the tables below.

Oslo

This trial included 1115 patients entered from 1964 to 1972, all of whom received a Halsted radical mastectomy; half were randomly allocated to receive immediate radiotherapy (Host and Brennhovd 1975, 1977). Again, two different types of radiotherapy were used. In the first half of the trial, 200-kV photons were used, whereas during the latter half of accrual radiotherapy was from a cobalt source. The two halves are treated separately below and are designated Oslo I and Oslo II respectively. All patients received ovarian irradiation with a target dose of 6.5–9.0 Gy.

Heidelberg

This was a smaller unpublished trial in which 143 patients from a single center were randomized between 1967 and 1972. One patient died from sequelae of the mastectomy and was not included in the analysis. Some form of protocol violation was reported in 23 of the remaining 142 patients, but they have been included in the analysis. The apparent imbalance in the treatment allocation was due to a run in the random number table used. All patients were treated by radical mastectomy and if no distant metastases were found they were randomized for radiotherapy, to be initiated within 4–5 weeks after surgery at the latest. This consisted of a 6-week course, with a total tumor dose of about 65.0 Gy given by daily fractionation. A ^{60}Co source was used and radiotherapy was given to the supraclavicular area, the apex of the axilla, and the ipsilateral internal mammary chain.

Stockholm

From 1971 to 1976, 960 patients were entered in a three-arm trial (Wallgren 1977; De Schryver 1976). All patients received a modified radical mastectomy which spared both pectoral muscles but removed the pectoral fascia. This is not strictly a radical mastectomy, but on balance the trial is probably more closely allied to radical mastectomy trials than to those employing a simple mastectomy. One arm consisted of preoperative radiotherapy and the 316 patients in this group are not included below. The remaining 644 patients received a modified radical mastectomy and half were then randomized to be given postoperative megavoltage (^{60}Co and electron) radiotherapy.

Following the trials of radical mastectomy with or without radiotherapy there followed a period in which the relative merits of simple mastectomy with radiotherapy were compared against radical mastectomy without radiotherapy. These trials were based on the therapeutic ideas of McWhirter, and the results in terms of long-term survival are presented by Cuzick et al. (1987).

Simple Mastectomy with of Without Radiotherapy

Around 1970 the next generation of local therapy trials began. The value of radiotherapy was assessed in the context of simple mastectomy as primary surgery.

King's/Cambridge CRC

Twenty-eight hundred patients were randomized between 1970 and 1975 from 80 centers in this large multicenter trial (Cancer Research Campaign Working Party 1976, 1980). A total of 557 of these patients were considered to be noneligible because of protocol violations, but a recent analysis (Cancer Research Campaign Working Party 1980) suggests that these patients have fared similarly to the remainder in the trial, and consequently all randomized patients have been included in the analysis below.

Manchester Regional

A total of 714 patients with clinical stage-I disease entered between 1970 and 1975 are included in this part of the trial (Lythgoe and Palmer 1982; Lythgoe and Swindell 1978). Clinical stage-II patients are reported on by Cuzick et al. (1987). Premenopausal patients and women <3 years after menopause were offered oophorectomy or ovarian ablation by radiotherapy.

NSABP-B04

Clinically node-negative patients were randomized three ways to radical mastectomy, total mastectomy with radiotherapy, or total mastectomy without radiotherapy (Fisher et al. 1977, 1981, 1985b). Clinically node-positive patients were allocated to either radical mastectomy or total mastectomy with radiotherapy. Only those patients with clinically negative nodes who were treated by total mastectomy with or without irradiation can be considered here. Between 1971 and 1974, 717 such patients were randomized. All of the patients randomized for either radical mastectomy or total mastectomy with irradiation are considered in Cuzick et al. (1987). This means that 352 patients with N_0 disease who were randomized for total mastectomy and postoperative radiotherapy are included in both analyses. A total of 100 of the 1765 patients in the entire trial (5.7%) were judged to be ineligible and were not followed up.

Edinburgh I

From 1974 to 1979, 348 patients with stage-I and -II breast cancer were entered in this trial (Duncan et al. 1975). All patients were considered not to have node involvement, either because the sampled nodes proved histologically to be negative or because none were identified by the surgeon for examination. Patients with positive nodes identified by this procedure were included in a parallel chemotherapy trial and are not included here.

Trials Not Included

We are aware of two trials which would have been included had the data been available. The largest of these is an early NSABP trial (B02) comparing radical mastectomy with or without radiotherapy. A total of 1882 patients were entered from 1961 to 1968, of whom 1103 were deemed to be eligible. Survival figures were presented in 1970 (Fisher et al. 1970), but further follow-up has not been possible. We are also aware of a small trial of 150 patients started in Southampton in 1973 (Turnbull et al. 1978) comparing simple mastectomy alone and simple mastectomy with radiotherapy. Further follow-up information is not available.

The more recent trials of breast conservation (Veronesi et al. 1981; Fisher et al. 1985a) as well as several trials in which radiotherapy was a randomized option within chemotherapy trials, e.g., the Mayo Clinic trial (Ahmann et al. 1978), have not been included because they are not sufficiently mature to provide useful information on long-term survival. However, it will be important to include them in future overviews. Trials including radiotherapy but which compare surgical methods, such as the Cape Town trial (Helman et al. 1972) and the Cardiff trial (Forrest et al. 1982) have also been excluded because they did not contain a randomized comparison of radiotherapy.

Data Collected and Statistical Methods

This report stems from a meeting held in Edinburgh in June 1981 under the auspices of the Breast Cancer Trial Co-ordinating Subcommittee of the (United Kingdom) Co-ordinating Committee on Cancer Research and was funded by the Cancer Research Campaign. Because of the diversity of the material available both in country of origin and in the decade of recruitment, this overview has necessarily been kept as simple as possible. We have collected only survival data, and the only subgroups that have been examined are based on age (<50 or >50 years) and clinical nodal status.

We have striven to include all randomized patients without exclusion. In some cases this has meant that we have reported on larger numbers than in previous publications.

Individual patient information was made available in an anonymous form for all trials except NSABP-B04, where summary tables were provided. This meant that this trial was excluded from a summary survival curve illustration (Fig. 1), but the trial is fully represented in all statistical calculations. In many cases the follow-up reported here extends that available from previous published accounts of these trials.

A summary log-rank (Mantel-Haenszel) statistic is obtained by adding together across trials the differences between observed and expected deaths. The variance of this statistic is obtained since the sum of the variances of each of the trials, and a chi-squared statistic on one degree of freedom is obtained by squaring the sum of the observed minus expected differences and dividing by the overall variance. This procedure is optimal when the true differences in the mortality ratio across all trials are the same, but it is valid more generally and, in the absence of further specific information about the likely differences in the trials, is the appropriate test for a shift in survival rates that is in the same *direction* for all trials. Methodologically, the approach is similar to an analysis of a multicenter trial which has been stratified by center both in random allocation and at analysis. The statistical procedures are formally identical, but variation from trial to trial is likely to be greater than from center to center because of the lack of a uniform protocol. The statistical issues associated with combining trials have been discussed more fully by Yusulf et al. (1985).

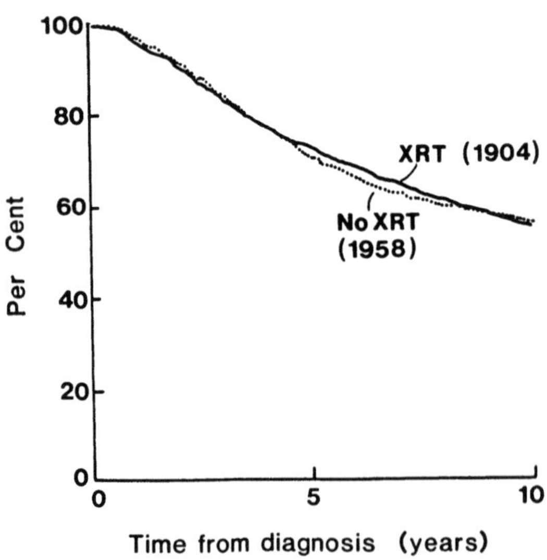

Fig. 1. Combined 10 year survival according to allocated treatment for trials employing a simple mastectomy. *Curves* do not include material from NSABP-B04 trial. *Numbers in parentheses* represent total patients at risk in each arm (excluding NSAPB)

Table 3. Patients at risk in each treatment arm and no. of deaths in the two major types of trials for different follow-up periods[a]

Type of trial	Patients		No. of patients		All deaths		No. of deaths at				No. alive at 10 years		No. of deaths at			
							0–5 years		5–10 years				10–15 years		>15 years	
	Age (years)	Nodes	With XRT	Without XRT	With XRT	Without XRT	With XRT	Without XRT	With XRT	Without XRT	With XRT	Without XRT	With XRT	Without XRT	With XRT	Without XRT
Radical mastectomy ±XRT	<50	Negative	292	314	114	115	49	41	19	33	169	198	13	15	33	26
	<50	Positive	346	317	244	221	159	136	35	39	130	118	17	22	33	24
	≧50	Negative	532	550	289	270	105	108	91	80	244	249	46	35	47	47
	≧50	Positive	509	502	386	393	211	230	93	97	140	126	37	29	45	37
	All		1679	1683	1033	999	524	515	238	249	683	691	113	101	158	134
Simple mastectomy ±XRT	<50	Negative	696	687	260	252	149	157	96	86	251	223	15	9	0	0
	<50	Positive	150	133	72	67	47	45	20	18	61	45	5	4	0	0
	≧50	Negative	1165	1238	549	605	304	357	198	199	358	398	47	49	0	0
	≧50	Positive	245	265	157	154	94	99	52	48	65	98	11	7	0	0
	All		2256	2323	1038	1078	594	658	366	351	735	764	78	69	0	0
All	<50	Negative	988	1001	374	367	198	198	115	119	420	421	28	24	33	26
	<50	Positive	496	450	316	288	206	181	55	57	191	163	22	26	33	24
	≧50	Negative	1697	1788	838	875	409	465	289	279	602	647	93	84	47	47
	≧50	Positive	754	767	543	547	305	329	145	145	205	224	48	36	45	37
	All		3935	4006	2071	2077	1118	1173	604	600	1418	1455	191	170	158	134

[a] *XRT*, radiotherapy.

Differences in the logarithms of hazard ratios between the two arms were estimated by the approximation $\Delta = (O - E)/\text{var}(O - E)$ and 95% confidence limits for the difference were approximated by $\Delta \pm 1.96\ (\text{var}(O - E))^{-1/2}$. Here, O and E refer to observed and expected deaths in the subset of interest. A value of Δ equals zero means no overall differences in the survival between the two arms. For small values of Δ, 100 Δ gives an estimate of the percentage difference in the mortality between the two arms. More generally, 100 (exp (Δ)-1) gives the percentage increase or decrease in mortality as compared with the reference arm.

Results

The numbers of patients and deaths which have occurred in different time periods are shown for each treatment arm for the major subgroups of each type of trial in Table 3. Details for individual trials are given in Appendixes A–C. A total of 7941 patients have been treated and followed up in these trials and 4148 deaths have been recorded. A total of 2873 patients survived for at least 10 years and of these, 653 have died after ≥10 years of follow-up. Most of the deaths in this period (506 total) have come from trials of the type radical mastectomy with or without radiotherapy. This is due to their greater follow-up time. In Table 4 the log-hazard ratios (Δ) and their associated chi-square values are given for the two types of trials over the different time periods. As anticipated by the results already published on individual trials, there is little difference in the first 5 years. Also, little difference is seen in the period 5–10 years after diagnosis. The combined survival curves for the first 10 years of follow-up are shown for trials of the form radical mastectomy with or without radiotherapy in Fig. 2 and for simple mastectomy with or without radiotherapy in Fig. 1 (excluding NSABP-B04). Estimates of the log-hazard ratio and 95% confidence intervals on a trial-by-trial basis are plotted for the entire follow-up period in Fig. 3 and for the first 10-year follow-up in Fig. 4. Ten-year survival rates were 54% in each arm of the combined radical mastectomy trials and 57% in each arm of the combined simple mastectomy trials. These dif-

Table 4. Estimate of log-hazard ratios for each type of trial and 5-year follow-up period[a]

Type of trial	Years					
	0–5	5–10	10–15	15+	10+	All
Radical mastectomy ±XRT	0.02 (0.14)	-0.06 (0.40)	0.14 (0.97)	0.39 (10.61)	0.28 (9.61)	0.07 (2.22)
Simple mastectomy ±XRT	-0.05 (0.90)	0.08 (1.02)	0.37 (4.52)	0.00 (0.00)	0.37 (4.52)	0.02 (0.15)
All	-0.02 (0.20)	0.02 (0.14)	0.23 (4.40)	0.39 (10.61)	0.30 (13.94)	0.04 (1.75)

[a] Data have been stratified by age and clinical nodal status. Negative value favors radiotherapy. χ^2 values are given in *parentheses*. Ratios are given by $\Delta = O - E/\text{var}\ (O - E)$.
XRT, radiotherapy.

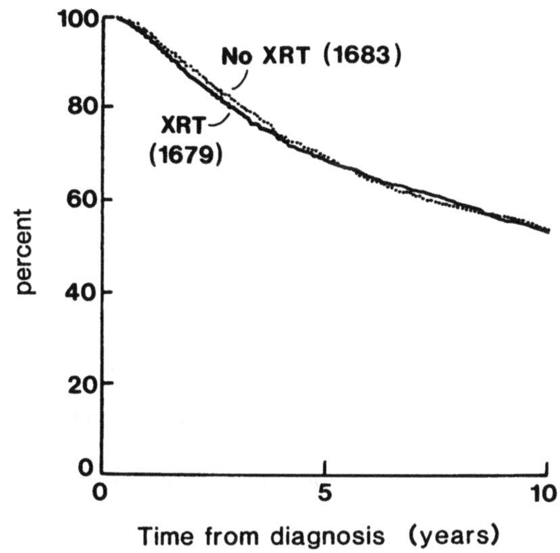

Fig. 2. Combined 10 year survival according to allocated treatment for all trials employing a radical mastectomy. *Numbers in parentheses* represent total patients at risk in each arm

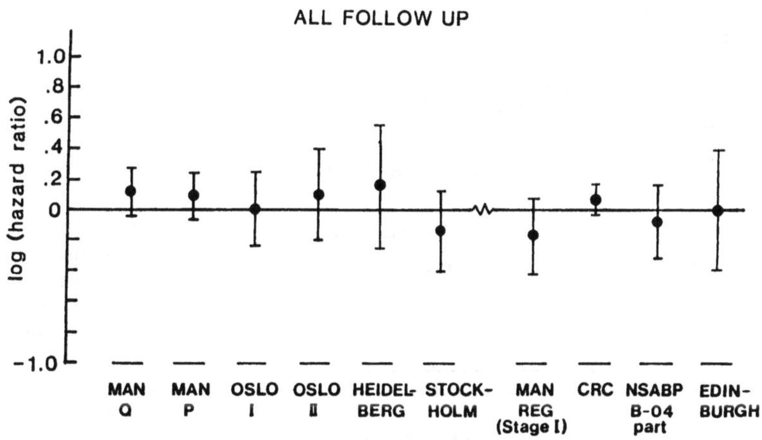

Fig. 3. Log-hazard ratios and 95% confidence intervals for entire follow-up period by trial

ferences are probably due to changes in referral patterns, earlier diagnosis, and patient selection. The nonrandomized comparison cannot be taken to offer any evidence for differences in survival according to the type of surgery used.

However, a significant difference showing poorer survival in the group receiving adjuvant radiotherapy is seen in the period after a 10-year survival ($\chi^2 = 13.94$; $P < 0.001$) Table 3). This was apparent in both the simple mastectomy trials ($\chi^2 = 4.52$; $P = 0.04$) and the radical mastectomy trials ($\chi^2 = 9.61$; $P = 0.002$). Only the trials employing radical mastectomy have follow-up after 15 years, but the results continue to hold in this period ($\chi^2 = 10.16$; $P = 0.001$). Subsequent survival for 10-year survivors in this group of trials is shown in Fig. 5. The differences correspond to a 26% reduction in the hazard of death in the nonirradiated arm in

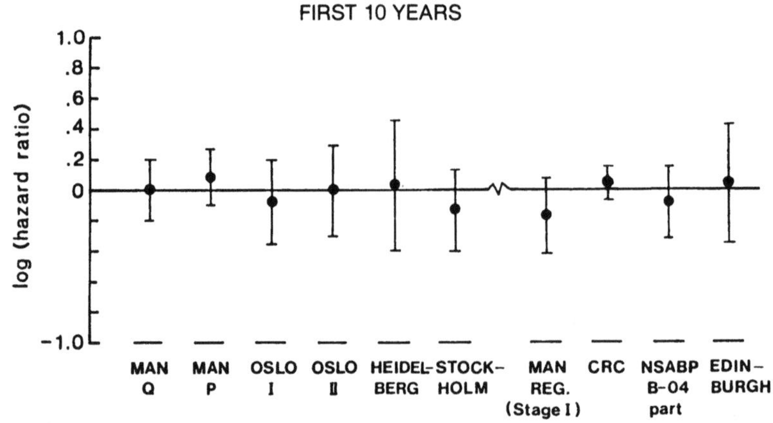

Fig. 4. Log-hazard ratios and 95% confidence intervals for first 10 years of follow-up by trial

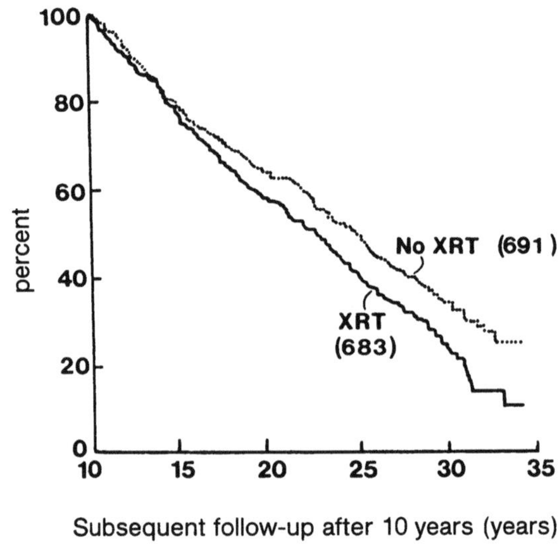

Fig. 5. Subsequent survival in patients surviving 10 years who were in a trial employing radical mastectomy. There is a significant difference favoring patients treated by radical mastectomy alone ($P = 0.002$). *Numbers in parentheses* represent total patients at risk in each arm

the period after 10 years of follow-up. The 25-year survival rate among 10-year survivors treated by radical surgery alone was 51%, whereas it was 42% among those who also received radiotherapy. A plot of the estimated log-hazard ratio and 95% confidence intervals for each trial for 10-year survivors is shown in Fig. 6. This shows that individual trial results are all consistent with the overall result and that increased mortality is seen in all trials except that from Stockholm. The results from the Manchester Q trial, the Oslo II trial, and the CRC trial are individually significant.

In Table 5 these results are given separately according to clinical nodal status, in Table 6 separately for women >50 or <50 years of age. The advantage in the nonirradiated arm on survival after 10-year (and 15-year) follow-up appears to be somewhat greater in the node-negative group (estimated reduction in hazard ratio

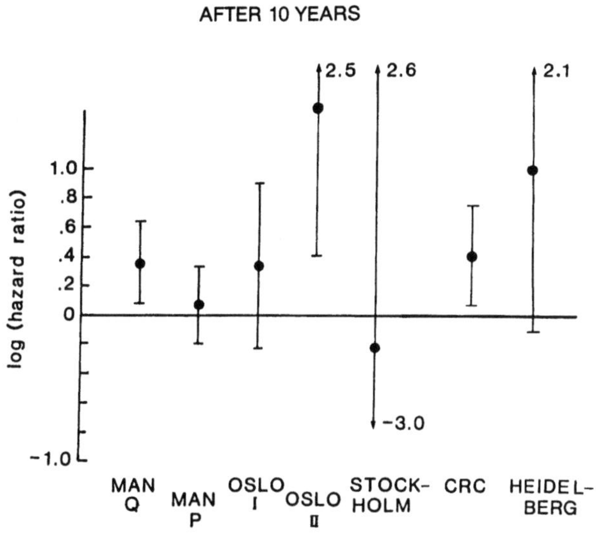

Fig. 6. Log-hazard ratios and 95% confidence intervals for subsequent 10-year survival by trial

32% vs 16%) and in the women aged >50 years at diagnosis (estimated reduction in hazard ratio 30% vs 18%). However, neither of these interactions is even near statistical significance ($\chi^2 = 1.82$ for nodal status; $\chi^2 = 0.78$ for age), and in view of the post hoc nature of this comparison, this could very likely be due to chance alone.

Complete details regarding survival are given on a trial-by-trial basis in Appendix C. This allows the interested reader to look at any combination of trials he may wish.

Discussion

The considerations in this overview have been limited to an evaluation of *randomized* trials. Where the differences between treatments are thought to be relatively small (i.e., <20%-30%), we believe that this is the only viable approach and that the biases involved in trying to compare nonrandomized series with historical controls or concurrent controls from different institutions are too large to draw reliable conclusions. Unfortunately, the methods of randomization used in some of the older trials would not be considered satisfactory by current standards (Table 2). This is particularly worrisome for the Manchester Q series, where a significant imbalance in treatment allocation is observed ($\chi^2 = 5.87$; $P = 0.02$) and the largest differences in long-term survival are seen. Nevertheless, any bias in allocation would be more likely to make itself manifest in the first 10 years of follow-up and is less likely to affect long-term mortality when there are no differences in the first 10 years.

The overview has confirmed the general belief that when a mastectomy is performed the use of radiotherapy has little effect on survival in the first 5-10 years after treatment. What is surprising is the suggestion of a detrimental impact on

Table 5. Estimate of log-hazard ratios in separate categories of trials to clinical nodal status[a]

Nodes	Treatment arm	Years					
		0–5	5–10	10–15	15+	10+	All
Negative	Radical mastectomy ±XRT	0.10 (0.68)	0.03 (0.06)	0.34 (3.02)	0.51 (9.05)	0.43 (11.63)	0.19 (6.65)
Negative	Simple mastectomy ±XRT	-0.08 (1.68)	0.06 (0.44)	0.30 (2.44)	0.00 (0.00)	0.30 (2.44)	-0.01 (0.04)
Negative	Total	-0.04 (0.53)	0.05 (0.48)	0.32 (5.45)	0.51 (9.05)	0.39 (13.73)	0.05 (1.69)
Positive	Radical mastectomy ±XRT	-0.01 (0.01)	-0.13 (1.15)	-0.07 (0.13)	0.27 (2.49)	0.12 (0.89)	-0.01 (0.02)
Positive	Simple mastectomy ±XRT	0.05 (0.15)	0.16 (0.87)	0.66 (2.74)	0.00 (0.00)	0.66 (2.74)	0.12 (1.49)
Positive	Total	0.01 (0.02)	-0.03 (0.10)	0.07 (0.17)	0.27 (2.49)	0.17 (1.99)	0.03 (0.26)

[a] Data have been stratified by age and are given for each 5-year follow-up period. Negative value favors radiotherapy. χ^2 values are given in *parentheses*. Ratios are given by $\Delta = O - E/\text{var}(O - E)$

XRT, radiotherapy.

Table 6. Estimate of log-hazard ratios for different categories of trials given separately for women < and > 50 years of age[a]

Age (years)	Treatment arm	Years					
		0–5	5–10	10–15	15+	10+	All
<50	Radical mastectomy ±XRT	0.18 (2.92)	-0.25 (1.97)	-0.16 (0.44)	0.38 (4.03)	0.18 (1.42)	0.10 (1.65)
<50	Simple mastectomy ±XRT	-0.05 (0.29)	-0.01 (0.01)	0.29 (0.65)	0.00 (0.00)	0.29 (0.65)	-0.02 (0.10)
<50	All	0.06 (0.66)	-0.10 (0.89)	-0.02 (0.01)	0.38 (4.03)	0.20 (1.99)	0.04 (0.50)
≧50	Radical mastectomy ±XRT	-0.07 (0.70)	0.01 (0.01)	0.27 (2.68)	0.40 (6.58)	0.34 (8.94)	0.05 (0.83)
≧50	Simple mastectomy ±XRT	-0.05 (0.61)	0.12 (1.65)	0.39 (3.92)	0.00 (0.00)	0.39 (3.92)	0.04 (0.46)
≧50	All	-0.06 (1.30)	0.07 (1.08)	0.32 (6.40)	0.40 (6.58)	0.35 (12.82)	0.04 (1.26)

[a] Data have been stratified by clinical nodal status and are given for each 5-year follow-up period. Negative value favors radiotherapy. χ^2 values are given in *parentheses*. Ratios are given in $\Delta = O - E/var(O - E)$

XRT, radiotherapy

long-term survival. It is difficult to know how to interpret this result. Is it due to an excess of deaths from breast cancer and if so, were these deaths caused by metastases from the original tumor or second primary neoplasms? A recent survey of 14000 women treated for breast cancer has found no relationship between use of radiotherapy and contralateral breast cancer (Basco et al. 1985). Is some other specific cause of death elevated? Unfortunately, we were given details of the cause of death and whether or not breast cancer was present at death in the patients in only some of these trials, so these questions cannot be answered at present. We hope to be able to complete this information for future analyses.

The combined analysis of trials comparing radical mastectomy without radiotherapy against simple mastectomy with radiotherapy (Cuzick et al. 1987) also shows less mortality after 15 years of follow-up in the group not given radiotherapy ($\chi^2=3.06$; $P=0.08$). However, this is balanced by a trend in the opposite direction in the 10- to 15-year follow-up period, so that survival after a 10-year follow-up is similar in both arms ($\chi^2=0.09$; not significant).

The only mature trial of appreciable size missing from this overview is the NSABP-B02 trial. It has not been possible to trace patients in the trial. The reported mortality at 10 years was similar in the irradiated and nonirradiated groups (Fisher et al. 1970), which agrees with the results reported herein. If follow-up information were to become available on all randomized patients, this would add considerably to our knowledge of long-term differences in survival and make the results less dependent on the Manchester Christie experience.

The relevance of these results to current practice also requires careful consideration. The majority of the information on survival after a 10-year follow-up comes from the older trials, especially the Manchester Christie and Oslo I series, where kilovoltage irradiation was used; this produced many more acute side effects than modern megavoltage irradiation. While it is generally accepted that the benefits resulting from the use of megavoltage rather than orthovoltage therapy relate more to method of administration and tissue reaction than to biological effectiveness, the higher dose absorbed by underlying and surrounding tissues with kilovoltage irradiation may also be important for late effects. However, the magnitude of the survival differences after 10 years is similar in the trials employing simple mastectomy and is of borderline statistical significance, but none of these trials have follow-up >15 years.

With onset dates spanning 25 years, it is not surprising that treatment schedules for the patients given irradiation have varied not only between the trials studied but also within some trials (Table 1). However, the doses used fall within the levels generally accepted as adequate for postoperative radiotherapy today, and a recently published analysis of the postoperative radiotherapy given within the large CRC trial (Brinkley et al. 1984) generally supports the view that local and regional recurrence rates within this range are similar.

The current trials in primary therapy are evaluating surgical procedures which remove less material in combination with radiotherapy, and the results from this overview indicate that the long-term implications of this policy must be monitored carefully. The results of these trials and other more recent trials of radiotherapy in conjunction with chemotherapy should be subjected to a similar overview in about 5 years, when the results will be more mature.

Appendix A. Patients and deaths for different time periods and subgroups for individual trials of radical mastectomy ± XRT

Patients		No. of patients		All deaths		No. of deaths at 0–5 years		No. of deaths at 5–10 years		No. alive at 10 years		No. of deaths at 10–15 years		No. of deaths at >15 years	
Age (years)	Nodes	With XRT	Without XRT	With XRT	Without XRT	With XRT	Without XRT	With XRT	Without XRT	With XRT	Without XRT	With XRT	Without XRT	With XRT	Without XRT
Manchester Q															
<50	Negative	37	60	31	41	10	12	2	8	25	40	1	5	18	16
<50	Positive	113	105	104	94	63	60	11	14	39	31	10	8	20	12
≧50	Negative	68	82	66	72	16	20	20	16	32	46	10	13	20	23
≧50	Positive	109	146	107	138	58	81	21	28	30	36	9	10	19	19
All		327	393	308	345	147	173	54	66	126	153	30	36	77	70
Manchester P															
<50	Negative	58	64	37	33	15	12	4	6	39	46	4	5	14	10
<50	Positive	102	84	86	70	58	35	11	11	33	38	4	12	13	12
≧50	Negative	81	78	77	71	23	22	18	16	40	40	12	10	24	23
≧50	Positive	141	133	136	127	70	72	27	24	44	37	14	13	25	18
All		382	359	336	301	166	141	60	57	156	161	34	40	76	63
Oslo I															
<50	Negative	79	72	20	15	10	6	7	5	62	61	2	4	1	0
<50	Positive	41	37	18	19	9	9	6	8	26	20	3	2	0	0
≧50	Negative	95	101	38	39	7	13	17	18	71	70	12	8	2	0
≧50	Positive	70	57	51	41	28	22	13	15	29	20	9	4	1	0
All		285	267	127	114	54	50	43	46	188	171	26	18	4	0
Oslo II															
<50	Negative	61	66	13	11	4	3	4	7	25	37	5	1	0	0
<50	Positive	36	44	15	16	12	14	3	2	14	18	0	0	0	0
≧50	Negative	117	121	39	25	17	13	17	10	49	52	4	1	1	1
≧50	Positive	64	54	28	31	11	17	14	13	17	9	3	1	0	0
All		278	285	95	83	44	47	38	32	105	116	12	3	1	1
Heidelberg															
<50	Negative	10	9	6	5	4	2	1	3	5	4	1	0	0	0
<50	Positive	10	8	6	7	6	6	0	1	4	1	0	0	0	0
≧50	Negative	34	22	26	12	14	8	5	2	15	12	7	2	0	0
≧50	Positive	30	19	25	16	19	11	4	4	7	4	2	1	0	0
All		84	58	63	40	43	27	10	10	31	21	10	3	0	0
Stockholm															
<50	Negative	47	43	7	10	6	6	1	4	13	10	0	0	0	0
<50	Positive	44	39	15	15	11	12	4	3	14	10	0	0	0	0
≧50	Negative	137	146	43	51	28	32	14	18	37	29	1	1	0	0
≧50	Positive	95	93	39	40	25	27	14	13	13	20	0	0	0	0
All		323	321	104	116	70	77	33	38	77	69	1	1	0	0

Appendix B. Patients and deaths for different time periods and subgroups for individual trials of simple mastectomy ± XRT

Patients		No. of patients		All deaths		No. of deaths at				No. alive at 10 years		No. of deaths at			
						0–5 years		5–10 years				10–15 years		> 15 years	
Age (years)	Nodes	With XRT	Without XRT	With XRT	Without XRT	With XRT	Without XRT	With XRT	Without XRT	With XRT	Without XRT	With XRT	Without XRT	With XRT	Without XRT
King's/CRC															
< 50	Negative	392	382	169	152	89	89	66	56	194	184	14	7	0	0
< 50	Positive	132	118	69	62	44	42	20	16	58	43	5	4	0	0
≧ 50	Negative	641	689	345	360	167	203	133	115	272	304	45	42	0	0
≧ 50	Positive	211	235	142	143	83	94	48	42	57	90	11	7	0	0
All		1376	1424	725	717	383	428	267	229	581	621	75	60	0	0
Manchester Regional (I)															
< 50	Negative	132	137	33	39	25	31	8	8	7	2	0	0	0	0
< 50	Positive	0	0	0	0	0	0	0	0	0	0	0	0	0	0
≧ 50	Negative	223	222	85	99	65	79	20	20	8	9	0	0	0	0
≧ 50	Positive	0	0	0	0	0	0	0	0	0	0	0	0	0	0
All		355	359	118	138	90	110	28	28	15	11	0	0	0	0
NSABP-B04															
< 50	Negative	117	118	43	50	24	30	18	19	37	28	1	1	0	0
< 50	Positive	0	0	0	0	0	0	0	0	0	0	0	0	0	0
≧ 50	Negative	235	247	102	120	63	65	37	49	67	77	2	6	0	0
≧ 50	Positive	0	0	0	0	0	0	0	0	0	0	0	0	0	0
All		352	365	145	170	87	95	55	68	104	105	3	7	0	0
Edinburgh															
< 50	Negative	55	50	15	11	11	7	4	3	13	9	0	1	0	0
< 50	Positive	18	15	3	5	3	3	0	2	3	2	0	0	0	0
≧ 50	Negative	66	80	17	26	9	10	8	15	11	8	0	1	0	0
≧ 50	Positive	34	30	15	11	11	5	4	6	8	8	0	0	0	0
All		173	175	50	53	34	25	16	26	35	27	0	2	0	0

XRT, radiotherapy.

Appendix C. Differences between observed and expected deaths for different time periods and subgroups on a trial-by-trial basis

Patients		Years														
Nodes	Age (years)	0–5			5–10			10–15			15+			All		
		O - E	var	χ^2	O - E	var	χ^2	O - E	var	χ^2	O - E	var	χ^2	O - E	var	χ^2
Manchester Q																
Negative	< 50	1.87	5.10	0.69	−1.61	2.30	1.13	−1.39	1.44	1.34	5.00	7.91	3.16	3.87	16.75	0.89
Negative	≧ 50	−0.14	8.87	0.00	4.27	8.79	2.07	0.45	5.56	0.04	5.76	9.11	3.64	10.34	32.33	3.31
Positive	< 50	0.44	30.22	0.01	−2.35	6.16	0.90	0.15	4.43	0.01	2.39	7.76	0.74	0.63	48.57	0.01
Positive	≧ 50	−1.22	33.38	0.04	−0.56	11.96	0.03	0.68	4.65	0.10	4.65	8.73	2.48	3.55	58.72	0.21
Negative	All	1.73	13.97	0.21	2.66	11.09	0.64	−0.94	7.00	0.13	10.76	17.02	6.80	14.21	49.08	4.11
Positive	All	−0.78	63.60	0.01	−2.91	18.12	0.47	0.83	9.08	0.08	7.04	16.49	3.01	4.18	107.29	0.16
All	< 50	2.31	35.32	0.15	−3.96	8.46	1.85	−1.24	5.87	0.26	7.39	15.67	3.49	4.50	65.32	0.31
All	≧ 50	−1.36	42.25	0.04	3.71	20.75	0.66	1.13	10.21	0.13	10.41	17.84	6.07	13.89	91.05	2.12
All		0.95	77.57	0.01	−0.25	29.21	0.00	−0.11	16.08	0.00	17.80	33.51	9.46	18.39	156.37	2.16
Oslo I																
Negative	< 50	1.72	3.99	0.74	0.87	3.00	0.25	−1.01	1.50	0.68	0.52	0.25	1.08	2.10	8.74	0.50
Negative	≧ 50	−2.83	5.00	1.60	−0.53	8.75	0.03	2.27	4.98	1.03	0.99	0.49	2.00	−0.10	19.22	0.00
Positive	< 50	−0.67	4.47	0.10	−1.28	3.49	0.47	0.18	1.23	0.03	0.00	0.00	0.00	−1.77	9.19	0.34
Positive	≧ 50	1.45	12.44	0.17	−2.46	6.92	0.87	1.28	3.13	0.52	0.00	0.00	0.00	0.27	22.49	0.00
Negative	All	−1.11	8.99	0.14	0.34	11.75	0.01	1.26	6.48	0.25	1.51	0.74	3.08	2.00	27.96	0.14
Positive	All	0.78	16.91	0.04	−3.74	10.41	1.34	1.46	4.36	0.49	0.00	0.00	0.00	−1.50	31.68	0.07
All	< 50	1.05	8.46	0.13	−0.41	6.49	0.03	−0.83	2.73	0.25	0.52	0.25	1.08	0.33	17.93	0.01
All	≧ 50	−1.38	17.44	0.11	−2.99	15.67	0.57	3.55	8.11	1.55	0.99	0.49	2.00	0.17	41.71	0.00
All		−0.33	25.90	0.00	−3.40	22.16	0.52	2.72	10.84	0.68	1.51	0.74	3.08	0.50	59.64	0.00
Oslo II																
Negative	< 50	0.67	1.75	0.26	−1.19	2.74	0.52	2.97	1.34	6.58	–	–	–	2.45	5.83	1.03
Negative	≧ 50	2.40	7.49	0.77	4.30	6.72	2.75	1.52	1.25	1.85	–	–	–	8.22	15.46	4.37
Positive	< 50	−0.28	6.47	0.01	0.81	1.23	0.53	0.00	0.00	0.00	–	–	–	0.53	7.70	0.04
Positive	≧ 50	−4.89	6.87	3.48	−2.43	6.41	0.92	0.61	0.96	0.39	–	–	–	−6.71	14.24	3.16
Negative	All	3.07	9.24	1.02	3.11	9.46	1.02	4.49	2.59	7.78	–	–	–	10.67	21.29	5.35
Positive	All	−5.17	13.34	2.00	−1.62	7.64	0.34	0.61	0.96	0.39	–	–	–	−6.18	21.94	1.74
All	< 50	0.39	8.22	0.02	−0.38	3.97	0.04	2.97	1.34	6.58	–	–	–	2.98	13.53	0.66
All	≧ 50	−2.49	14.36	0.43	1.87	13.13	0.27	2.13	2.21	2.05	–	–	–	1.51	29.70	0.08
All		−2.10	22.58	0.20	1.49	17.10	0.13	5.10	3.55	7.33	–	–	–	4.49	43.23	0.47

Appendix C *(continued)*

Patients		Years														
Nodes	Age (years)	0–5			5–10			10–15			15+			All		
		O - E	var	χ^2	O - E	var	χ^2	O - E	var	χ^2	O - E	var	χ^2	O - E	var	χ^2
Manchester P																
Negative	< 50	2.78	6.65	1.16	−0.60	2.48	0.15	−0.24	2.23	0.03	3.55	5.87	2.15	5.49	17.23	1.75
Negative	≧ 50	0.15	11.17	0.00	0.33	8.40	0.01	1.37	5.44	0.35	2.03	11.58	0.36	3.88	36.59	0.41
Positive	< 50	11.87	22.82	6.17	0.69	5.44	0.09	−3.78	3.98	3.59	−0.85	6.14	0.12	7.93	38.38	1.64
Positive	≧ 50	−5.89	34.87	0.99	−0.30	12.53	0.01	−0.92	6.61	0.13	2.90	10.59	0.79	−4.21	64.60	0.27
Negative	All	2.93	17.82	0.48	−0.27	10.88	0.01	1.13	7.67	0.17	5.58	17.45	1.78	9.37	53.82	1.63
Positive	All	5.98	57.69	0.62	0.39	17.97	0.01	−4.70	10.59	2.09	2.05	16.73	0.25	3.72	102.98	0.13
All	< 50	14.65	29.47	7.28	0.09	7.92	0.00	−4.02	6.21	2.60	2.70	12.01	0.61	13.42	55.61	3.24
All	≧ 50	−5.74	46.04	0.72	0.03	20.93	0.00	0.45	12.05	0.02	4.93	22.17	1.10	−0.33	101.19	0.00
All		8.91	75.51	1.05	0.12	28.85	0.00	−3.57	18.26	0.70	7.63	34.18	1.70	13.09	156.80	1.09
Heidelberg																
Negative	< 50	0.92	1.49	0.57	−0.92	1.00	0.85	0.44	0.25	0.77	-	-	-	0.44	2.74	0.07
Negative	≧ 50	0.85	5.28	0.14	0.94	1.70	0.52	2.71	2.21	3.32	-	-	-	4.50	9.19	2.20
Positive	< 50	−0.90	2.90	0.28	−0.67	0.22	2.04	0.00	0.00	0.00	-	-	-	−1.57	3.12	0.79
Positive	≧ 50	1.59	7.27	0.35	−0.76	1.92	0.30	−0.05	0.65	0.00	-	-	-	0.78	9.84	0.06
Negative	All	1.77	6.77	0.46	0.02	2.70	0.00	3.15	2.46	4.03	-	-	-	4.94	11.93	2.05
Positive	All	0.69	10.17	0.05	−1.43	2.14	0.96	−0.05	0.65	0.00	-	-	-	−0.79	12.96	0.05
All	< 50	0.02	4.39	0.00	−1.59	1.22	2.07	0.44	0.25	0.77	-	-	-	−1.13	5.86	0.22
All	≧ 50	2.44	12.55	0.47	0.18	3.62	0.01	2.66	2.86	2.47	-	-	-	5.28	19.03	1.46
All		2.46	16.94	0.36	−1.41	4.84	0.41	3.10	3.11	3.09				4.15	24.89	0.69
Stockholm																
Negative	< 50	−0.34	2.99	0.04	−1.78	1.23	2.58	0.00	0.00	0.00	-	-	-	−2.12	4.22	1.07
Negative	≧ 50	−0.93	14.98	0.06	−2.33	7.98	0.68	−0.11	0.49	0.02	-	-	-	−3.37	23.45	0.48
Positive	< 50	−1.45	5.71	0.37	0.21	1.74	0.03	0.00	0.00	0.00	-	-	-	−1.24	7.45	0.21
Positive	≧ 50	−1.15	13.00	0.10	0.46	6.74	0.03	0.00	0.00	0.00	-	-	-	−0.69	19.74	0.02
Negative	All	−1.27	17.97	0.09	−4.11	9.21	1.83	−0.11	0.49	0.02	-	-	-	−5.49	27.67	1.09
Positive	All	−2.60	18.71	0.36	0.67	8.48	0.05	0.00	0.00	0.00	-	-	-	−1.93	27.19	0.14
All	< 50	−1.79	8.70	0.37	−1.57	2.97	0.83	0.00	0.00	0.00	-	-	-	−3.36	11.67	0.97
All	≧ 50	−2.08	27.98	0.15	−1.87	14.72	0.24	−0.11	0.49	0.02	-	-	-	−4.06	43.19	0.38
All		−3.87	36.68	0.41	−3.44	17.69	0.67	−0.11	0.49	0.02	-	-	-	−7.42	54.86	1.00

King's/CRC																
Negative	< 50	−1.32	44.48	0.04	3.36	30.46	0.37	3.06	5.24	1.79	–	–	–	5.10	80.18	0.32
Negative	≧ 50	−10.42	92.32	1.18	12.40	61.95	2.48	6.20	21.46	1.79	–	–	–	8.18	175.73	0.38
Positive	< 50	0.13	21.48	0.00	0.81	8.95	0.07	−0.26	2.18	0.03	–	–	–	0.68	32.61	0.01
Positive	≧ 50	0.24	44.04	0.00	6.82	22.29	2.09	4.42	4.14	4.72	–	–	–	11.48	70.47	1.87
Negative	All	−11.74	136.80	1.01	15.76	92.41	2.69	9.26	26.70	3.21	–	–	–	13.28	255.91	0.69
Positive	All	0.37	65.52	0.00	7.63	31.24	1.86	4.16	6.32	2.74	–	–	–	12.16	103.08	1.43
All	< 50	−1.19	65.96	0.02	4.17	39.41	0.44	2.80	7.42	1.06	–	–	–	5.78	112.79	0.30
All	≧ 50	−10.18	136.36	0.76	19.22	84.24	4.39	10.62	25.60	4.41	–	–	–	19.66	246.20	1.57
All		−11.37	202.32	0.64	23.39	123.65	4.42	13.42	33.02	5.45	–	–	–	25.44	358.99	1.80
Manchester Regional (clinically node negative)																
Negative	< 50	−3.03	14.00	0.66	−0.26	3.99	0.02	–	–	–	–	–	–	−3.29	17.99	0.60
Negative	≧ 50	−7.60	35.98	1.61	−0.17	9.94	0.00	–	–	–	–	–	–	−7.77	45.92	1.31
Negative	All	−10.63	49.98	2.26	−0.43	13.93	0.01	–	–	–	–	–	–	−11.06	63.91	1.91
NSABP-B04 (simple mastectomy ± XRT)																
Negative	< 50	2.62	12.32	0.56	−4.07	6.80	2.44	–	–	–	–	–	–	−6.69	19.12	2.34
Negative	≧ 50	2.73	29.46	0.25	−1.46	17.91	0.12	–	–	–	–	–	–	1.27	47.37	0.03
Negative	All	0.11	41.78	0.00	−5.53	24.71	1.24	–	–	–	–	–	–	−5.42	66.49	0.44
Edinburgh																
Negative	< 50	1.71	4.49	0.65	0.55	1.75	0.17	−0.56	0.25	1.25	–	–	–	1.70	6.49	0.45
Negative	≧ 50	0.56	4.69	0.07	−2.51	5.69	1.11	−0.55	0.25	1.21	–	–	–	−2.50	10.63	0.59
Positive	< 50	0.25	1.49	0.04	−1.17	0.48	2.85	0.00	0.00	0.00	–	–	–	−1.42	1.97	1.02
Positive	≧ 50	3.16	3.99	2.50	−1.00	2.50	0.40	0.00	0.00	0.00	–	–	–	2.16	6.49	0.72
Negative	All	2.27	9.18	0.56	−1.96	7.44	0.52	−1.11	0.50	2.46	–	–	–	−0.80	17.12	0.04
Positive	All	2.91	5.48	1.55	−2.17	2.98	1.58	0.00	0.00	0.00	–	–	–	0.74	8.46	0.06
All	< 50	1.46	5.98	0.36	−0.62	2.23	0.17	−0.56	0.25	1.25	–	–	–	0.28	8.46	0.01
All	≧ 50	3.72	8.68	1.59	−3.51	8.19	1.50	−0.55	0.25	1.21	–	–	–	−0.34	17.12	0.01
All		5.18	14.66	1.83	−4.13	10.42	1.64	−1.11	0.50	2.46	–	–	–	−0.06	25.58	0.00

XRT, radiotherapy

References

Ahmann DL, Payne WS, Scanlon PW et al. (1978) Repeated adjuvant chemotherapy with phenylalanine mustard or 5-fluorouracil, cyclophosphamide, and prednisone with or without radiation, after mastectomy for breast cancer. Lancet i: 893-896

Basco VE, Coldman AJ, Elwood JM et al. (1985) Radiation dose and second breast cancer. Br J Cancer 52: 319-325

Brady LW, Fletcher GH, Levitt SH (1977) Cancer of the breast: the role of radiation therapy after mastectomy. Cancer 39: 2868-2874

Brinkley D, Haybittle JL, Houghton J et al. (1984) The cancer research campaign (King's/Cambridge) trial for early breast cancer: an analysis of the radiotherapy data. Br J Radiol 57: 309-316

Calle R, Pilleron JP, Schlienger P et al. (1978) Conservative management of operable breast cancer. Cancer 42: 2045-2053

Cancer Research Campaign Working Party (1976) Management of early cancer of the breast. Br Med J 1: 1035-1038

Cancer Research Campaign Working Party (1980) Cancer research campaign (King's/Cambridge) trial for early breast cancer. Lancet ii: 55-60

Cuzick J, Stewart H, Peto R et al. (1987) Overview of randomized trials comparing radical mastectomy without radiotherapy against simple mastectomy with radiotherapy in breast cancer. Cancer Treat Rep 71: 7-14

De Schryver A (1976) The Stockholm breast cancer trial: preliminary report of a randomised study concerning the value of pre-operative or post-operative radiotherapy in operable disease. Int J Radiat Oncol Biol Phys 1: 601-609

Duncan W, Forrest APM, Gray N et al. (1975) New Edinburgh primary breast cancer trials. Br J Cancer 32: 628-630

Easson EC (1968) Post-operative radiotherapy in breast cancer. In: Forrest APM, Kunkler PB (eds) Prognostic factors in breast cancer. Livingstone Edinburgh. pp 118-127

Ellis F (1965) Dose, time and fractionation: a clinical hypothesis. Clin Radiol 20: 1-7

Fisher B, Slack NH, Cavanaugh PJ et al. (1970) Postoperative radiotherapy in the treatment of breast cancer. Ann Surg 172: 711-732

Fisher B, Montague E, Redmond C et al. (1977) Comparison of radical mastectomy with alternative treatments for primary breast cancer. Cancer 39: 2827-2839

Fisher B, Wolmark N, Redmond C et al. (1981) Comparison of radical mastectomy with alternative treatments. II. The clinical and biologic significance of medial-central breast cancers. Cancer 48: 1863-1872

Fisher B, Bauer M, Margolese R et al. (1985a) Five-year results of a randomized clinical trial comparing total mastectomy and segmental mastectomy with or without radiation in the treatment of breast cancer. N Engl J Med 312: 664-673

Fisher B, Redmond C, Fisher E et al. (1985b) Ten-year results of a randomized clinical trial comparing radical mastectomy and total mastectomy with or without radiation. N Engl J Med 312: 674-681

Fletcher GH, Montague ED (1978) Does adequate irradiation of the internal mammary chain and supraclavicular nodes improve survival rates? Int J Radiat Oncol Biol Phys 4: 481-492

Forrest APM, Stewart HJ, Roberts MM et al. (1982) Simple mastectomy and axillary note sampling in the management of primary breast cancer. Ann Surg 196: 371-378

Helman P, Bennette MB, Louw JH et al. (1972) Interim report on trial of treatment for operable breast cancer. S Afr Med J 46: 1374-1375

Hellman S, Harris JR, Levene MB (1980) Radiation therapy of early carcinoma of the breast without mastectomy. Cancer 46 [Suppl 4]: 988-994

Host H, Brennhovd IO (1975) Combined surgery and radiation therapy versus surgery alone in primary mammary carcinoma. Acta Radiol Ther Phys Biol 14: 25-32

Host H, Brennhovd IO (1977) The effect of post-operative radiotherapy in breast cancer. Int J Radiat Oncol Biol Phys 2: 1061-1067
Levitt SH, McHugh RB (1975) Early breast cancer and postoperative irradiation. Lancet ii: 1258-1259
Levitt SH, McHugh RB (1977) Radiotherapy in the postoperative treatment of operable cancer of the breast. Cancer 39: 924-932
Levitt SH, McHugh RB (1978) Reply to rebuttal letter by Drs. Stjernsward and Day. Cancer 40: 382-383
Lythgoe JP, Palmer MK (1982) Manchester regional breast study - 5- and 10-year results. Br J Surg 69: 693-696
Lythgoe JP, Swindell R (1978) Manchester regional breast study, preliminary results. Lancet i: 744-747
Palmer MK, Ribeiro CG (1985) Thirty-four-year follow-up of patients with breast cancer in a clinical trial of postoperative breast cancer. Br Med J 291: 1088-1091
Paterson R (1962) Breast cancer: a report of two clinical trials. J R Coll Surg Edinb 7: 243-254
Paterson R, Russell MH (1959) Breast cancer: evaluation of post-operative radiotherapy. J Fac Radiol 10: 174-180
Ribeiro GC (1979) Thirty years' experience with breast cancer clinical trials at the Christie Hospital in Manchester - clinical aspects. In: Scheurlen H, Weckesser G, Armbruster I (eds) Clinical trials in early breast cancer. Springer, Berlin Heidelberg New York (Lecture notes in medical informatics, vol 4)
Stjernsward J (1974) Decreased survival related to irradiation postoperatively in early operable breast cancer. Lancet ii: 1285-1286
Stjernsward J (1977a) Adjuvant radiotherapy trials in breast cancer. Cancer 39: 2846-2867
Stjernsward J (1977b) Can survival be decreased by postoperative irradiation? Int J Radiat Oncol Biol Phys 2: 1171-1175
Stjernsward J, Day N (1978) Rebuttal of two articles by Dr. Levitt et al., Cancer 1977. Cancer 40: 381
Stjernsward J, Muenz LR, von Essen CF (1978) Postoperative radiotherapy and breast cancer. Lancet i: 749
Timothy AR, Overgaard J, Overgaard M et al. (1979) Treatment of early carcinoma of the breast. Lancet ii: 25-26
Turnbull AR, Turner DTL, Chant ADB et al. (1978) Treatment of early breast cancer. Lancet ii: 7-9
Watson TA (1977) Can survival be increased by post-operative irradiation? Int J Radiat Oncol Biol Phys 2: 1181-1183
Wallgren A (1977) A controlled study: pre-operative versus post-operative irradiation. Int J Radiat Oncol Biol Phys 2: 1167-1169
Veronesi U, Saccozzi R, Del Vecchio M et al. (1981) Comparing radical mastectomy with quadrantectomy, axillary dissection, and radiotherapy in patients with small cancers of the breast. N Engl J Med 305: 6-11
Yusuf S, Peto R, Lewis J et al. (1985) Beta-blockade during and after myocardial infarction: an overview of the randomised trials. Prog Cardiovasc Dis 27: 335-371

*Combining Randomized and Nonrandomized Patients in the Statistical Analysis of Clinical Trials**

M. Schumacher and K. Davis**

Institut für Medizinische Biometrie und Informatik, Universität Freiburg,
Stefan-Meier-Straße 26, 7800 Freiburg, FRG

Introduction

Randomized clinical trials are widely accepted as the definitive method of comparing treatments. In a well-designed trial, the treatment comparison has internal validity since the treatment groups are randomly selected. The trial may not be of practical use, however, unless it also has external validity. The patients who are studied in the trial are only a small portion of the patients who satisfy the trial entry criterion. Eligible patients may not be approached for consent if their physician feels they will not benefit from participation. Patients may be excluded because they prefer their therapy to be chosen based on their own or their physician's judgement, because they don't like the protocol requirements of the trial, or simply because they are not in an area where a trial is being conducted. To have external validity, the trial results must be applicable to eligible patients who were not enrolled.

To assess the external validity, the researcher first needs to know whether or not the patients who agreed to be randomized were different from the patients who declined randomization. If there are measurable differences, the effect of these differences on the conclusions of the trial should be examined. The researcher must also examine the results of therapy in the nonrandomized population. Even if the randomized and nonrandomized groups are similar, it is possible that therapy assigned by physician judgement and delivered in an usual clinic setting may have a different outcome from therapy which was randomly assigned and delivered in the setting of a clinical trial. Patients in a randomized trial may have a different outcome because the care given to patients in the trial is not the same as care given to patients not in the trial. Also, it is possible that physicians are able to select patients who will benefit from treatment by using informed judgement, which cannot be quantified as data. If physician judgement alone is the major fac-

* Dedicated to Prof. Dr. med. Herbert Immich on the occasion of his 70th birthday.

** We would like to thank Manfred Olschewski, Freiburg, and Hans Scheurlen, Heidelberg, for their valuable contributions and Rolf Dietl, Dortmund, and Andrzej Kosinski, Seattle, for computational assistance.

Recent Results in Cancer Research, Vol. 111
© Springer-Verlag Berlin · Heidelberg 1988

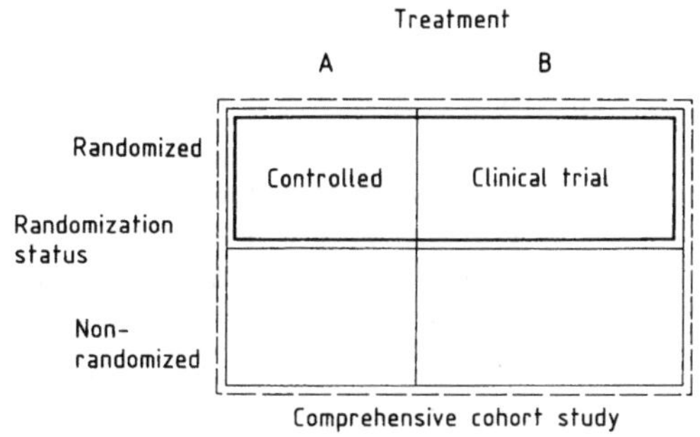

Fig. 1. Schematic representation of the comprehensive cohort study design

tor, then patients assigned to surgery on a physician's decision will have better average results than apparently comparable patients randomized to surgery.

The comprehensive cohort study design proposed by Scheurlen et al. (1984) and Olschewski and Scheurlen (1985) provides a framework for studying the external validity of a clinical trial. In this design, all available eligible patients are enrolled whether or not they consent to randomized treatment assignment. The design is essentially a prospective cohort study with a randomized subcohort, as illustrated in Fig. 1. In this paper we will explore the use of the Cox model for survival analysis (Cox 1972) in the context of a comprehensive cohort design to examine the external validity of a randomized clinical trial and to strengthen the trial results.

Methods

It is the aim of this section to provide a sound statistical methodology for a simultaneous analysis of randomized and nonrandomized patients in a clinical trial comparing two treatments, let us say A and B, when the survival time is the criterion.

As a first step toward a statistical model we assume that the relative risk of treatment A to B is equal to some quantity a in the nonrandomized patients, and equal to some quantity $a \cdot c$ in the randomized patients. The latter can be seen as the internal "gold standard" since it is based on a randomized comparison. Similarly, we can assume that the relative risk of randomized to nonrandomized patients is equal to some quantity b in patients treated with B and to some quantity $b \cdot c$ in patients treated with A. These relative risks can simply be derived by taking ratios in the following 2×2 table:

	Treatment	
	A	B
Randomized	$a \cdot b \cdot c$	b
Nonrandomized	a	1

The quantity c can be referred to as the treatment-randomization status interaction which allows for the relative risks of treatment A to B being different in randomized and in nonrandomized patients.

This simple model enables us to define more precisely the term "stable conditions" in a comprehensive cohort study which has been suggested by Olschewski and Scheurlen (1985): We consider conditions to be stable if $c=1$, i.e., if there is no interaction between treatment and randomization status. In this case we have equal relative risks of treatment A to B in randomized and in nonrandomized patients. Note, however, that even under stable conditions the randomized patients are allowed to be different from the nonrandomized ones.

Thus, estimating the quantity c and testing the hypothesis "$c=1$" of no treatment-randomization status interaction takes a central part in the statistical analysis of a comprehensive cohort study. This analysis can be carried through in the framework of a Cox regression model (Cox 1972) with the treatment indicator, the randomization indicator, and a multiplicative interaction term as binary covariates.

This model, however, will be too simple in almost all practical applications since patients' heterogeneity has to be taken into account (Schumacher et al. 1987). This can be done by including several other prognostic factors as covariates into an extended Cox model and, if necessary, by considering also the treatment-covariate interactions. In addition, a logistic regression model (Cox 1971) should be set up relating the odds of accepting randomization to these prognostic factors.

The Coronary Artery Surgery Study

The Coronary Artery Surgery Study (CASS) was initiated in 1972 by the National Heart, Lung, and Blood Institute to compare coronary bypass surgery with conventional medical therapy for coronary artery disease. Complete details of the CASS design and protocol have been published previously (Principal Investigators of CASS and Their Associates 1981). The study was carried out at 15 participating medical centers in the United States and Canada. CASS was designed as a randomized trial within a larger registry. For the registry, every patient who underwent coronary angiography for evaluation of suspected ischemic coronary disease at one of the 15 centers during the period of enrollment from 1974 to 1979 was asked to participate. Patients were enrolled following informed consent. The 24 959 registry patients comprise 94% of the eligible patients. Eligible patients for the randomized trial were defined to be those who had mild angina, Canadian Heart classification I or II, or who were asymptomatic following a myocardial infarction. These patients were asked to accept random assignment to medical or surgical therapy. Of the 2099 eligible patients, 780 accepted randomized therapy assignment and 1319 declined. These 2099 patients form a comprehensive cohort study. The entire registry was followed annually through November 1982; follow-up of the comprehensive cohort continues. Follow-up for vital status for patients in the rest of the registry is done through the National Death Index (Davis et al. 1985).

In keeping with the principle of analysis by intent to treat, treatment group is defined by the original randomized assignment for the randomized patients. A substantial number of patients assigned randomly to medicine later had surgery when their angina became more severe. Of the 390 patients randomized to medical therapy, 23.5% underwent bypass surgery within 5 years. In order to define a similar "intent-to-treat" cohort within the nonrandomized patients, surgical patients were defined as those who had early elective surgery and medical patients were defined as those who did not have surgery or had late surgery. Specifically, surgery was defined to be "early" if it occurred within 90 days of enrollment or within the time period for each hospital within which 95% of the surgeries were done in the first year of the CASS study. Cut-off time ranges from 90 to 240 days; the average is 125 days. For randomized patients, survival is dated from the time of randomization. For nonrandomized patients, surgical survival is dated from the time of surgery and medical survival is dated from the average time to surgery at the patient's particular hospital within the first year. Average times to surgery range from 20 to 96 days; the average is 53 days. Four of the 1319 nonrandomized patients who died before their hospital's average time to surgery were excluded from the analysis. More details are given by Davis (this volume).

Results

Covariate values for the 735 randomized and 988 nonrandomized patients in the comprehensive cohort for whom baseline ejection fraction was available are given in Table 1. There were no significant differences in these covariates between the two groups.

About 45% of the nonrandomized patients received bypass surgery; the other 55% had medical treatment. So there was only a slight imbalance in treatment allocation in the nonrandomized patients compared with the 1:1 allocation in the randomized ones. Table 2 comprises the estimated coefficients in the simple version of the Cox regression model taking only the treatment and the randomization status into account. The coefficients correspond to the logarithms of the quantities *a*, *b* and *c* introduced in the Methods section. It should be noted that in the pres-

Table 1. Covariate percents for the comprehensive cohort

Covariate	Randomized (n=735)	Nonrandomized (n=988)	*p*1	*p*2
Age >median	50.5	49.0	0.54	0.60
Class-II angina	62.9	66.1	0.17	0.32
History of MI	59.7	57.2	0.30	0.96
Proximal LAD >70%	31.7	34.2	0.27	0.21
LV score >10	22.3	18.8	0.07	0.40
Number of vessels diseased:				
1	28.4	32.5	0.10	0.10
2	39.2	34.7		
3	32.4	32.8		
Ejection fraction <0.50	21.8	19.0	0.16	0.68

*p*1 is the *P*-value associated with the univariate chi-square statistic; *p*2 is the chi-square *P*-value associated with logistic regression with all covariates in the model.

Table 2. Results of a simple Cox regression analysis for the comprehensive cohort

Covariate	Estimated coefficient	Standard error	*P*-value
Treatment	−0.06	0.18	
Randomization status	0.16	0.17	
Treatment × randomization status	−0.15	0.26	0.57

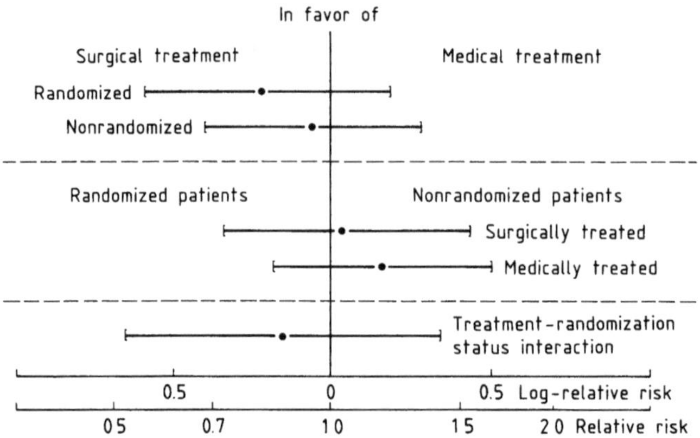

Fig. 2. Estimated relative risks (x) with 95% - confidence intervals ([x]) on a logarithmic scale for CASS patients with ejection fraction measured

ence of an interaction term the other coefficients cannot be interpreted directly as the treatment effect or the effect of the randomization status. However, in the present example it can be seen that the treatment-randomization status interaction can be neglected.

Thus, in general, from the figures in Table 2, estimates of the relative risks can be derived in a very simple and straightforward manner. For the CASS patients, these are displayed in Fig. 2 on a logarithmic scale jointly with 95%-confidence intervals. There is a slight indication of a superiority of bypass surgery but by no means of a significant magnitude.

For an extended analysis, the most important other prognostic factors already listed in Table 1 as well as the treatment-covariate interactions have been considered. From the results presented in Table 3 it can be concluded that the treatment-randomization status interaction can be neglected. In a second step, the relevance of the remaining seven treatment-covariate interactions is examined by the likelihood ratio criterion, yielding a *P*-value less than 0.01. This shows the heterogeneity of the treatment effect in the different prognostic subgroups defined by the values of the covariates. The distribution of these estimated relative risks is displayed - again on a logarithmic scale - in Fig. 3. It is interesting to note that the extreme on the right side of the histogram refers to the subgroup of patients who are

Table 3. Results of an extended Cox regression analysis for the comprehensive cohort

Covariate	Estimated coefficient	Standard error	−2*Log likelihood
Treatment	−1.04	0.63	
Randomization status	0.07	0.18	3481
Age	0.23	0.18	
Angina	−0.12	0.18	
Prior MI	0.47	0.23	
LAD disease	0.39	0.19	
LV-score	0.64	0.22	
Diseased vessels	0.01	0.12	
Ejection fraction	−0.86	0.22	3400
Treatment × age	0.17	0.27	
Treatment × angina	0.10	0.28	
Treatment × prior MI	−0.38	0.32	
Treatment × LAD disease	−0.54	0.27	
Treatment × LV score	−0.34	0.35	
Treatment × diseased vessels	0.41	0.19	
Treatment × ejection fraction	0.62	0.35	3381
Treatment × randomization status	0.001	0.27	3381

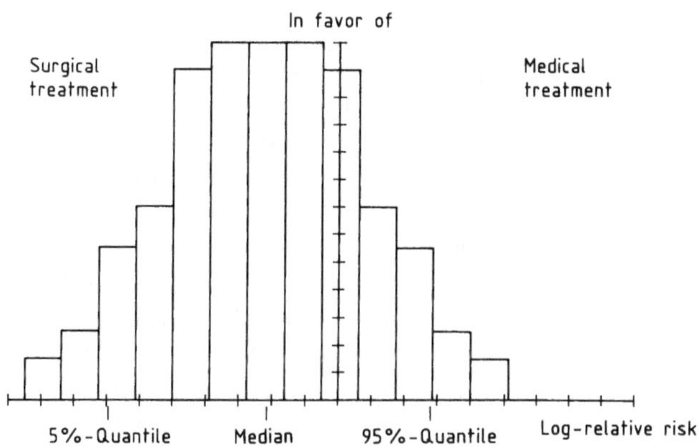

Fig. 3. Distribution of estimated relative risks in various prognostic subgroups on a logarithmic scale for CASS patients with ejection fraction measured

young, have no or at least class-I angina, only one vessel diseased, and a high ejection fraction. In contrast, the subgroup of patients belonging to the extreme on the left side of the histogram consists of patients who are old, have class-II angina, a history of MI, and a low ejection fraction. In general, it can be seen that the relative risks of treatment A to B are uniformly equal for randomized and nonrandomized patients but are rather heterogeneous through the range of prognostic subgroups. Thus, there might be some doubt that a global measure for the relative risk as the median or some weighted average should be of substantial value.

Discussion

Although the example used in this paper is from cardiovascular disease, the consideration of randomized as well as of nonrandomized patients is at least as important in the statistical analysis of many cancer clinical trials. This is especially true when the treatments under study differ substantially in a qualitative way, e.g., breast preservation vs. mastectomy in a breast cancer trial or aggressive chemotherapy vs a moderate hormone therapy. The reason for using the data of the CASS patients in this context is that these data have been completely available for the randomized and for the nonrandomized patients.

In ongoing and future cancer clinical trials where randomization is not accepted by all eligible patients, it should be a must to have these data available too. This implies that all eligible patients have to be followed up with the same care, which is actually done in the West German breast cancer trials sponsored by the Federal Government.

It should be kept in mind, however, that the comprehensive cohort design cannot substitute for a randomized comparison. It is rather - as already indicated in the introduction - a necessary complement to a controlled clinical trial to ensure external validity. From this it follows that the controlled clinical trial itself must be large enough to ensure a valid treatment comparison (CASS Principal Investigators and Their Associates 1984). A sufficient number of patients in the randomized part of the comprehensive cohort is also necessary for a high power of the test for a treatment-randomization status interaction, i.e., so that a substantial difference in the relative risks for randomized patients and nonrandomized patients can be detected with a sufficiently high probability.

The methodology proposed in this paper allows a simultaneous analysis of the impact of therapy, randomization status, and other prognostic factors. This is new and in contrast to common practice, where only the comparability of entry characteristics is investigated or at most a comparison of randomized to nonrandomized patients' survival experience is made within each therapy (CASS Principal Investigators and Their Associates 1984). The advantage of the methods proposed is that all these factors are analyzed simultaneously and that under certain circumstances - what one could define as "stable conditions" - a combination of the results in the randomized and in the nonrandomized patients can be obtained. For the more technical details of the statistical methods used for this purpose and for further statistical analyses as model checking, the reader should be referred to a separate, forthcoming paper of the authors.

The results obtained for CASS are in agreement with recent CASS publications. In the initial report of the CASS randomized trial, no overall difference between the two treatments could be found (CASS Principal Investigators and Their Associates 1983). However, trends which indicated a possible heterogeneity of results among subgroups were noted. In a later analysis of further follow-up, a significant difference in favor of surgery was noted for patients with low ejection fraction, the right side extreme in Fig. 3 (Passamani et al. 1985). In comparing results in the randomized and nonrandomized patients, it was concluded that survival rates were similar in both medical and both surgical groups (CASS Principal Investigators and Their Associates 1984). This is in agreement with the present analysis. Thus, in this particular study, the interpretation of the results is relatively easy and the results of CASS might be thought to be too nice to serve as a realistic example for many cancer clinical trials where other scenarios could be expected. But even if the results are not as concordant as in CASS, the methodology of a comprehensive cohort study including the simultaneous statistical analysis of all important factors influencing patients' survival provides a powerful tool for a valid treatment comparison.

References

CASS Principal Investigators and their Associates (1983) Coronary Artery Surgery Study (CASS): a randomized trial of coronary artery bypass surgery. Survival data. Circulation 68: 939-950

CASS Principal Investigators and Their Associates (1984) Coronary Artery Surgery Study (CASS): a randomized trial of coronary artery bypass surgery. Comparability of entry characteristics and survival in randomized patients and non-randomized patients meeting randomization criteria. JACC 3: 114-128

Cox DR (1971) Analysis of binary data. Methuen, London

Cox DR (1972) Regression models and life tables (with discussion). J R Stat Soc B 34: 187-220

Davis KB, Fisher L, Gillespie MJ, Pettinger M (1985) A test of the National Death Index using the Coronary Artery Surgery Study (CASS). Controlled Clin Trials 6: 179-191

Olschewski M, Scheurlen H (1985) Comprehensive cohort study: an alternative to randomized consent design in a breast preservation trial. Methods Inf Med 24: 131-134

Passamani E, Davis KB, Gillespie MJ, Killip T, CASS Principal Investigators and Their Associates (1985) A randomized trial of coronary artery bypass surgery. Survival of patients with a low ejection fraction. N Engl J Med 312: 1665-1671

Principal Investigators of CASS and Their Associates (1981) The National Heart, Lung and Blood Institute Coronary Artery Surgery Study (CASS). Circulation 63 [Suppl I]: I - 1-81

Scheurlen H, Olschewski M, Leibbrand D (1984) Zur Methodologie kontrollierter klinischer Studien über die Primärbehandlung des operablen Mammakarzinoms. Strahlentherapie 160: 459-468

Schumacher M, Olschewski M, Schmoor C (1987) The impact of heterogeneity on the comparison of survival times. Stat Med 6: 773-784

The Comprehensive Cohort Study: The Use of Registry Data to Confirm and Extend a Randomized Trial

K. Davis

Department of Biostatistics, CASS Coordinating Center, University of Washington, 1107 N. E. 45th Street, Room 530, Seattle, WA 98105, USA

Introduction

The randomized clinical trial is usually the best method of comparing treatment modalities because it is unbiased. However, there is sometimes concern that the patients in the trial are not representative of all patients who could be treated. Thus, the trial results may be unbiased but not generalizable. A means of verifying the external validity of the trial is given by the comprehensive cohort study design (Olschewski and Scheurlen 1985). In this design, all available eligible patients are enrolled whether or not they consent to randomized treatment assignment. The design is essentially a prospective cohort study with a randomized subcohort.

This paper presents an example of a comprehensive cohort study and discusses the use of this design in studying the generalization and extension of the trial results. Particular problems in defining treatment groups among the nonrandomized patients are also discussed.

The Coronary Artery Surgery Study

The Coronary Artery Surgery Study (CASS) was designed to compare coronary bypass surgery with conventional medical therapy for coronary artery disease (Principal Investigators of CASS and Their Associates 1981). The study was carried out at 15 participating medical centers in the United States and Canada. CASS was designed as a randomized trial within a larger registry. For the registry, every patient who had angiographic evaluation for suspected ischemic cardiac disease at one of the 15 centers was asked to participate. Following informed consent, patients were enrolled in the registry. Very few patients (6%) declined to be enrolled, since registry participation did not involve any change in medical treatment and only required permission for telephone follow-up at annual intervals. Eligible patients for the randomized trial were defined as those who had mild angina, i.e., angina brought on only by rather marked exertion such as climbing stairs or walking rapidly. The registry patients who were not eligible for the trial consisted of patients whose disease was so advanced that surgery could not be

Recent Results in Cancer Research, Vol. 111
© Springer-Verlag Berlin · Heidelberg 1988

considered and patients who were found to have totally normal coronary arteries, as well as a broad spectrum of other patients. Eligible patients were asked to accept random assignment to medical or surgical therapy. From this process a total of 24959 registry patients was obtained. Of these, there were 780 randomized patients and 1319 "randomizable" patients. "Randomizable" patients are defined as eligible patients who did not enter the randomized trial. The term does not include patients actually randomized.

The planning phase for the study was 1973-1974. Enrollment in the registry began in July 1974 and continued to June 1979. Patients were enrolled in the randomized trial from August 1975 to June 1979. The entire registry was followed annually through November 1982. Follow-up of the randomized and randomizable patients is scheduled to continue through 1993. Follow-up for vital status for most patients in the rest of the registry is continued through the National Death Index, a centrally maintained record of all deaths which occur in the United States (Davis et al. 1985). The investigators were given the results of the trial only at the time of the first major report from the randomized trial in late 1983 (CASS Principal Investigators et al. 1983a, b, 1984a, b). The treatment itself, open heart surgery, could not be blinded.

Figure 1 is a survival curve from the randomized study. These data are for the randomized patients who had an ejection fraction greater than 50%, i.e., at most a modest impairment of function. For these patients there is little difference in outcome for medicine and surgery. There is perhaps a slight difference beginning to appear at 8 years. Other studies have shown that the vein used to do the bypass graft begins to deteriorate after about 8 years (Campeau et al. 1983). Figure 2 is a

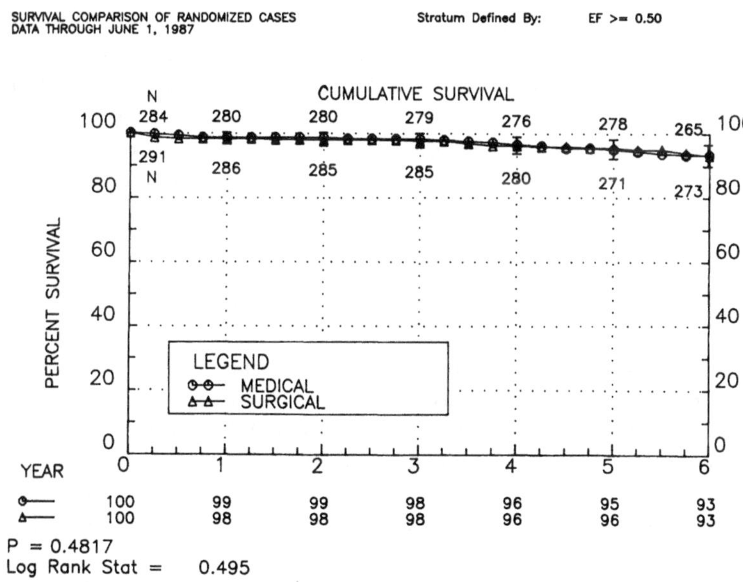

Fig. 1. Cumulative survival rates for CASS randomized patients with ejection fraction of at least 0.50

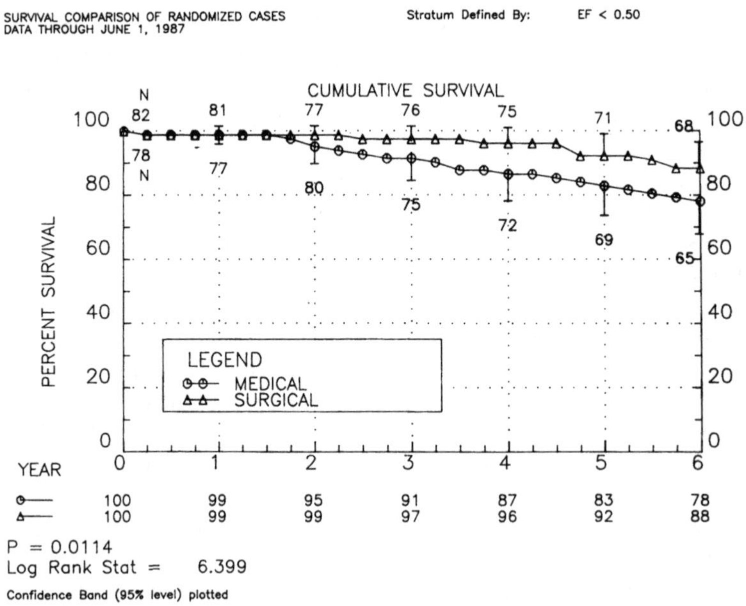

Fig. 2. Cumulative survival rates for CASS randomized patients with ejection fraction less than 0.50

survival curve for randomized patients with ejection fraction less than 50%, which indicates some impairment of ventricular function. For these patients, there is a marked benefit from bypass surgery.

As these curves illustrate, patients with cardiovascular disease often have very low event rates. However, coronary disease is a major source of morbidity and mortality, so small differences in these rates can have major implications for public health. Thus, very large sample sizes are often necessary for meaningful studies.

The CASS data base is somewhat different from other large studies of coronary disease, such as Framingham, in that all patients initially underwent angiography, so the amount of coronary disease present was known at the time of enrollment.

CASS as an Example of a Comprehensive Cohort Study

The CASS randomized and randomizable patients together are an example of a comprehensive cohort study. The data can be used to examine the differences in baseline characteristics and in the outcome of therapy between eligible patients who did and did not accept randomization. The CASS study design has the added benefit that data were also collected on patients who were not eligible for the trial. These data can be used to investigate the extension of the trial results to other populations.

Characteristics of the randomized and randomizable populations were compared in an early CASS publication (CASS Principal Investigators et al. 1984a). It was established that the two groups were indeed fairly similar. There were some

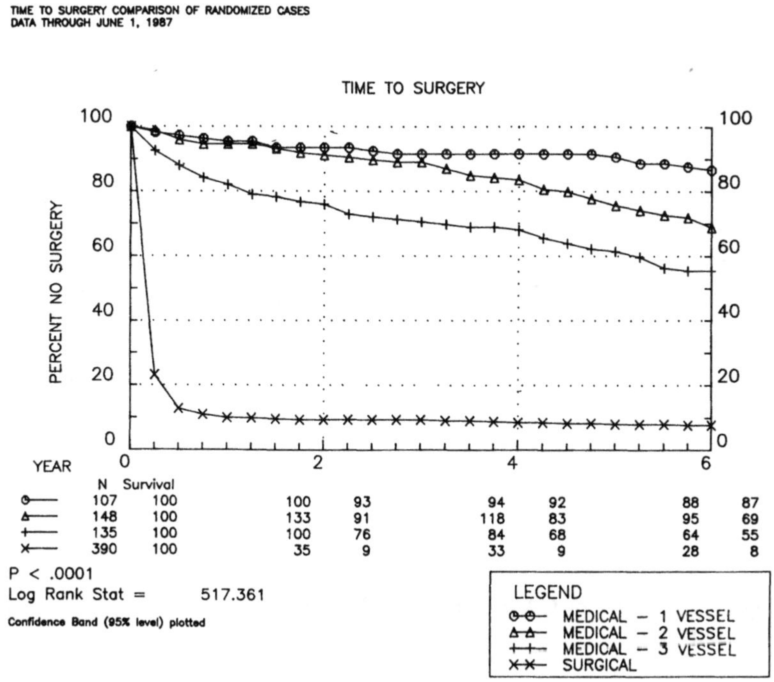

Fig. 3. Percentage of patients in the CASS randomized trial in the surgical group and medical groups with single-, double-, and triple-vessel disease who had not yet had surgery at various time intervals

differences – for instance, the patients who declined randomization were more likely to be taking beta-blockers, which are prescribed to relieve chest pain – but most of them were minor and the differences were described. The methodology for these comparisons is straightforward.

Comparison of the results of treatment presents a more interesting analysis problem. In order to make this comparison, equivalent definitions of "surgically treated" and "medically treated" must be made for randomized and randomizable patients. The randomized patients are analyzed by "intent to treat." Those patients assigned to either treatment are analyzed as part of their assigned treatment group, regardless of their actual therapy. Figure 3 is an actuarial curve showing time to first surgery for randomized patients separated according to treatment assigned. The bottom curve for patients assigned to surgery shows that some of these patients did not undergo the procedure immediately. The top three curves are for patients assigned to medical therapy. There was a differential rate for patients with one-, two-, and three-vessel disease. Since surgery usually relieves chest pain, medically assigned patients tended to switch to surgery when their chest pain became intolerable. Patients with three-vessel disease have more extensive involvement and are more likely to have increasing angina. Thus, CASS was essentially a trial of immediate surgery versus surgery delayed until symptoms warranted it.

It is difficult to define comparable treatment groups for the randomizable pa-

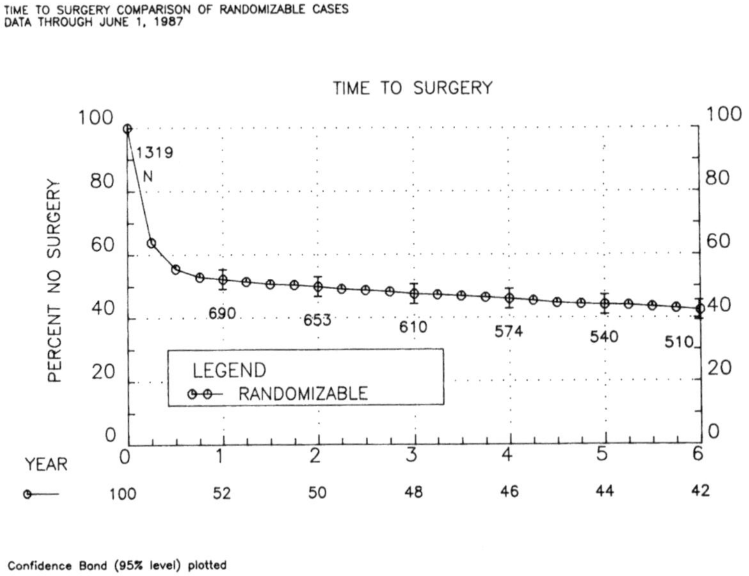

Fig. 4. Percentage of CASS randomizable patients who had not yet had surgery at various time intervals

tients. Figure 4 is an actuarial curve showing time to surgery for the randomizable patients over 6 years of follow-up. After the first year, patients were still receiving first surgery at the rate of about 2% per year. Patients eligible for the trial have only moderate disease and live a relatively long time, and disease progression is a dynamic process over all the long follow-up period. In order to study survival time following surgery, a decision must be made as to which surgeries to include. For example, should patients who had surgery 8 years after enrollment be included? These patients must of course survive 8 years on medical treatment first.

Four methods of defining the groups were considered.

1. All patients may be defined as in the medically treated group initially. In the survival analysis, survival for medically treated patients would date from the time of enrollment and patients would be censored at the time of surgery. Patients would be defined as surgically treated if they have surgery at any time. Survival would be dated from the date of surgery. With this method, medical therapy is credited with keeping patients alive until surgery, but medical therapy is also credited with all early deaths, even for patients who died 1 h before scheduled surgery. Unlike the group definition for the randomized patients, therapy is "locked in." All patients in the surgical group have surgery, and all those in the medical group never have surgery. The survival following surgery for medical patients who have late surgery is not included as "medical" survival as it is for the randomized patients.
   The use of this method was discussed in a study of "medically treated" patients from the CASS registry (Chaitman et al. 1983). The study concerned nonrandomized patients who had mid left anterior descending artery disease, com-

bined proximal left anterior descending and proximal circumflex artery disease, or left main coronary disease. The actuarial survival curve in Fig. 5a illustrates a problem with method 1. The left main patients are a subgroup for which surgery is almost always recommended. In this subgroup the estimates start out based on 858 patients and quickly drop at the first year to 68 patients because most patients had early surgery. In this case, the printed initial sample size of 858 is not the effective sample size.

There is also a problem in contrasting the baseline characteristics of the medically and surgically treated patients, since the same surgery patients are in both groups. On the same basis, the power of the Cox model would be affected since a surgery patient's baseline covariates would be used twice.

2. The groups may be defined as in method 1, but all patients who have surgery within a defined early period would be excluded from the medically treated group. With this method, the printed sample size is more reasonable, but therapy is still locked in and there is still the problem that all early deaths are attributed to medical therapy. Since the early denominator is reduced, the early deaths have a large influence on the early mortality. The effect is illustrated in Fig. 5b. These data are from the same patients used for Fig. 5a. For these patients, there was a high early mortality and the change in denominator markedly changed the early survival estimates. This method is not recommended.
3. Patients may be classified into groups according to what therapy was recommended at baseline. This was considered in planning CASS, and a box was included on the eligibility form to check which therapy was recommended for nonrandomized patients. Using this, surgical patients could be defined as those for whom surgery was recommended, and medical patients could be defined as those for whom medical therapy was recommended.

   Unfortunately, recommended therapy may not bear much relation to reality. In CASS, the enrolled patients were being seen on referral. There were several physicians involved, with several different opinions, and the physician who filled out the form was not necessarily the one who had the greatest influence with the patient. Some hospitals, possibly in recognition of this problem, routinely left the box blank. In CASS this has not been a useful classification rule.
4. Surgical patients may be defined as those patients having "early" surgery. Surgery may be defined as "early" if it occurred within 90 days of enrollment or within the time period for each hospital within which 95% of the surgeries were done in the first year. The hospital-specific method is preferable to a fixed time point such as 90 days. At hospitals with long waiting lists for surgery a fixed time point would eliminate many patients who were actually scheduled for surgery at the time of enrollment. For example, in CASS the Montreal Heart Institute, which is under a different system of national medical care, had an average time to surgery of almost 3 months as compared with that of the Mayo Clinic, in the U.S., which was 14 days. The average cut-off time in CASS is 4 months. Survival time would be dated from the date of surgery.

All other patients would be defined as medically treated. Survival for medically treated patients would be dated from the average time to surgery at each hospital. In CASS, the range is 20-96 days; the average is 53 days.

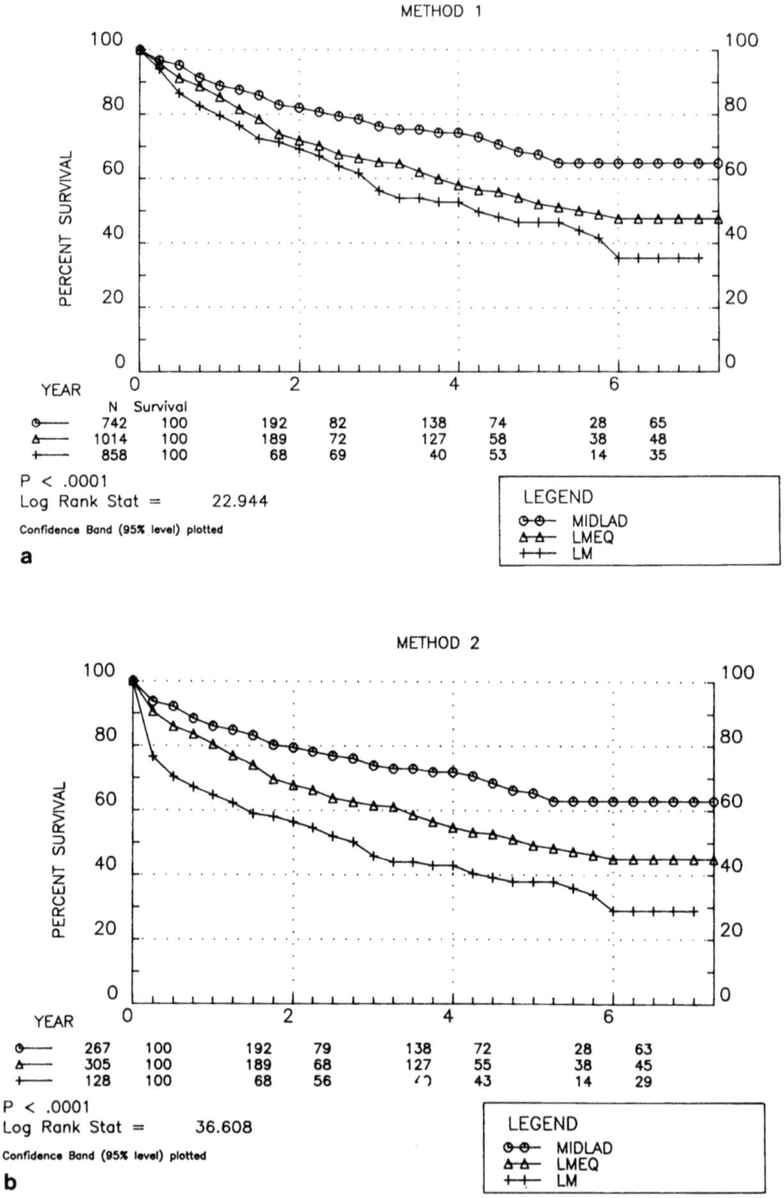

Fig. 5a-c. Cumulative survival rates using three methods of analysis for CASS patients with mid left anterior descending artery disease *(MIDLAD)*, combined proximal left anterior descending and proximal left circumflex artery disease *(LMEQ)*, and left main coronary disease *(LM)*. **a** All patients in medical group initially, censored at the time of surgery. All patients with surgery in surgical group. **b** All patients except those with surgery during the first 6 months in medical group. Medical survival censored at the time of surgery. All patients with surgery in surgical group. **c** Patients without early surgery (see text) in medical group; survival starts at average time to surgery. Patients with early surgery in surgical group (see p. 145)

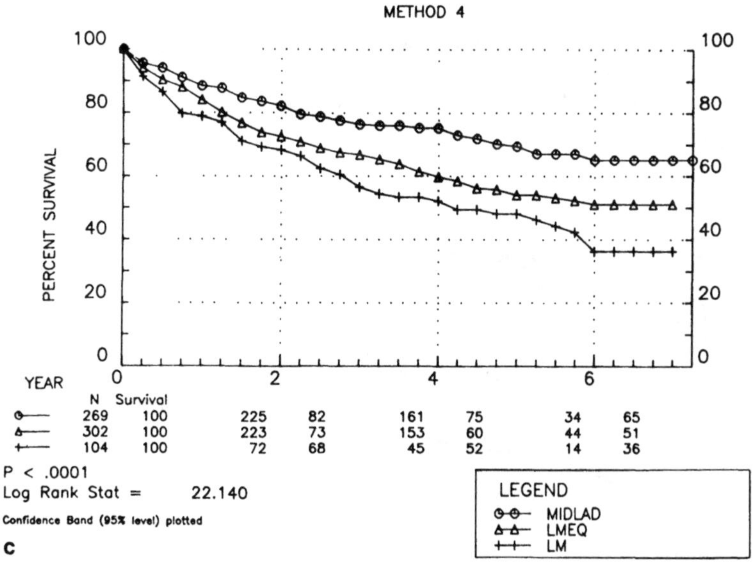

c

Fig. 5c. Legend see p. 144

This method solves a number of problems. Therapy is not locked in. Although all surgical patients have surgery, medically treated patients who have late surgery remain in the medical group. The printed sample size is easy to interpret, and the medical and surgical patients form two distinct groups. It must be noted that patients who die early are completely excluded from the analysis. For the CASS, this removed four of the 1319 randomizable patients.

Using this method, survival based on the previously displayed data for medically treated patients in the CASS registry is illustrated in Fig. 5c. The primary difference in the estimates is in the early period. Method 1 includes the early deaths, but the denominator is so large for the short period before surgery occurs that the estimated early mortality rates remain very low. Method 2 includes the early deaths but drastically reduces the denominator, with the effect that the estimated early mortality rates are much higher. Method 4 excludes some of the early deaths but also reduces the denominator, so the estimated early mortality rates for these patients are between the estimates for methods 1 and 2. For the longer term, there may be more difference with further follow-up as more people switch over to surgery, because patients remain in the medically treated group in method 4, but are removed from the medically treated group in methods 1 and 2.

Method 4 has been used for the randomizable patients in all published analyses of the CASS randomized and randomizable patients. An example of these comparisons is given in Fig. 6a and b. Figure 6a shows survival for the medically treated patients. For these groups, the survival curves are virtually superposable. The rate of switch-over to surgery, displayed at the bottom of the figure, was also the same for both groups. Surgical results are shown in Fig. 6b. In this group of patients there appears to be no "third factor" of physician judgement that selected patients who would benefit from surgery, unless physician judgement and differ-

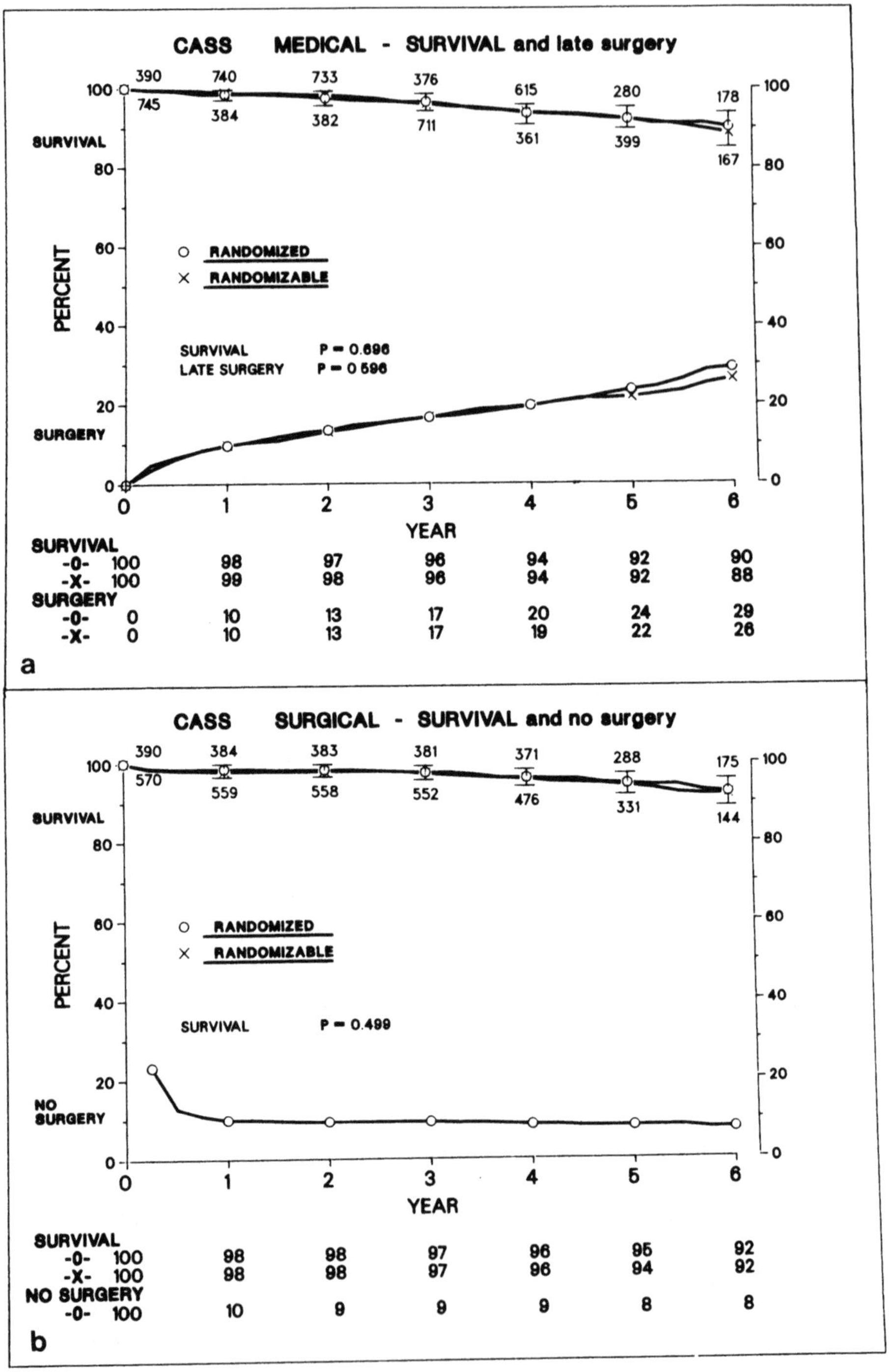
CASS MEDICAL - SURVIVAL and late surgery
390 740 733 376 615 280 178
745 384 382 711 361 399 167
SURVIVAL
SURGERY
PERCENT
RANDOMIZED
RANDOMIZABLE
SURVIVAL P = 0.696
LATE SURGERY P = 0.596
YEAR
SURVIVAL
-0- 100 98 97 96 94 92 90
-X- 100 99 98 96 94 92 88
SURGERY
-0- 0 10 13 17 20 24 29
-X- 0 10 13 17 19 22 26
a
CASS SURGICAL - SURVIVAL and no surgery
390 384 383 381 371 288 175
570 559 558 552 476 331 144
SURVIVAL
NO SURGERY
PERCENT
RANDOMIZED
RANDOMIZABLE
SURVIVAL P = 0.499
YEAR
SURVIVAL
-0- 100 98 98 97 96 95 92
-X- 100 98 98 97 96 94 92
NO SURGERY
-0- 100 10 9 9 9 8 8
b

ent treatment somehow canceled each other. There is no switch-over curve for the randomizable patients because all of them had surgery by definition.

In the comparison of CASS randomized and randomizable patients there is a slight inconsistency in the starting date, in that survival for randomized patients begins a little earlier, at the time of randomization, instead of at the time of surgery. It is possible to correct this. At the time of randomization, before the assignment was made, the surgical department was called and a date of scheduled surgery was obtained. This gave a comparable date of scheduled surgery for both medically and surgically treated patients which could be used for analysis. Since the CASS papers published from the randomized trial alone were done using date of enrollment, it was decided to do the same for the comparison papers so that the numbers would be consistent from paper to paper.

Extension of the Randomized Trial to Other Populations

Since CASS included a complete registry of angiographically evaluated patients who were not eligible for randomization, the extension of the results from the randomized trial to other patient groups could be explored. There is so much difficulty in making comparable definitions of surgical and medical treatment groups in the randomized and nonrandomized population, that the contrast of the randomized patients to patients who were not eligible for the trial and who had self-selected treatment is interesting but somewhat tenuous. The randomizable patients are a more natural comparison group, because the group definitions are comparable. Since the randomized trial studied patients with mild angina, it was of natural interest to compare results in the patients with more severe angina. A CASS registry study showed that if angina is more severe - brought on by only mild exertion - then bypass surgery appears to prolong survival (Kaiser et al. 1985). Another registry study explored the extension of trial results to patients older than 65 years, since these patients were excluded from randomization (Gersh et al. 1985).

Summary

There are distinct advantages to the comprehensive cohort design for randomized clinical trials. The design allows the researcher to systematically compare the trial participants and the trial results with the characteristics and results in the population of eligible patients who were not randomly assigned to treatment. There are some problems with this design. The added costs of enrollment and follow-up for the nonrandomized cohort can add substantially to the cost of a trial. As the

◁ **Fig. 6. a** Cumulative survival rates and rates of late surgery in the 390 patients randomized to medical management and the 745 patients meeting criteria for randomization but not accepting randomization who were medically managed. **b** Cumulative survival rates and rates of no surgery in the 390 patients randomized to surgical management and cumulative survival in the 570 surgical randomizable patients, all of whom had surgery. (Reprinted with permission from the Journal of the American College of Cardiology 3: 114-128, 1984)

CASS example illustrates, careful attention must be given to definition of the treatment groups in the nonrandomized cohort. For the randomized patients, group assignment by "intention to treat" is preferred in most cases. The definition of "intention to treat" in the nonrandomized cohort may be difficult, since the patient may receive recommendations from several sources and, in the case of chronic disease, the decision may be postponed for a long period. This problem is not specific to the comprehensive cohort design, however, and a comparison group of concurrently enrolled and followed patients is almost always preferred over a comparison group found elsewhere.

References

Campeau L, Enjalbert M, Lesperance J, Vaislic C, Grondin CM, Bourassa MG (1983) Atherosclerosis and late graft closure of aortocoronary saphenous vein grafts: sequential angiographic studies at 2 weeks, 1 year, 5 to 7 years, and 10 to 12 years after surgery. Circulation 68 [Suppl II]: II-1

CASS Principal Investigators and Their Associates: Coronary Artery Surgery Study (CASS) (1983a) A randomized trial of coronary artery bypass surgery, survival data. Circulation 68: 939-950

CASS Principal Investigators and Their Associates: Coronary Artery Surgery Study (CASS) (1983b) A randomized trial of coronary artery bypass surgery. Quality of life in patients randomly assigned to treatment groups. Circulation 68: 951-960

CASS Principal Investigators and Their Associates: Coronary Artery Surgery Study (CASS) (1984a) A randomized trial of coronary artery bypass surgery. Comparability of entry characteristics and survival in randomized and nonrandomized patients meeting randomization criteria. J Am Coll Cardiol 3: 114-128

CASS Principal Investigators and Their Associates (1984b) Myocardial infarction and mortality in the Coronary Artery Surgery Study (CASS) randomized trial. N Engl J Med 310: 750-758

Chaitman BR, Davis K, Fisher LD, Bourassa MG, Mock MB, Lesperance J, Rogers WJ, Fray D, Tyras DH, Judkins MP, Ringqvist I, Killip T (1983) A life-table and Cox regression analysis of patients with combined proximal left anterior descending and proximal circumflex coronary artery disease: non-left main equivalent lesions (CASS). Circulation 68: 1163-1170

Davis KB, Fisher L, Gillespie MJ, Pettinger M (1985) A test of the National Death Index using the Coronary Artery Surgery Study (CASS). Controlled Clin Trials 6: 179-191

Gersh BJ, Kronmal RA, Schaff HV, Frye RL, Ryan TJ, Mock MB, Myers WO, Athearn MW, Gosselin AJ, Kaiser GC, Bourassa MG, Killip T (1985)

Comparison of coronary artery bypass surgery and medical therapy in patients 65 years of age or older. N Engl J Med 313: 217-224

Kaiser GC, Davis KB, Fisher LD, Myers WO, Foster ED, Passamani ER, Gillespie MJ (1985) Survival following coronary artery bypass grafting in patients with severe angina pectoris (CASS). J Thorac Cardiovasc Surg 89: 513-524

Olschewski M, Scheurlen H (1985) Comprehensive cohort study: an alternative to randomized consent design in a breast preservation trial. Meth Inf Med 24: 131-134

Principal Investigators of CASS and Their Associates (Killip T, editor, Fisher LD, Mock MB, associate editors) (1981) National Heart, Lung, and Blood Institute Coronary Artery Surgery Study (CASS). Circulation 63 [Suppl I]: I-1-81

Subjective Opinions and Informed Consent

Treatment Decisions in Breast Cancer

S. M. Gore, A. O. Langlands, D. J. Spiegelhalter, and H. J. Stewart

MRC Biostatistics Unit, 5 Shaftesburry Road, Cambridge CB2 2BW, Great Britain

Introduction

Past surveys (Forrest et al. 1969; Nemoto 1973) of surgical opinion, albeit using diverse methods of inquiry, have suggested international differences in the extent of mastectomy for early breast cancer. A 1983 questionnaire (Gazet et al. 1985) to British surgeons about their treatment of primary breast cancer reported no consensus in respect of primary surgery, pattern of referral for postoperative radiotherapy or the use of adjuvant systemic treatment. This lack of consensus could, however, have derived from differences in disease presentation, as seen by different surgeons.

Our report concerns closely contemporaneous surveys, using one questionnaire, of clinical opinion in Scotland (November 1984, March 1985) and in Australia (December 1984) on how to treat two particular paper-patients (a standardisation device), Mrs. Martin and Mrs. O'Neill. The two patient profiles, selected from a set of eight which we have piloted, were chosen to explore treatment decisions in early breast cancer against the backdrop of (a) past consensus conferences (Stewart 1977; Moxley et al. 1980) on combinations of surgery and radiotherapy, the subject also of meta-analyses in preparation, (b) increased interest in and evaluation of breast conservation (Peckham et al. 1984; Taylor et al. 1984; Fisher et al. 1985) - the trial everybody needs and nobody wants, and (c) forthcoming formal overviews of randomised controlled trials of adjuvant chemotherapy and tamoxifen (Anon 1984; Blamey 1985; Peto 1985). The two (hypothetical) patients were of roughly the same age (early fifties) with tumours 4 cm in size but different prognoses.

The questionnaire (see Appendix A) probes the two main areas of judgement that could lead to a lack of consensus about appropriate treatment - *beliefs* and *values*, which together determine decision *structure*. As well as being asked about their treatment of choice for the described patient, doctors were asked to rank given treatment options and to comment on how acceptable the options seemed to the respondent for the particular patient (decision structure: the range of possible, noncontraindicated, options may vary from doctor to doctor). Respondents were then asked whether, and if so how, they distinguished their own and the given

Recent Results in Cancer Research, Vol. 111
© Springer-Verlag Berlin · Heidelberg 1988

treatment options in respect of survival, local disease control and morbidity (both acute and long-term). Ranking the given treatment options compares doctors' beliefs - judgements about likely prognosis following particular therapies, while the rank assigned to their own treatment indirectly assesses differences in doctors' values; for example, interest in avoiding side effects or trade-offs between quality and length of life.

Materials and Methods

Content, wording and layout of the questionnaire - including definition of the type of mastectomy, precoding of treatment components and of morbidity, the use of qualifiers to indicate sequencing of primary treatment (for example, the use of adjuvant therapy contingent upon nodal involvement, N+) - had been successively refined in three pilot studies.

In Scotland, a postal census of surgical opinion was scheduled for 5 November 1984. The census documents, which referred to one or the other of two patients, were sent by first-class mail on Thursday 1 November 1984, to all surgeons in Scotland who treat primary breast cancer and who were listed with the Scottish Cancer Trials Office. The address list of 151 surgeons was alphabetic; alternate surgeons received the questionnaire for Mrs. Martin (see Appendix A).

In Australia, 120 members of the breast group in the Clinical Oncological Society of Australia (COSA) and all radiotherapists (17) and medical oncologists (9) in Sydney who were not members of the breast group were sent the survey documents on 12 December 1984. On 15 January 1985, when only 30 replies had been received, there was a second posting to request the return of completed or partially completed questionnaires as soon as possible.

Later, in March 1985, to allow comparison with Australian counterparts, the questionnaire for Mrs. Martin only (anticipating 35% effective response rate) was mailed to 27 radiotherapists listed with the Scottish Cancer Trials Office.

Results

Response Rate

In Scotland, the response rate was 37%; 59 completed or partially completed questionnaires were returned (28 for Mrs. Martin, 31 for Mrs. O'Neill); three surgeons noted that they did not treat breast cancer and three others wrote to us about difficulties in the questionnaire, which they had therefore not completed, and one radiotherapist declined to complete the questionnaire because his treatment recommendation would be made after discussion with the patient and her spouse, not on purely clinical data and a paper profile.

In Australia, the response rate was 41%; 56 completed or partially completed questionnaires were returned (34 for Mrs. Martin, 22 for Mrs. O'Neill) and one was returned blank by a surgical pathologist to whom it had been sent inappropriately. Three correspondents commented upon the questionnaire: "Somewhat frustrated by its tortuosity and also because I find a paper profile a poor substitute for the real patient", or "I spent nearly an hour trying to fill in that (questionnaire)", or "I must say it took me approximately two hours to do. Towards the end of the profile ... I found my enthusiasm and fine sense of intellectual nicety rather dulled ... Nevertheless I thank you for your invitation to be a part of an interesting project and look forward to reading the results."

Only one respondent was female.

Mrs. Martin

Case Summary

Mrs. Martin is probably the standard patient with breast cancer - a middle-aged woman with the goals of family life largely achieved. The features which could lead to a separation of treatment plans are her menopausal status (adjuvant chemotherapy?), a large tumour which is probably node positive on histology (breast conservation?) and her negative receptor status (adjuvant endocrine therapy?). Mrs. Martin prefers to leave it all to the doctor. How well will she cope with treatment morbidity?

Recommended Treatment Plan

Sixty-two respondents nominated 36 treatment plans. Table 1 summarises the distribution of different components of the treatments selected for Mrs. Martin, while Table 2 describes broad treatment structure.

There is a strong Australian preference for Patey mastectomy, with which radiotherapists associate radiotherapy, oncologists associate chemo- or endocrine therapy and surgeons offer alone or in combination. Scottish surgeons chose chemotherapy significantly less often than their Australian counterparts ($\chi^2_{(1)}=8.0$, $P\sim0.01$). Simple mastectomy, axillary node sampling and radiotherapy was a feature of seven of 19 treatment plans by Scottish surgeons, and tied with wide local excision, axillary node sampling and radiotherapy plus boost to primary as the modal choice by Scottish radiotherapists. Neither chemo- nor endocrine therapy was advised by Scottish radiotherapists.

Tamoxifen was a component of 12 plans overall (19%), in spite of the patient being receptor negative.

Overall Rank

Australian doctors differentiated clearly ($P\sim0.001$) amongst the given treatment options for Mrs. Martin (see Table 3). Patey mastectomy, which scored best, was graded as an acceptable alternative to their own treatment plan by as many respondents (47%) as found the last option - simple mastectomy, axillary node sampling and six cycles CMF if positive node histology - contraindicated for Mrs. Martin.

Table 1a. Recommended treatment plan for Mrs. Martin

Treatment code	Number of respondents						
	Scotland			Australia			
	S	R	total	S	R	O[a]	total
Surgery to breast							
B2 Patey mastectomy	4	1	5	12	5	4	25
B3 simple mastectomy	10	3	13	·	2	·	3
B4 quadrantectomy	1	1	2	1	·	·	1
B5 wide local excision	4	4	8	1	2	1	4
B9 other	·	·	·	1	·	·	1
	19	9	28	15	9	5	34
Surgery to axilla							
A0 none	·	·	·	·	·	·	1
A1 full dissection: same incision	7	1	8	13	5	4	26
A2 sampling of nodes	11	8	19	2	4	·	6
A3 full dissection: separate incision	1	·	1	·	·	1	1
	19	9	28	15	9	5	34
Radiotherapy							
X0 none	4	·	4	9	·	4	14
X1 chest-wall + axilla + fossa	11N+	5	16N+	1N+	6N+N+	·	9N+N+N
X2 as above plus boost to primary	4N+	4	8N+	1	1	·	3
X3 primary site only	·	·	·	·	·	1	1
9 other	·	·	·	4	2	·	7
	19	9	28	15	9	5	34
Chemotherapy							
C0 none	18	9	27	8	8	1	21
C1 six cycles CMF	1	·	1	6N+ N+	·	3N+N+	9N+N+N N+
C9 other	·	·	·	1	1	1	4
	19	9	28	15	9	5	34
Endocrine therapy							
E0 none	12	9	21	13	7	3	28
E1 tamoxifen	7	·	7	2	1	1	4
E2 ovarian ablation	·	·	·	·	1	·	1
E9 other	·	·	·	·	·	1N+	1N+
	19	9	28	15	9	5	34

S, surgeons; *R*, radiotherapists; *O*, oncologists.
[a] Australian total includes five respondents who did not record speciality.

Table 1b. Recommended treatment plan for Mrs. O'Neill

Treatment code	Number of respondents				
	Scotland	Australia			
	surgeons	S	R	O[a]	total
Surgery to breast					
B2 Patey mastectomy	6	7	2	4	15
B3 simple mastectomy	16	2	1	·	3
B4 quadrantectomy	1	·	·	·	·
B5 wide local excision	7	1	1	1	3
B9 other	1R+	1	·	·	1
	31	11	4	5	22
Surgery to axilla					
A0 none	5	·	·	·	1
A1 full dissection: same incision	7	7	2	3	13
A2 sampling of nodes	18	3	1	1	5
A3 full dissection: separate incision	1R+	1	1	·	2
A9 other	·	·	·	1	1
	31	11	4	5	22
Radiotherapy					
X0 none	13	8	1	3	12
X1 chest-wall + axilla + fossa	9N+N+N+N+ N+N+	·	2	1N+	3N+
X2 as above plus boost to primary	5N+N+	1	·	·	1
X3 primary site only	2	·	·	1	1
X9 other	2	2	1	·	5
	31	11	4	5	22
Chemotherapy					
C0 none	27	7	3	2	14
C1 six cycles CMF	2N+N+	3N+ N+	1	2N+	6N+N+N+
C9 other	2	1	·	1	2
	31	11	4	5	22
Endocrine therapy					
E0 none	15	9	2	4	17
E1 tamoxifen	13N+N+	2N+	1	1	4N+
E2 ovarian ablation	1	·	1	·	1
E9 other	2	·	·	·	·
	31	11	4	5	22

S, surgeons; *R*, radiotherapists; *O*, oncologists.
[a] Australian total includes two respondents who did not record speciality.

Table 2. Recommended treatment plans: broad structure

Surgery to breast	Scotland				Australia			
	Radiotherapy	Adjuvant systemic therapy			Radiotherapy	Adjuvant systemic therapy		
		Chemo-	Endocrine	Neither		Chemo-	Endocrine	Neither
Mrs. Martin								
(Adjuvant systemic totals)		1	7	20		11	5	16
Patey mastectomy	2 no	1	1	·	13 no	7	2	4
	3 yes	·	1	2	12 yes	2	1	9
Simple mastectomy	2 no	·	1	1	0 no	·	·	·
	11 yes	·	1	10	3 yes	·	·	3
Conservation	0 no	·	·	·	0 no	·	·	·
	10 yes	·	3	7	4 yes	2	2	·
Mrs. O'Neill								
(Adjuvant systemic totals)		2	14	13		7[a]	3	11
Patey mastectomy	6 no	1	3	2	9 no	4	·	5
	0 yes	·	·	·	6 yes	2[b]	1	3
Simple mastectomy	5 no	·	2	3	2 no	·	1	1
	10 yes	1	4	5	1 yes	·	·	1
Conservation	1 no	·	1	·	0 no	·	·	·
	7 yes	·	4	3	3 yes	1	1	1

[a] Two Australian plans for Mrs. Martin were not classifiable; likewise one Australian and two Scottish plans for Mrs. O'Neill.
[b] Two plans included endocrine as well as chemotherapy.

In contrast, the given options did not differ significantly in overall rank according to Scottish doctors, whose more tentative ordering of options favoured Patey mastectomy somewhat less than did Australian opinion.

Within speciality, the five Australian medical oncologists notably ranked last the option which entailed radiotherapy, whilst radiotherapists (Australian and Scottish) were firm, more so than surgeons, in contraindicating the option which included CMF if node histology was positive.

Survival

Thirteen (including four of the five medical oncologists) of 34 Australian doctors distinguished treatments for Mrs. Martin in terms of survival, as did six of 25 Scottish doctors: in all, 32% of respondents. Eighteen of the 19 doctors who ranked treatments for survival ranked their own treatment as best or equal best, but the average assigned rank did not differ significantly for the three given treatment options, being 1.7, 2.2 and 2.1 for options a, b and c respectively ($\chi^2_{(2)}=2.53$, $P=0.30$).

Table 3. Treatment options for Mrs. Martin and Mrs. O'Neill: overall rank and acceptability

Treatment option	Scotland									Australia											
Mrs. Martin	Surgeons			Radio-therapists			Total			Surgeons			Radio-therapists			Oncologists			Total		
Differentiating	(17)			(7)			(24)			(15)			(9)			(5)			(34)		
Missing data	(2)			(2)			(4)			(0)			(0)			(0)			(0)		
	Av. rank	A	C	Av. rank	A	C	Av. rank	A	C	Av. rank	A	C	Av. rank	A	C	Av. rank	A	C	Av. rank	A	C
a Patey mastectomy (B2,A1)	1.7	7	2	2.0	4	0	1.8	11	2	1.4	8	1	1.8	2	1	1.2	4	0	1.5	16	3
b Simple mastectomy radiotherapy (B3,A0,X1)	2.0	7	0	1.4	5	0	1.8	12	0	2.2	6	1	1.4	4	1	2.8	1	1	2.0	13	3
c Simple mastectomy, axillary node sampling plus 6 cycles CMF if node-positive ($B3,A2,C1^{N+}$)	2.3	7	4	2.6	1	3	2.4	8	7	2.4	4	5	2.7	0	7	2.0	3	2	2.5	7	16
Comparison of ranks $\chi^2_{(2)}$ (P-value)	2.68 (0.30)			5.79 (0.08)			5.08 (0.10)			8.23 (0.02)			7.72 (0.03)			6.40 (0.04)			14.60 (0.001)		

Table 3 *(continued)*

Treatment option	Scotland			Australia											
Mrs. O'Neill	Surgeons			Surgeons			Radio-therapists			Oncologists			Total		
Differentiating	(28)			(11)			(4)			(5)			(22)		
Missing data	(3)			(0)			(0)			(0)			(0)		
	Av. rank	A	C	Av. rank	A	C	Av. rank	A	C	Av. rank	A	C	Av. rank	A	C
a Patey mastectomy + 6 cycles CMF (B2,A1,C1)	3.2	7	9	1.8	8	0	4.3	1	1	2.3	2	1	2.5	11	3
b Patey mastectomy, post-op. radiotherapy + 6 cycles CMF (B2,A1,X1,C1)	3.6	6	12	2.9	4	3	3.1	3	1	2.7	2	2	2.8	9	7
c Simple mastectomy + post-op. radiotherapy (B3,A0,X1)	1.9	15	1	3.4	3	2	2.8	3	0	3.8	0	2	3.2	7	4
d Patey mastectomy, post-op. radiotherapy + bilateral oophorectomy (B2,A1,X1,E2)	2.9	14	6	3.4	3	5	2.8	3	1	3.6	2	2	3.2	8	9
e Local excision and axillary node sampling, radiotherapy + 6 cycles CMF (B5,A2,X2,C1)	3.4	10	6	3.5	3	3	2.9	2	2	2.6	1	1	3.3	6	8
Comparison of ranks $\chi^2_{(4)}$ (*P*-value)	19.7 (0.005)			9.3 (0.06)			3.8 (0.55)			3.5 (0.51)			3.5 (0.51)		

A, the number of respondents who graded treatment option as acceptable alternative to their own treatment plan for the patient; *C*, the number of respondents who graded the treatment option as contraindicated for this patient.

Significantly, fourteen of the 19 respondents who distinguished treatments for Mrs. Martin in terms of survival included some form of adjuvant therapy in the recommended treatment plan, compared with only 12 of the 42 doctors who claimed no survival differential ($\chi^2_{(1)} = 10.89$, $P \sim 0.001$).

Local Control

Eighty percent of the respondents were of the opinion that treatments could be distinguished in terms of local disease control.

Twenty-eight of 34 Australian doctors differentiated treatments for Mrs. Martin in respect of local disease control, all but two of whom ranked their own treatment as best or equal best for local control. They also distinguished clearly ($P \sim 0.001$) amongst the given treatment options: simple mastectomy, axillary node sampling and CMF if node positive on histology - option c - offered the poorest prospect for local control. The distinction, in terms of rank and acceptability for local control, between Patey mastectomy and simple mastectomy plus radiotherapy was not pronounced (see Table 4).

The ranking by 11 Scottish surgeons coincided with Australian opinion, but it was less definite and did not achieve statistical significance. Six of eight Scottish radiotherapists differentiated treatments in respect of local control, with five of them assigning ranks which favoured simple mastectomy plus radiotherapy ($P \sim 0.04$). Of the 16 Scottish respondents who assigned ranks in respect of local control, 14 ranked their own treatment plan as best or equal best.

Acute Morbidity

Twenty-eight Australian doctors convincingly ranked ($P \sim 0.001$) the three given treatment options for Mrs. Martin in respect of acute morbidity (see Table 4), the same ranking being offered by 21 Scottish doctors. The acute morbidity associated with Patey mastectomy was felt to be less than that from simple mastectomy and radiotherapy - for example, 15 of 21 Scottish respondents took this view, four were neutral and only two disputed it. The worst option in terms of acute morbidity was certainly the one which included CMF. In respect of acute morbidity, their own treatment plan was ranked best or equal best by only 42% of respondents: by nine of 16 Scottish surgeons, by two of five Scottish radiotherapists, by six of 11 Australian surgeons, by one of eight Australian radiotherapists and by one of the five oncologists. The major side effects associated with each option are recognised: breast disfigurement and body image compromised by mastectomy, and arm lymphoedema in association with Patey mastectomy or radiotherapy, for which skin reactions, nausea and anxiety are also cited; nausea, hair loss and bone marrow suppresion are the dominant concerns in relation to CMF.

Table 4. Treatment options for Mrs. Martin: local control, acute and long-term morbidity average rank

Treatment option	a	b	c	Comparison of ranks $\chi^2_{(2)}$ (P-value)	No. ranking	% own plan best/equal	No. with missing data
	Average rank						
Local control							
Scotland	2.2	1.4	2.4	9.1 (0.02)	16	94	7
Australia	1.8	1.5	2.7	23.0 (0.001)	26	88	2
Acute morbidity							
Scotland	1.2	1.8	2.9	5.1 (0.001)	21	52	5
Australia	1.1	2.0	2.8	39.5 (0.001)	28	36	5
Long-term morbidity							
Scotland	1.4	2.1	2.4	9.3 (0.01)	18	67	5
Australia	1.3	2.3	2.4	15.8 (0.001)	20	60	4

Treatment options for Mrs. O'Neill: local control, acute and long-term morbidity average rank

Treatment option	a	b	c	d	e	Comparison of ranks $\chi^2_{(4)}$ (P-value)	No. ranking	% own plan best/equal	No. with missing data
	Average rank								
Local control									
Scotland	3.1	2.6	2.4	2.8	4.0	7.9 (0.10)	13	77	4
Australia	3.4	2.4	3.1	2.1	4.1	16.8 (0.005)	17	35	1
Acute morbidity									
Scotland	2.6	4.0	1.6	3.3	3.4	29.4 (0.001)	22	91	7
Australia	2.6	3.9	1.3	3.3	3.8	33.1 (0.001)	18	61	3
Long-term morbidity									
Scotland	2.6	3.2	2.1	3.5	3.1	8.1 (0.08)	17	94	8
Australia	2.5	4.2	2.1	3.3	3.0	12.4 (0.02)	11	36	9

Long-term Morbidity

Ten Australian doctors (five of them surgeons) claimed no differentiation of treatments in respect of long-term morbidity, whereas 20 respondents ranked the given treatment options (see Table 4) and associated significantly less long-term morbidity with Patey mastectomy - a view which was also held by Scottish respondents. The ranking for options b and c, which include radiotherapy and six cycles of CMF respectively, is similar. If equal ranks are imputed for the ten Australian and five Scottish doctors who assessed long-term morbidity equally for the three given treatment options, then options a, b and c still rank significantly differently (Australian ranks: $\chi^2_{(2)}=10.52$, $P \sim 0.01$; Scottish ranks: $\chi^2_{(2)}=7.30$, $P \sim 0.05$).

Treatment Aspects: Summary

The overall ranking of the three given treatment options is consistent with the views expressed on four separate aspects of treatment. Acceptable local control and least acute as well as long-term morbidity are associated with Patey mastectomy, whereas option c, which includes six cycles of CMF, is marked down on these aspects. There is, however, a strong association between belief in differential survival and inclusion of chemo- or endocrine therapy in one's own treatment plan.

Since the acute morbidity associated with either radiotherapy or six cycles of CMF in association with simple mastectomy is believed to be more grave than for Patey mastectomy, the traditional Scottish treatment plan of simple mastectomy, axillary node sampling and radiotherapy may derive from a belief in better local control (offsetting morbidity). Either option b reflects poorly the traditional Scottish plan because it omits axillary node sampling, or the Scottish tradition is an inconsistent choice of therapy for the average expressed belief; alternatively, value judgements make the perceived acute morbidity acceptable.

In terms of one's own treatment plan, the Australian tendency to invoke chemotherapy underplays the associated morbidity but is associated with a belief in improved survival.

Mrs. O'Neill

Case Summary

Mrs. O'Neill, who is premenopausal and has a moderately well differentiated, receptor-positive adenocarcinoma, appears, at first, to be a much less difficult case than Mrs. Martin. It may be reasonable to assume that the patient's breast size would allow a good cosmetic result with a local excision, but such conservative management requires a degree of consent and participation in the decision that may not be forthcoming, and so a more orthodox simple or Patey mastectomy might be agreed upon. The evidence points towards negative-node histology and hence a good prognosis.

Recommended Treatment Plan

Fifty-three respondents nominated 42 treatment plans. Table 1 reveals a broadly similar pattern to that observed for Mrs. Martin: (a) a strong Australian preference for Patey mastectomy (entailing full dissection of the axilla) compared with a Scottish tendency towards simple mastectomy and sampling of axillary nodes and (b) preference for associated treatment being appropriate to the speciality of the respondent.

Tamoxifen was a component of 17 plans (33%) for Mrs. O'Neill. Whereas endocrine therapy was recommended significantly more often for Mrs. O'Neill than for Mrs. Martin ($\chi^2_{(1)}=4.78$, $P \sim 0.03$), radiotherapy was more often omitted from recommended treatments (see Table 2) for Mrs. O'Neill ($\chi^2_{(1)}=4.02$, $P \sim 0.05$).

Overall Rank

Fifty respondents ranked the options according to overall quality. The Scottish surgeons expressed a preference for plan c (simple mastectomy plus radiotherapy), while Australian surgeons consistently ranked plan a (Patey mastectomy plus six cycles of CMF) highly and graded it 'acceptable' in contrast to nine Scottish surgeons who found it 'contraindicated.' Australian radiotherapists, on the other hand, were averse to plan a, with the result that, taken overall, the Australian respondents showed no significant pattern in their rankings (see Table 3). As with Mrs. Martin, there was considerable evidence of strong disagreement; for example, option b for Mrs. O'Neill (Patey mastectomy, radiotherapy and six cycles of CMF) was found acceptable by 16 of 50 respondents, and contraindicated by 19 (38%).

Survival

Eleven of 22 Australian respondents (including four of the five medical oncologists) distinguished treatments in terms of survival. They assigned ranks which differed significantly from chance expectation ($\chi^2_{(4)}=20.1$, $P \sim 0.001$), tending to believe that options a and b for Mrs. O'Neill, both of which include six cycles of CMF, lead to better survival (average ranks 1.7 and 2.0 respectively).

In contrast, only six of 29 Scottish surgeons believed the treatment options could be distinguished in terms of survival, and no consistent ranking of options emerged as a consequence.

Only ten of the 17 respondents who assigned survival ranks ranked their own treatment plan as giving the best or equal best survival prospect - in contradistinction to the poor-prognosis case, Mrs. Martin.

Local Control

Fifteen Scottish surgeons of 29 respondents distinguished between the treatments with regard to local control but with little evidence of consistent preference (see Table 4). However, 17 of 21 Australian respondents differentiated in this respect, with a strong preference for options b and d. Plan e (local excision, axillary node sampling, radiotherapy and six cycles of CMF) was ranked low by both groups, but there was still considerable disagreement, 12 doctors finding it an acceptable treatment in respect of local control, ten finding it contraindicated.

Nine of 13 Scottish respondents who ranked treatments considered their own plan best or equal best for local control compared with seven of 17 Australians - the Australian seven included all four radiotherapists.

Acute Morbidity

There was a strong similarity between the 22 Scottish and 18 Australian respondents who considered that treatments differed with respect to acute morbidity; plan c, the only one without adjuvant chemo- or endocrine therapy, consistently ranked high (see Table 4). However, the Australian respondents were less liable to consider a treatment contraindicated due to acute morbidity. Respondents were generally agreed as to the important side effects (see Mrs. Martin). Twenty of 22 Scottish respondents and 12 of 18 Australians ranked their treatment plan as best or equal best with regard to acute morbidity.

Long-term Morbidity

As with acute morbidity, there was a similar pattern for Scottish and Australian physicians, with plan c (simple mastectomy plus radiotherapy) again ranking high. "Carcinogenic risk" was mentioned as a major cause of concern by only two of 21 Scottish respondents, compared with eight of 12 Australians, of whom, however, only two were surgeons. Their own treatment plan was ranked best or equal best by 16 of 17 Scottish respondents but by only five of 11 Australians ($P \sim 0.02$).

Treatment Aspects: Summary

The chosen treatment plans for Mrs. O'Neill, the better-prognosis patient, reflect a strong desire to minimise morbidity, and although there is a consensus that this could be achieved by simple mastectomy and radiotherapy (option c), there is a strong Australian view that more radical surgery but minimal additional therapy can also achieve this, and that local recurrences can be dealt with if and when they arise. Although the doctors in general did not choose treatments intended to maximise local control, it appears that for this patient, disagreement about this aspect of treatment may provide some of the basis for choice between treatments which are similar in more important considerations - for this patient - of morbidity.

Discussion

A treatment census in Scotland - possible because the Scottish Cancer Trials Office maintains a current list of surgeons and radiotherapists who treat primary breast cancer - was not, in fact, realised because of nonresponse; in Australia - the obvious choice for international comparison because of the residence there of one of us - a census was not attempted, questionnaires being posted instead to COSA members who had a major interest in breast cancer and to radiotherapists or medical oncologists in Sydney who were not members of the COSA breast group.

The health services in the two countries are different: the National Health Service in Scotland provides the vast majority of medical expertise in public hospitals, whereas in Australia, although the majority of surgeons are in private practice, radiation therapy and chemotherapy are mostly provided by full-time specialists in public hospitals who have limited rights of private practice. There is a greater tendency in Australia for patients not to be referred prior to primary surgery for consultation with a radiotherapist or medical oncologist.

The vagaries of the British and Australian postal systems conspired to make the initial posting in the two countries different by 1 month, during which was published a preliminary review (Anon 1984a) of mortality results in randomised trials testing either (a) tamoxifen or (b) long-term cytotoxic chemotherapy in early breast cancer. The vagary of the authors was responsible for delayed circulation to the 27 Scottish radiotherapists. This was turned to advantage, however; only Mrs. Martin's profile was sent, for whom the replies by Australian radiotherapists were more numerous. Return of 35% of questionnaires completed or partially completed in so detailed a postal inquiry compares not unfavourably with upward of 66% effective response rates for much simpler questionnaires (Gazet et al. 1985; Baber et al. 1984). Responders were not confined to those currently collaborating in controlled trials of how to manage primary breast cancer, as can happen if surveys are associated with scientific meetings or established trials (Baum and Houghton 1980) - 54 of the 115 respondents were trialists. The unexpressed opinions of nonresponders may, of course, differ importantly from the views of doctors who took the time and trouble to answer, and can only add further to the diversity of recommended treatment.

Prespecified treatment options were not designed formally to study the main effects and interaction of treatment components, as would be the case in conjoint analysis (Richardson et al. 1984), but anticipated likely treatments. The multiplicity of recommended treatment plans (36 for Mrs. Martin, 42 for Mrs. O'Neill) shows how difficult this was, with considerable heterogeneity in even gross treatment structure (see Table 2). Yet some success can be claimed, because the specified options with worst overall assigned rank were still described as an acceptable alternative to their own plan by a quarter of the respondents. This diversity of recommended treatment plan for a particular patient, even in terms of gross treatment structure, highlights the problem of choosing the best primary strategy and could mean that there is no perceived best choice. Yet respondents (grouped by country or speciality) showed significant discrimination in their ranking of the prespecified treatment options, overall and for particular treatment aspects. Such beliefs are testable - by formal (Collins et al. 1985; Gore and Oldham 1986) statistical review of published and unpublished treatment comparisons so as to pool information without bias across methodologically sound studies, or, in principle, by the design of appropriate randomised trials. Note that value judgements by patients or doctors may limit or preclude randomisation, as shown by reported difficulties of accrual to randomised breast conservation trials (Peckham et al. 1984; Taylor et al. 1984; Stewart and Robinson 1984; Angell 1984; Ellenberg 1984).

There is still a considerable preference in the Scottish experience for radiotherapy when local control is at issue. The choice of surgery is predominantly between simple mastectomy and some form of breast conservation - even for Mrs. Martin, who had poor-prognosis disease, a third of the Scottish respondents opted for some kind of breast conservation.

Patey mastectomy, radiotherapy and chemotherapy were more commonly features of Australian than Scottish treatment plans. Doctors who distinguished treatments in terms of survival were significantly more likely to have included chemo- or endocrine therapy in their own treatment plan than doctors who did not differentiate treatments in respect of survival. Acute morbidity may be more acceptable (value judgement) if the doctor believes that the treatment with which it is associated increases survival.

For acute morbidity, only 42% of doctors who differentiated treatments on this aspect ranked their own treatment plan for Mrs. Martin as best or equal best, whereas for the good-prognosis patient, Mrs. O'Neill, 80% of doctors ranked their own treatment plan best or equal best in respect of acute morbidity. Thus, acute morbidity, in association with radiotherapy or chemotherapy, for example, may be more accepted in poor-prognosis patients (value judgement).

Major side effects of treatment, both acute and long-term, were clearly recognised, including a long-term carcinogenic risk associated with chemotherapy. Breast disfigurement and body image were more frequently cited than the favourable ranking of associated treatments, especially Patey mastectomy, might have led one to expect (value judgement).

There was still strong support for treatment options which appeared to us to have little support in the literature. For example, Patey mastectomy with postoperative radiotherapy was commonly recommended in Australia, in spite of considerable data from clinical trials showing that the combination is not superior in terms of survival or disease control at death but *is* associated with increased morbidity (Easson 1968; Lipsett 1981).

Similarly, the preference for adjuvant endocrine therapy in a receptor-negative patient (19% of recommended plans for Mrs. Martin) is surprising in view of considerable data suggesting that it will not be of benefit. Its use in receptor-negative patients is supported by preliminary data from only one trial (Baum et al. 1983) and may represent greater willingness to integrate "positive" rather than "negative" outcomes into treatment strategies compared, for example, with discontinuation of routine postoperative radiotherapy.

Have breast cancer clinical trials, designed and reported as heretofore, affected treatment decisions? If so, it is difficult to see how different geographical and speciality-dependent strategies can be reconciled with the enormous literature in a common language on breast cancer management. Alternatively, reference to that literature is made only selectively, allowing opinion and editorial licence (Correspondence [Breast Cancer] 1985; Hughes and Courtney 1985) to dominate data.

The solution is threefold. Major questions in the treatment of breast cancer need to be addressed in the first instance by formal review of accumulated, relevant studies. Two such meta-analyses were reported in outline recently (Anon 1984a): overviews of short-term mortality by allocated treatment in almost all of the randomised trials of tamoxifen (43 trials) and of prolonged cytotoxic therapy (37 trials) in early breast cancer – for each adjuvant systemic therapy, there is highly significant evidence of a delay of death, the net effect of cytotoxic therapy on early mortality among women diagnosed under the age of 50 appearing to be almost twice as great as in the older groups (Peto 1985). Secondly, unresolved issues, highlighted in surveys such as ours, should be tackled prospectively, so that beliefs are put to the test once and for all. Finally, values, on the other hand, are neither right nor wrong and differ legitimately between individuals. When value judgements determine treatment, it is important that doctor and patient are in accord for there to be truly informed consent to the recommended plan (Anon 1984b).

Response rate, responder bias, restriction to two paper-patients and to two countries, different survey times (before and after a *Lancet* publication reviewing mortality results in randomised trials in early breast cancer; Anon 1984a) and our choice of (prespecified) treatment options impose different limitations on the inferences to be drawn from this survey of treatment decisions in breast cancer. It seems clear that the survey has significant implications, however:

1. Practical application of the literature on breast cancer has not lead to uniformity of treatment recommendations.
2. International, speciality, prognosis-dependent differences in belief exist and are testable against soundly accumulated data: for example, chemotherapy and increased survival; radiotherapy in association with mastectomy in poor-prognosis patients.
3. Values differ legitimately between individuals; they influence recommended treatment and so may need to be made explicit between doctor and patient.

References

Angell M (1984) Patients' preferences in randomized clinical trials. N Engl J Med 310: 1385–1387

Anon (1984a) Review of mortality results in randomized trials in early breast cancer. Lancet ii: 1205

Anon (1984b) Consent: how informed? Lancet i: 1445–1447

Baber NS, Julian DG, Lewis JA, Rose G (1984) β-blockers after myocardial infarction: have trials changed practice? Br Med J 289: 1431–1432

Baum M, Houghton J (1980) Current and future management of "early" breast cancer: attitude survey amongst participants in Cancer Research Campaign trial. Lancet i: 929

Baum M, Brinkley DM, Dossett JA et al. (1983) Improved survival amongst patients treated with adjuvant tamoxifen after mastectomy for early breast cancer. Lancet ii: 450

Blamey RW (1985) Cytotoxic chemotherapy in breast cancer. Lancet i: 459

Collins R, Jusuf S, Peto R (1985) Overview of randomized trials of diuretics in pregnancy. Br Med J 290: 17-23

Correspondence (Breast Cancer) (1985) Br Med J 290: 855-856

Easson EC (1968) Post-operative radiotherapy in breast cancer. In: Forrest APM, Kunkler P (eds) Prognostic factors in breast cancer. Livingstone, Edinburgh, pp 118-127

Ellenberg SS (1984) Randomization designs in comparative clinical trials. N Engl J Med 310: 1404-1408

Fisher B, Bauer B, Margolese R et al. (1985) Five-year results of a randomized trial comparing total mastectomy and segmental mastectomy with or without radiation in the treatment of breast cancer. N Engl J Med 312: 665-673

Forrest APM, Burn JI, Hayward JL et al. (1969) Breast cancer symposium. Points in the practical management of breast cancer. Br J Surg 63: 569-575

Gazet JC, Rainsbury RM, Ford HT, Powles TJ, Coombes RC (1985) Survey of treatment of primary breast cancer in Great Britain. Br Med J 290: 1793-1795

Gore SM, Oldham JA (1986) Randomized trials of high- versus low-dose steroids in renal transplantation: does the evidence favour a consensus? Transplantation 41: 319-327

Hughes LE, Courtney SP (1985) Follow-up of patients with breast cancer. Br Med J 290: 1229-1230

Lipsett MB (1981) Post-operative radiation for women with cancer of the breast and positive axillary lymph nodes. Should it continue? N Engl J Med 304: 112-114

Moxley JH, Allegra JG, Henney J et al. (1980) Treatment of primary breast cancer. Summary of National Institutes of Health consensus development conference. JAMA 244: 797-800

Nemoto T (1973) Treatment of early breast cancer. NY State J Med 73: 1901-1904

Peckham MJ, Tobias JS, Houghton J et al. (1984) Recruitment to breast cancer trials. Lancet ii: 1460-1461

Peto R (1985) Cytotoxic chemotherapy in breast cancer. Lancet i: 459

Richardson DK, Gabbe SG, Wind Y (1984) Decision analysis of high-risk patient referral. Obstet Gynecol 63: 496-501

Stewart HJ (1977) Controlled trials in the treatment of "early" breast cancer: a review of published results. World J Surg 1: 309-313

Stewart HJ, Robinson SM (1984) Recruitment to breast cancer trials. Lancet ii: 1096-1097

Taylor KM, Margolese RG, Soskiline CL (1984) Physicians' reasons for not entering eligible patients in a randomized clinical trial of surgery for breast cancer. N Engl J Med 310: 1363-1367

Appendix A

Please read the profile of Mrs. Martin and then complete the attached questionnaire.

Profile of Mrs. Martin:

Aged 53, married with three children aged 29, 20, 18
Menopause at age 50
Housewife
Comfortably well off, married to a bank manager
Interested in the church, local community affairs
Has a normal harmonious relationship with husband and family
Is ignorant of basic aspects of health and disease and prefers to 'leave it all to the doctor'
Family history is negative and past medical history is not significant.

Clinical data:

Weight 10 st/71 bs, height 5 ft, 4 in.
Breasts large; 4-cm carcinoma upper outer quadrant R breast with partial fixation of overlying skin but none to deeper structures; 5 cm from areolar margin; nipple normal; two rounded, mobile, clinically significant nodes R axilla
Mammogram confirms clinical diagnosis of carcinoma and presence of axillary lymphadenopathy.
T2a N1b M0
Moderately well differentiated adenocarcinoma
Grade II
ER -ve PR -ve

Questionnaire

1. With reference to the primary treatment codes (see Appendix B), please describe the treatment plan that you would recommend for Mrs. Martin.

Recommended treatment plan	*Code*	*Further specification for code 9*
Surgery to the breast	B ☐	....
Surgery to the axilla	A ☐	....
Radiotherapy	X ☐	....
Chemotherapy	C ☐	....
Endocrine therapy	E ☐	....

2. Please comment on what considerations determined your primary treatment plan for Mrs. Martin.
3. In Table 1 please rank the primary treatment options for Mrs. Martin (rank 1 indicates highest order of preference, rank 2 being assigned to the treatment option which you rank next and so on; use = to designate equal ranks, for example 1=, 1=, 3 etc.)

Table 1

Treatment option	Rank	Grade
Your treatment plan	[1]	[–]
Patey mastectomy (B2,A1)	☐	☐
Simple mastectomy (B3,A0) and radiotherapy (X1)	☐	☐
Simple mastectomy and axillary node sampling (B3,A2) plus six cycles of CMF chemotherapy if node-positive ($C1^{N+}$)	☐	☐

4. In Table 1 please give your overall assessment of each treatment option by grading it as
   A (treatment you consider as **A**cceptable **A**lternative to the plan you recommend for Mrs. Martin)
   I (treatment you consider **I**nferior for this patient)
   C (treatment you consider **C**ontraindicated for Mrs. Martin)

5. Please comment on what considerations determined your ranking of the above treatment options and their grades.

Please answer questions 6–12 assuming that nodal pathology for Mrs. Martin is 2/20 nodes involved.

6. Do you think that the following four treatments
   1 Your treatment plan
   2 Patey mastectomy (B2,A1)
   3 Simple mastectomy and radiotherapy (B3,A0,X1)
   4 Simple mastectomy and axillary node sampling plus six cycles of CMF chemotherapy if node-positive (B3,A2,C1^{N+})

   are distinguishable in terms of survival for Mrs. Martin? N = no ☐ Y = yes

   If yes: in Table 2 please rank the treatments according to your beliefs about survival (rank 1 indicates highest believed survival; use = to designate equal ranks, for example 1 =, 1 =, 3, etc.). Please also grade treatments relative to the treatment you ranked first for survival (grade A = Acceptable Alternative, I = Inferior, C = Contraindicated for Mrs. Martin in respect of survival).

Table 2

Treatment	Survival		Control of local disease	
	Rank	Grade	Rank	Grade
1	☐	☐	☐	☐
2	☐	☐	☐	☐
3	☐	☐	☐	☐
4	☐	☐	☐	☐

7. Do you think that treatments 1–4 differ in terms of local disease control for Mrs. Martin? N = no ☐ Y = yes

   If yes: in Table 2 please rank the treatments according to your beliefs about local disease control (rank 1 indicates best local control; use = to designate equal ranks). Please also grade treatments relative to the treatment you ranked first for control of local disease (grade A = Acceptable Alternative, I = Inferior, C = Contraindicated for Mrs. Martin in respect of control of local disease).
8. For Mrs. Martin, do you think that treatments 1–4 differ in terms of acute morbidity? N = no ☐ Y = yes

   If yes: in Table 3 please rank the treatments according to your beliefs concerning acute morbidity, i.e. morbidity from start of treatment to 1 month after completion of primary treatment (rank 1 indicates the treatment you believe entails least acute morbidity for Mrs. Martin; use = to designate equal ranks). Please also grade treatments relative to the treatment which you believe entails least acute morbidity (grade A = Acceptable Alternative, I = Inferior, C = Contraindicated for Mrs. Martin in respect of acute morbidity).

Table 3

Treatment	Acute morbidity		Acute morbidity codes
	Rank	Grade	
1	☐	☐	☐☐ ☐☐ ☐☐ ☐☐
2	☐	☐	☐☐ ☐☐ ☐☐ ☐☐
3	☐	☐	☐☐ ☐☐ ☐☐ ☐☐
4	☐	☐	☐☐ ☐☐ ☐☐ ☐☐

9. In Table 3 please list for each treatment up to four acute side effects (see Appendix B) which were uppermost in your mind when you assessed the treatment for Mrs. Martin and gave its rank for acute morbidity.
10. For Mrs. Martin, do you think that treatments 1-4 differ in terms of long-term morbidity? N = no ☐
Y = yes

If yes: in Table 4 please rank the treatments according to your beliefs about long-term morbidity, i.e. morbidity from 1 month after completion of primary treatment (rank 1 indicates the treatment you believe entails least long-term morbidity for Mrs. Martin; use = to designate equal ranks). Please also grade treatments relative to the treatment which you believe entails least long-term morbidity (grade A = Acceptable Alternative, I = Inferior, C = Contraindicated for Mrs. Martin in respect of long-term morbidity).

Table 4

Treatment	Long-term morbidity		Long-term morbidity codes
	Rank	Grade	
1	☐	☐	☐☐ ☐☐ ☐☐ ☐☐
2	☐	☐	☐☐ ☐☐ ☐☐ ☐☐
3	☐	☐	☐☐ ☐☐ ☐☐ ☐☐
4	☐	☐	☐☐ ☐☐ ☐☐ ☐☐

11. In Table 4 please list for each treatment up to four long-term side effects (see Appendix B) which were uppermost in your mind when you assessed the treatment for Mrs. Martin and gave its rank for long-term morbidity.
12. Consider only those aspects which you identified above as differentiating between treatment options. Please rank in order of their importance to you for determining how Mrs. Martin should be treated (rank 1 indicates the most important of the four aspects).

Treatment aspect	Rank
Survival	☐
Control of local disease	☐
Acute morbidity	☐
Long-term morbidity	☐

Appendix B

Codes for acute treatment-related and long-term morbidity:

1. Operative mortality
2. Breast disfigurement
3. Body image and self-esteem
4. Arm movement restricted to less than 90°
5. Lymphoedema of the arm (more than 2 cm increased girth over untreated side)
6. Skin reaction which requires dressing by a nurse
7. Pneumonitis
8. Spontaneous fracture of ribs or clavicle
9. Carcinogenic risk
10. Premature menopause
11. Pain
12. Nausea and vomiting
13. Stomatitis
14. Hair loss necessitating the wearing of a wig
15. Bone marrow suppression leading to dose modification, inpatient treatment or the abandoning of treatment
16. Depressive illness
17. Anxiety
18. Insomnia
19. Loss of normal sex life
20. Inability to continue at work
99. Other (if code 99 is used, please specify other morbidity)

Definition of Mastectomies

Halsted radical mastectomy (B1,A1): implies removal of the whole breast, the sternal origin of pectoralis major muscle, pectoralis minor muscle and all of the nonessential contents of the axilla.

Patey mastectomy (B2,A1): implies removal of the whole breast but preservation of pectoralis major muscle. Pectoralis minor muscle may be removed or not removed, and all the nonessential contents of the axilla are removed.

Simple mastectomy: implies removal of the whole breast without any axillary dissection. The pectoral muscles are preserved.

Primary Treatment Codes

Please code surgery to the breast as:
B0. No surgical treatment
B1. Halsted radical mastectomy (B1,A1)
B2. Patey mastectomy (B2,A1)

Please code surgery to the axilla as:
A0. No surgical treatment
A1. Full dissection at time of treating breast
A2. Axillary node sampling at time of treating breast

B3. Simple mastectomy

B4. Quadrantectomy

B5. Wide local excision

B9. Other (if code 9 is used, please specify other surgery)

A3. Full dissection through separate incision

A9. Other (if code 9 is used, please specify other surgery)

Please code radiotherapy as:

X0. No radiotherapy

X1. Radiotherapy to chest wall, axilla and supraclavicular fossa

X2. Radiotherapy to chest-wall, axilla and supraclavicular fossa plus boost to primary site

X3. Radiotherapy to the primary site only

X9. Other (if code 9 is used, please specify other radiotherapy)

Please code chemotherapy as:

C0. No chemotherapy

C1. Chemotherapy of six cycles CMF (with or without prednisolone)

C2. Chemotherapy of six cycles AC

C9. Other chemotherapy (if code 9 is used, please specify other sequences of chemotherapy)

Please code endocrine therapy as:

E0. No endocrine therapy

E1. Tamoxifen

E2. Ovarian ablation

E9. Other adjuvant endocrine therapy (if code 9 is used, please specify other adjuvant endocrine therapy)

Please use qualifiers to indicate sequencing of primary treatment

N+ (node positive)

Thus $X1^{N+}$ means radiotherapy only if node positive

R+ (response positive)

Thus $B2^{R+}$,$A1^{R+}$ means Patey mastectomy only if patient responded to first line therapy

Similar definitions for

R− (response negative)

N− (node negative)

Two examples of coding:

Simple mastectomy plus axillary node sampling and radiotherapy to chest wall, axilla and supraclavicular fossa if node-positive (B3,A2,$X1^{N+}$)

Chemotherapy then radiotherapy then chemotherapy (X2,C9) where C9 = AC × 3 cycles then XRT then CMF × 6 cycles

Randomization and Follow-up Care of Patients in a Breast Cancer Clinical Trial: Personal Experience

V. Unbehaun

Städtisches Krankenhaus, Frauenklinik, Röntgenstraße 2, 7990 Friedrichshafen, FRG

I should like to report here on practical experience of my own resulting from daily clinical work and colored by local factors. I work in a medium-sized hospital on the southern border of the Federal Republic of Germany in a beautiful area which has a high density of physicians. We treat about 50 new cases of breast cancer in women a year. At present 45 patients are being treated or receiving care in the context of clinical studies. Our noncentral position makes it especially important for us to check our breast cancer therapy in order to carry out our work in accordance with modern standards and to assess it in comparison with the results of larger hospitals and centers. We can discipline our thinking and make a contribution to answering critical questions only on the basis of participation in clinical studies.

Clear, incontestable randomization is present when a patient consents to the randomization decision in full knowledge of the disease and the forms of treatment available and agrees to accept the decision. Women suffering from cancer must arrive at this decision in a state of the most profound inner agitation. Announcement of the diagnosis "breast cancer" negates at a stroke all prior conscious and unconscious notions about the further course of life. The patient is confronted directly and dramatically with the finiteness of life. She must arrive at a new orientation with regard to herself and the rest of her life. Various familiar reaction forms such as aggressive revolt against the diagnosis and against the people who had to communicate it, desperate searching for the causes, ideas of sin and punishment, a feeling of the absolute meaninglessness of all treatment measures, to mention only a few, are intensively experienced.

In this life-determining situation, the physicians who have the task of helping her evidently do not know themselves precisely what to do. On the contrary, they select the measures determining the patient's future existence on a random basis. This is how the question of randomization may appear in the eyes of the patient concerned.

How can the patient be helped in coming to terms psychologically with her fate, in the outlook on the new future, and in the measures to shape this future, one of which is therapy in accordance with the protocol of a clinical study? Patent recipes of general validity cannot be given here. Naturally, the informative and at the same time therapeutic discussion with the patient must be carried out on a basis appropriate to the individual patient.

Recent Results in Cancer Research, Vol. 111
© Springer-Verlag Berlin · Heidelberg 1988

The most crucial and important point can actually be stated in a single sentence: it is a matter of gaining the trust of the patient! This confidence must be so stable that it outlasts the patient's doubts that arise in the course of therapy. It must also stand up to the uninformed and insensitive gossiping of neighbors, irresponsible reporting in the media, and the treatment suggestions and requests of other physicians. Trust must be the basis for the patient's decision, and must be her protection in the subsequent weeks of therapy and the years of follow-up treatment which follow.

How can the trust of the cancer patient be gained and consolidated? Again, the solution can be stated in a few words: by the repeated, intensive talks with an experienced and competent physician, talks which combine information and therapy from the beginning. I should like here to mention a few key points. On first contact, the woman should be given factual and straightforward information on the suspicion of cancer or the probability of cancer diagnosis. This should be followed by detailed explanation of the measures required, and then a detailed description of the basic principles of treatment applied in the hospital in question. In my hospital these are:

- Exact substantiation of the cancer diagnosis, if necessary using a two-session procedure
- Concern on the one hand to treat the malignant and potentially fatal disease adequately according to the present state of knowledge, and on the other hand to proceed in a manner appropriate to the degree of disease in each individual
- Not to use the radical methods of surgery and irradiation previously practiced

Fears and worries can thus frequently be responded to and neutralized. If necessary, a further day should be given to allow time for reflection before continuation of the discussion. The wish to talk once more with another physician about the disease should be welcomed and supported. Before the operation, what was said earlier should be gone into in more detail, if possible in the presence of the husband or other relatives, and the information about a stage-related individualized therapy repeated. Fresh references to histological confirmation of the diagnosis and a two-session procedure in small tumors or with equivocal rapid-section findings give the patient the feeling of being secure from unnecessarily extensive operations.

There is then further discussion on the procedure. When all diagnostic results have been obtained and if the study's inclusion criteria are satisfied, the actual randomization discussion can then follow. It must be made clear that a clinical study is not a venture into unknown terrain but that, on the contrary, it entails careful registration, collection, and independent evaluation of the results of all patients during treatment. The duty of the physician to weigh up with the patient the advantages and disadvantages of various treatment procedures which are equivalent according to the general state of knowledge should be emphasized, and it should also be pointed out that our procedures are strictly controlled by our study management.

If trust has been created in the prior discussions, in particular on the basis of the caring attention which the patient has experienced in the previous days, consent to randomization may be obtained. The patient understands it as a part of the planned measures now beginning, providing hope for the orientation of future life. In principle, it is simpler to motivate the patient to make a random decision such as between several different kinds of chemotherapy than to renounce her right to decide whether the affected breast can be preserved or has to be removed. Reporting in the media ever more frequently represents preservation of a breast which has developed breast cancer as self-evident and mastectomy as superfluous. Thus, it will become increasingly more difficult for patients to weigh up objectively and without bias mastectomy on the one hand and breast-preserving radiotherapy on the other.

For the patient to arrive at a decision to accept randomization especially great emotional penetration and conviction are required of the physician in the discussion with the patient. This can only result from the absolute personal identification of physicians and nursing personnel of a hospital with the objectives and requirements of the study as laid down by the protocol. Inconstancy and halfheartedness of the part of the physician are no basis for an intensive talk which is to help the patient in a life situation which is unique and decisive for her.

If a patient were included in a clinical therapy study and the primary treatment carried out in accordance with the protocol, only consistent follow-up enables evaluation of therapy. Sloppiness in the continued observation or loss of contact with the patient render all the efforts and trouble futile. Under all circumstances the patient must continue to be observed by the institution which carried out the first treatment. Special local circumstances made it appear advisable to us that the additional diagnostic measures prescribed in the protocol should be largely transferred to doctors working in independent practices. This requires continuous, intensive written correspondence to ensure that the tests are performed and the findings communicated on time, but also promotes contact between the hospital and the doctors in independent practice. If the patient's trust was gained in primary treatment, she will be glad to return for regular checkups in the hospital. The close connection with the first-treating hospital is also important for the further psychological care of the patient. In the years following treatment, she will immediately associate a cold and any back or abdominal pain with breast cancer. It is the duty of the hospital to be available as the first port of call at any time. Worries and fears can then be reduced to the proper level. Above all, knowledge of the disease she has had can save the patient from overshoot diagnose and unnecessary treatment by other doctors. Exact scientific thinking and action must be complemented by warm-hearted care of and solicitude for the patient!

The intensive discussions with physicians and the encouragement and care from nursing staff during the highly sensitive phase in which the patient has to come to terms with her fate have not uncommonly meant that a deep emotional relationship has built up; this can make the presentation for examination an occasion on which friends meet again, although the relationship also has to prove its strength in the event of a relapse.

Alternative Treatments for Small Cancers of the Breast: Motives and Preferences of Patients Having to Choose

D. von Wrese

Evangelisches Krankenhaus, Postfach 100425, 4200 Oberhausen 1, FRG

In this paper I will report upon the experiences I have had during my preoperative talks with patients with a small carcinoma of the breast (T1 N0 M0).

For the patient these conversations concern the choice between two treatment modalities, namely modified radical mastectomy and breast-preserving measures like lumpectomy and radiotherapy. I do not intend to dwell upon the problem of randomizing patients who by definition have confidence in both measures mentioned above but no actual preference for one or the other. I will not, however, refrain from making some general remarks about death in our society.

In one of our medical bestsellers - a textbook for students - the female breast is almost exclusively described as an organ of sexual pleasure and a highly sensitive receiver of sexual stimuli. Under the heading "Breast cancer and its consequences," cancer is unilaterally discussed from the point of view of its interference with a happy sexual life. Identifying 12 psychometric characteristics, the author would have us believe that the loss of a breast is one of the worst blows destiny can deal out. Only a few words are devoted to the terror with which a patient is seized when the diagnosis of cancer is made. There is no indication that at the back of the patient's mind there is a passionate will to survive which far outweighs all thoughts of preserving the outward appearance of the body. In this way the book instills into the minds of young students a concept of the human being which is limited to sexual and reproductive functions and their corporal symbols.

Such a view is detrimental to the doctors' attitudes towards their future patients. Through such books prospective doctors are educated to believe that a patient will care more about her appearance than about her life. The patient's helplessness and her fears of terminal agony and death are pushed aside as if death were under a powerful taboo. One entertains the suspicion that in a world which is inclined to value only the superficial this neglect of the subject of death is no mere accident. There is method in it; all profit-oriented modes of thinking and living claim to be permanent and try to usurp a significance which they do not have.

Once the knowledge of the shortness of human life is gained by the patients, all the fashions and values of their time are unveiled as passing illusions. This revelation throws most patients into deep despair. They can find only poor consolation in the vague idea of another world to come, of a paradise the belief in which has

Recent Results in Cancer Research, Vol. 111
© Springer-Verlag Berlin · Heidelberg 1988

vanished along with the moral standards that went with this belief. Death is without meaning in our time, and so it is pointless for the doctor to speak about the seeming senselessness of dying and patients can only respect the doctor's not doing so. It is easier, and in some cases more lucrative, to speak about the impairment of the palpable and visible, about the faults and defects of the body which can be cured or redressed. This is not only in the interests of the patient herself, but also in the interests of the community; the patient feels a duty to have herself cured because members of the community do not want to be reminded of their own vulnerability and mortality by daily encounter with a visibly diseased person. Such an expectation becomes, for example, an evident disadvantage for an imbecile child whose physiognomy has been altered by cosmetic surgery. Such a child is deprived of those physical signals which are apt to evoke consideration and patience in his or her social environment. The confrontation with reality after such a cosmetic alteration is no longer mediated by the visible impairments, in this way making the encounter more abrupt and therefore more tragic too.

If a woman visits her doctor suspecting that she has breast cancer, she is filled with terror. All her thinking and feelings are dominated by the simple cruel fact that she too is mortal. The disease seems to have aroused in her this dormant fact. Pierced by a shiver of dismay she seeks somebody ready to lend a helping hand in her distress. But she does not express the fear of death openly, as if she were avoiding any worsening of her inner pain that might be caused by the echo of her voice. And without her uttering many words the common procedure of listening rather than talking and asking questions is reversed. The doctor has to take the initiative. Unconsciously patient and doctor both know that decisive information about the real nature and prognosis of her disease are conveyed to the patient by the modulation of the doctor's voice and the complex language of his gestures rather than by the mere contents of his words. Only when the words of the doctor beginn to correspond to his gestures will the patient become more accessible. Nevertheless, the conversation takes place against the background of a nearly suffocating fear. It is unfortunate that just at the time when logic is so important in weighing the arguments for and against the different methods of treatment of the carcinoma of her breast, mind and soul are haunted by innumerable anguishes. From this torrent of conflicting emotions emerges, as if it were the only logical thought, the thought of survival. In my experience the desire for safety occupies first place in the patient's considerations. Often this desire lies concealed behind her demand that any mutilating procedure be avoided, as if she were trying to offer the doctor a subject he can efficiently talk about as a technician well-versed in cosmetic surgery.

There remains, however, the conviction or perhaps instinct that survival as a human being counts far more than an unimpaired but possibly shortened lifetime as a complete woman. Without exploiting the jargon of the age too much it must be emphasized that through the modern media and their far-reaching penetration of society women are often defined only by their visible external features. Their deeper-rooted individual traits are under threat of being regarded as insignificant as a result of our visual age in which pictures dominate and a tendency prevails to only accept the palpable and visible and to ignore the incorporeal sides of a person. Before the invention of photography and its propagation it was not so easy to fix standards of external characteristics such as the ones to which a woman is nowadays more or less compelled to adapt. Sometimes it seems that women are typed in the same way a botanist types plants.

In my experience there is no question but that every woman would prefer radiotherapy to mastectomy if only equal therapeutic success could be guaranteed.

The fear of fibrosis induced by radiotherapy plays no important role in the decision in favor of or against breast-preserving measures. Even the hypothetical risk of a sarcoma of the breast developing with radiotherapy does not influence the choice of treatment decisively.

All the patient's thoughts revolve around the tormenting question: With what kind of therapy do I have the greatest likelihood of surviving this disease? The important thing is that the doctor gets rid of the idea that preserving the breast is the dominant wish of his patient. What fits the facts more precisely is that every patient is above all penetrated by an understandable fear of the possibly deadly consequences of her disease. When I am describing to a patient both methods of treating a small carcinoma of the breast, including technical details, because it is my duty to do so, I know that all these facts do not reach her while she is endeavoring to read what is in my face, to watch my gestures, to listen to the modulation of my voice. It goes without saying that all the time I am striving raise her spirits and to console her, and my words envelop her like a coat protecting her against the horrible coldness of her fear. At the same time, however, she is straining every nerve to discover my true opinion of the supposed equality of the cure rates of both treatments.

Under these circumstances it may be helpful to let the husband (or another confidant) take part in the conversation. In all probability he will have more distance from the disease and be able to evaluate both modalities of treatment more soberly. In his relative realism he does not hesitate to voice the true interests of his wife, wanting the maximal chance of success even if it means sacrificing her breast. For the husband, according to my experience, the loss of his wife's breast does not amount to the destruction of her femininity. Therefore the typical remark: "My wife and I don't care about the breast as long as she is going to be cured." Only too willingly does the patient acquiesce to the formulation of her will to survive by her husband. It seems to her to be a confirmation of his love that he does not insist on the doctor's preserving her unimpaired external appearance but rather places her existence in the foreground. And if she objects to amputation of the breast, pretending not to be able to live on because the loss of her breast means demanding too much of her husband, he is flattered too. He tacitly supposes that his wife is making all efforts to maintain her bodily integrity for him, even if before this time she had ceased to be of any significance in his sex life.

In studies of alternative treatments of small carcinomas of the breast the doctor is expected to refrain from making any recommendation. But during talks with my patients I have realized that it is impossible for me to escape the role of interpreter and guide.

It does not surprise me that a patient cannot easily understand that the doctor should not be recommending one of the forms of treatment offered by the study. It is a Sisyphean labor indeed to convince the patient that the doctor himself should not have any preference. It always puts me in a somewhat awkward situation if I am questioned about what kind of treatment I would recommend to my wife in case of breast cancer. There is always a trace of skepticism and incredulity in the patient's facial expression if I say that even my wife would have to decide for herself on the basis of all the arguments, both for and against, that I can offer as a so-called expert in breast cancer. Naturally my wife would wait for some key words, would be alert to nonverbal clues on my part to help her out of her dilemma: on the one hand mastectomy with the greatest chance of being cured, and on the other preserving her breast while exposing herself to an only potentially greater risk.

Preserving the breast is certainly not a goal in itself. Far from being of sexual importance, when cancer is diagnosed the preserved breast functions rather as a kind of prosthesis for the psyche, which is obviously positively influenced and stabilized by the daily perception of unimpaired corporal integrity. It helps the patient to combat the ever-present fear of approaching death by impeding her psyche from gathering visible and seemingly irrefutable proof of the legitimacy of her fear. Questions of self-esteem and self-assurance do not matter so much at the time of confrontation with the diagnosis of cancer.

After long hours of conversation with the patient the doctor will finally and unwittingly reveal to the patient his own preference of treatment, through his gestures, tone of voice, facial expressions, unconscious omissions, and so on. This preference has itself developed unconsciously from many components such as the age of the patient, the existence of dependent children, the profession the patient practices, her anxieties, and so on. And if the patient has at last come to the difficult decision, she and her doctor tacitly accept the self-deception that she has made the decision of her own free will. The absolute impartiality of the doctor can only be an illusion. He can never exclude himself from the process of finding the appropriate decision because he is an integral part of it. All his behavior is unconsciously goal oriented. Even if he tries to avoid any tendency to persuade or guide the patient he cannot resist it. Seldom will he be as objective as is required in a study, especially when cancer is concerned. In the framework of an objective study the doctor's suppressed conviction that he should take sides with the patient always forces its way up against his determination to be objective.

My description of preferences and motives in the choice of alternative treatment for small carcinomas of the breast must remain incomplete and occasionally a little superficial because it is nearly impossible to unravel the complex interrelationships between psyche and soma, disease and general sociocultural background. Some may find it disappointing that I am unable to draw up a list in which are catalogued all factors and circumstances which could make the decision of an individual patient almost predictable. There are, however, some situations in which the patient's decision may be explained and where the patient has a solid foundation for her preference for one treatment and does not waver or hesitate. The doctor's words in these cases just corroborate a preconceived idea about the necessity of amputation or preserving of the breast.

A 51-year-old patient, for example, wanted at the beginning of the conversation to know about the probable nature of her disease and the possible ways of treating it, including amputation of the breast. She did not want to run the slight risk connected with radiotherapy. On trying to discover the reasons for her implacable resolution to have her breast amputated in case of cancer, I learned that the patient was married to a man who had lost both legs in an accident. For several years he had been confined to a wheelchair. Both the patient and her husband were, as it were, chained to this wheelchair, her husband being completely dependent on her support. She could not bring herself to talk to her husband about the alternative treatment for small cancers of the breast, in her eyes the question of preserving the breast being a triviality in comparison to her husband's disability. Choosing radiotherapy, according to her, would have amounted to something like committing an offence against him, his quality and even duration of life being so inseparately linked with hers. This unequivocal decision for mastectomy was governed by familial considerations.

Another patient, a night club dancer, could not afford to sacrifice her breast, which was essential to her earning her living. She stated convincingly that she would even run the risk of a lower cure rate because she had no alternative to her present occupation. This decision was based on professional considerations.

As a last example I would like to mention a 45-year-old sister in a protestant nursing order. Friendly, but also somewhat unapproachable, she decided on mastectomy, avoiding in this way 6 weeks of radiotherapy which would have hindered her fulfillment of her daily duties. I presume that a kind of resignation to God's will influenced her decision and, I daresay, an aversion to making a fuss about such a worldly thing as a breast appears to have had its effect. These remarks, however, are only my own interpretation of her unvoiced deliberation.

The general conclusions that emerge from my experiences with patients who have had small cancers of the breast may be stated in the following terms:

1. Apart from a few cases, most patients demand the highest attainable degree of safety with regard to the treatment of cancer.
2. Because in our culture death is under a taboo (despite all appearances), the patient pretends to be primarily interested in the details of the possible preservation of her sick breast; however, during the conversations with the doctor all her thoughts and fears revolve around the question of survival.
3. The patient is not free to decide because free decisions in their original sense presuppose rational weighing of arguments for and against. This is impossible for a patient who is paralyzed by the idea of standing on the brink of an abyss into which she is sooner or later going to fall.
4. There is no impartiality on the doctor's part because it is impossible for the doctor to sever the ties which bind him to the patient and make him an integral part of the decision-making process.
5. As a consequence of the above, except for a few exceptional cases, the doctor unconsciously decides the method of treatment by his behavior towards and interaction with the patient.

A Final Remark. Among my patients who have had a small cancer of the breast the choice of the more radical surgery appears to be marginally preferred. This may be partly explained by the fact that the patient is offered the possibility of having her breast reconstructed by the application of a tissue-expander and the later insertion of a silicon prosthesis.

Subjective Theories on Etiology and Treatment of Cancer

R. Verres

Abteilung für Medizinische Psychologie, Universitäts-Krankenhaus Eppendorf, Martinistraße 52, 2000 Hamburg 20, FRG

In this paper I will present some results of an empirical study on subjective theories of lay people on cancer treatment. I would like to discuss the results of this study by focusing on the question of whether these theories are significant for the decisions people make about cancer treatment and for early detection of cancer.

What people think about diseases is not coherent nor without contradictions. The subjective theories are complex and subject to emotional influences. The impact of medical information on the early detection of cancer and on treatment methods will be better if experts have more detailed information on concepts of cancer held by the general public.

Personal theories of laymen on diseases and treatment possibilities do not automatically correspond to medical progress. Since emotional elements are also involved in people's subjective decision-making processes, opinions often appear to be more intuitive than rational-cognitive and do not primarily reflect the style of thinking that would be typical in a medical frame of reference. Elements of the individual's self-concept, for instance the individual life-style, the life goals, and body perception, affect these decision-making processes.

Psychological research on health motivation distinguishes between a (more compulsive-ascetic) "health discipline" and a (more hedonistic) "health preference." Individuals that tend to exercise "health discipline" are more likely to be "compliant" in regard to treatment recommendations made by medical authorities. On the other hand, we assume that individuals who have more hedonistic attitudes towards their body might present a more critical point of view if medical intervention is recommended that affects their body, and would be more likely to emphasize the importance of maintaining their self-perceived responsibility for their own body and life-style.

If we intend empirically to explore lay theories on the sense and usefulness of different treatment methods, we must first take into account the personal experiences on which the attitudes and opinions of individuals are based (Verres 1986). Here I am primarily thinking of the so-called vicarious experiences of human beings. This means that people usually observe in detail what happens to others (family members, neighbors, or colleagues) who get cancer, how their disease develops, and what kind of personal significance the observed medical intervention

Recent Results in Cancer Research, Vol. 111
© Springer-Verlag Berlin · Heidelberg 1988

has for the patient concerned. Since approximately one in four people gets cancer almost every healthy person knows at least one cancer patient. In our study, 87 out of 100 healthy individuals who were interviewed had experienced someone they knew getting cancer, and 49 had had this experience a couple of times.

Lay theories on cancer treatment may consist of knowledge and of sets of conclusions which can be right or wrong, such as "If I have a cancer checkup every year I will be protected against cancer." In 30% of our interviews with laymen we found a misunderstanding of early detection of cancer as a means of primary prevention. In addition, we need to take into account that as well as conscious thinking, associations and emotions are being processed; these appear as vivid pictures or memories of the fate of someone they knew with cancer. We call these phenomena affective connotations, which means that there are emotional meanings attached to thoughts. If these become intense enough they can interfere with logical thinking or even block it out altogether.

At this point I would like to present some results of our own study. In semi-structured interviews that lasted 90–120 min each we asked 101 subjects about their personal theories on cancer treatment. The people interviewed did not have cancer themselves and were recruited through general practitioners working in the southern part of Germany (Baden-Württemberg).

The complete transcripts of the interviews yielded 2446 pages of text and were evaluated by content analysis using a classification system which was developed by our group and consisted of 292 categories in total (Verres 1986).

The starting point was a content analysis of the unstructured reports our subjects gave us of their experiences when cancer had affected someone they knew. In total we recorded 83 case descriptions of cancer diseases according to the reports of our subjects who had witnessed the disease in someone else. Every one of the 102 154 words spoken by those interviewed was evaluated by content analysis by our team of six physicians and psychologists.

The most frequent statements with regard to the changing attitudes of cancer patients towards their life were ideas of resignation (33%) and social isolation (28%). One in three case descriptions contained spontaneous remarks about concealment and taboos increasing on the part of the patient. However, an increase in social support was reported by 49%.

The emotional connotations of the observed courses and treatments of disease were categorized by interviewer ratings performed at the end of each interview (see Table 1).

Table 1. Emotional connotations of observed courses and treatments of cancer ($n = 83$)

Medical Connotations	(%)	Psychosocial Connotations	(%)
Positive	8	Positive	25
Neutral/ambivalent	19	Neutral/ambivalent	25
Negative	68	Negative	38
No statement	5	No statement	12

The results show that when people recall what medical treatment and the disease meant for a cancer patient we must expect them to have mostly negative memories.

Compared with the medical course and treatment of cancer, its psychosocial course and treatment was described in a less negative way. This means that physical disease was not necessarily equated with resignation or social isolation, which are both indicators of a negative psychosocial development.

At a later point during the interview we asked specific questions relating to attitudes the subjects would have towards treatment if they themselves got cancer.

Table 2. Attitudes towards medical treatment for cancer of themselves ($n = 101$)

Attitude	(%)
Positive	27
Indifferent/ambivalent	48
Negative	25

This showed that although the majority of subjects consider the medical course of cancer to be unfavorable (Table 1), their attitudes to being medically treated themselves were more positive (Table 2). We also rated the attitudes towards medical treatment that were indicated during the unstructured reports of experiences with cancer diseases of others. The results (Table 3) were almost identical to the responses to questions about medical treatment of themselves for cancer (Table 2).

Table 3. Attitudes towards medical treatment of cancer patients ($n = 83$)

Attitudes	(%)
Positive	20
Indifferent/neutral/ambivalent	44
Negative	26

A comparison of Tables 2 and 3 shows that the attitudes were similar. Attitudes towards medical treatment are probably formed through experiences with disease courses of others. Since vivid memories function as anchors for these attitudes it is not easy for us as professionals to influence them by means of communication.

The attempts to reveal attitudes related to medical treatment of cancer gave the alarming result that merely 27% or 20% had a positive attitude. Evidently we medical professionals must deal with a considerable amount of distrust or at least ambivalence when we make treatment recommendations. This means that patients will seldom rely on medical recommendations alone when they have to decide about treatment possibilities. Instead they will utilize additional sources of information that are available within the lay system and which the doctor will know little of.

In regard to the communication about experiences among the general public another problem has to be considered: open communication about cancer is very difficult for many people. Of all subjects who participated in our study, 25% declared spontaneously during the interview (without a question from us about this) that fear of cancer could be a risk factor for cancer. They believed that talking as little as possible about cancer prevented them from going "crazy" and from becoming prone to cancer themselves. For this reason communication about cancer and treatment possibilities often remains fragmentary and as a consequence many ambivalences and doubts prevent the taking of clear decisions.

The observation that many people tend to avoid direct and consistent thinking about cancer can be illustrated with another example. During the interview we submitted two self-rating cards concerning the risk of getting cancer to each subject. The cards were shown one after the other. When the first card was presented the interviewer asked the subject: "How great do you think the risk is that *you* will get cancer at some point in your life?" When the second card was presented the question was: "If you look at this list, how many people do you think will get cancer?" Table 4 shows the response frequencies.

Table 4. Perceived risk of getting cancer ($n = 101$)

Own risk of cancer			General risk of cancer		
Response	(%)		Response	(%)	
Very high	5	24	Very many people	21	81
Quite high	19		Quite a lot of people	60	
Quite low	45	71	Only a few people	17	18
Very low	26		Almost none	1	
Don't know/ no response	5		Don't know/ no response	2	

Of course, the items in the two questions are not equivalent but at least in both self-rating cards a four-point rating scale from "low" to "high" was used. Although 81% estimated that the general risk for human beings of getting cancer was quite high or very high, only 24% estimated their own risk to be quite high or very high. This means that any communication about cancer is faced – when it refers to an individual's own risks – with a strong perceptive defense which must be taken into account. It makes rational logical thinking and clear decision making difficult for people. Out of those interviewed, 49% said that they usually repress their own fear of cancer. This means that they tend to change the topic when conversations focus on cancer issues.

Vicarious experiences concerning the treatment of others who have cancer will therefore probably not be thought through in most cases. Contradictory ideas can remain alongside each other in this way so that a subjective feeling of insecurity and lack of clarity will result.

Another impediment to undisturbed exchange of information between cancer patients and other people is that people are often afraid that cancer could be contagious. These fears are seldom admitted directly but they became evident when we asked concrete questions about behavior referring to different degrees of intimacy with cancer patients. Of the subjects, 18% would not want to eat something that a cancer patient had cooked, 32% would not want to drink from a glass that a cancer patient had used before, and 42% expressed resentment about direct physical contact with cancer patients in intimate situations.

One in three subjects declared that she or he would want to avoid an open dialogue with cancer patients or would at least expect to experience conflicts during communication. Of those who were willing to lead an open dialogue with a cancer patient at all, 50% expected the patient to initiate it.

In order to agree to treatment recommendations made by the physician it is necessary for the patient to have confidence in medicine and science. One of the questions we asked during our interview was: "How well is science informed about cancer today?" The response pattern is shown in Table 5.

Table 5. Perceived competence of science with regard to cancer ($n = 101$)

Response	(%)	
Science is ...		
Very well informed	4	47
Quite well informed	43	
Quite misinformed	47	51
Very misinformed	4	
No response	2	

We found that only half of the subjects we interviewed had confidence in medical science. This is another indication that patients are likely to be skeptical when they are faced with recommendations for medical treatment. Negative appraisals of cancer treatment mostly relate to procedures that are perceived to have aggressive qualities and do not so much refer to a perceived lack of effectiveness of cancer treatment.

In future, when giving information on cancer treatment, it seems important not only to point out treatment success in terms of prolonged life expectancy but also to explain openly the nature of the treatment and the quality of life that is linked to severe treatment methods. In response to our questions about whether an individual's behavior could influence the further course of the disease or even stop the progress of the disease, 88% emphasized the importance of the patient's own wish to recover. This indicates that we can assume that patients have strong inner motivation to actively take part in treatment decisions and treatment procedures and that they will not wish to be randomized in cancer clinical trials.

At the same rate that confidence in medicine decreases the probability that someone will - maybe behind our backs - seek so-called paramedical treatment increases. Of the subjects we interviewed, 50% stated that if they themselves got cancer they would "maybe" of "for sure" look for nonmedical help, for instance nonmedical practitioners, faith healers, diviners, or even drinking petroleum.

To sum up, it can be said that the results of this study support the idea that future information on cancer treatment should primarily focus on influencing the attitudes towards medicine in general in a positive direction. When a layperson assesses expectations and possible benefits of treatment of cancer the crucial point in the decision-making process is not only whether life can be prolonged but what the quality of life will be.

Reference

Verres R (1986) Krebs und Angst. Subjektive Theorien von Laien über Entstehung, Vorsorge, Früherkennung, Behandlung und die psychosozialen Folgen von Krebserkrankungen. Springer, Berlin Heidelberg New York

Individual Cases and the Scientific Method – A Conflict? Legal Aspects of Cancer Clinical Trials in the Federal Republic of Germany

W. H. Eberbach

Bundesministerium für Jugend, Familie, Frauen und Gesundheit, Koblenzer Straße 112, 5300 Bonn 2, FRG

In this paper I should like to approach the topic of cancer clinical trials from two directions. In the first part I will give an exposition of the current legal position. This part will contain information of a kind which in my opinion is absolutely necessary for all scientists involved in clinical trials. In the second part I will then try to approach the subject from a different and substantially more critical, perhaps even provocative, starting-point.

Problems Concerning the Duty to Give Information in Clinical Trials

The central legal questions relating to clinical trials are associated with the following keywords: information, alternative methods of treatment, randomisation.

The Physicians Duty to Give Information Before an Operation

Protection of Patient's Rights. The patient is an *autonomous subject* in the physician-patient relationship. When the physician performs an operation, the patient's life and health are affected. These interests of the patient are recognised legally by the constitution in the Federal Republic of Germany, as is the patient's "sovereignty of decision" (in Article 2 Paragraph 2, Article 1 Paragraph 1 and Article 2 Paragraph 1 of the Constitution, or *Grundgesetz*), and are protected against unauthorised encroachment. For this reason, where there is to be encroachment on the patient's physical integrity, the physician will, in principle, need the patient's "authorisation to have access", i.e. his consent. However, such consent amounts to a mere formalism if it is not based on the patient's conception and estimation of what he wants. The patient can only come to a decision that is truly his own decision if he is completely aware of the nature, importance and implications of the planned operation from information given to him by the physician concerned. Consequently, it follows from the patient's right to self-determination and from the freedom of decision to which everybody is entitled – and ultimately therefore from respect for human dignity – that physicians are under an obligation to give

© Springer-Verlag Berlin · Heidelberg 1988

their patients the information concerned. If a physician neglects this duty, the operation he performs is not justified by the consent given by the patient. In such a case the physician is criminally liable for inflicting bodily injury (under Section 223 et seq. of the Criminal Code). Moreover, the patient can bring forward claims under civil law for compensation from the physician for any damage caused and for pain and suffering (Section 823 et seq. and Section 847 of the Civil Code).

Contract with the Doctor. The duty incumbent on physicians to inform their patients also follows from the contract with the physician concerned. By virtue of the contract concluded the patient entrusts his person and thus his legal interests - his body, his dignity - to the physician. In the contract the physician assures the patient (without there having to be any explicit reference thereto) that he will protect the interests so entrusted and will assist the patient to make sensible use of his right to self-determination. The legal form this promise takes is that of the medical duty to inform and advise the patient. This duty obliges the physician to put the patient in the picture as regards his physical condition and, where necessary, to inform him about invasive operations as well as about the possibilities of medication or non-invasive treatment.

Information Concerning Alternative Methods of Treatment

At this point we must look into the aspect of it being possible for a particular disease to be treated in various ways, i.e. by various methods. As long as these methods are on an equal footing, i.e. as long as there are only immaterial differences between them with regard to the degree of intervention, the side effects and the prospects of success (as will frequently be the case in, for example, a conflict between different schools of thought), it will be for the physician, exercising his freedom of choice of therapy, to select the method he prefers. In cases like this, special information for the patient on a treatment that has not been selected is superfluous. Similarly, there is no need for the physician to inform the patient that there is another method of treatment if this is still untested and is used in only a few clinics.

On the other hand, according to the interpretation of the courts, the patient must be informed and advised of possible alternative methods of treatment where they differ in the degree of risk involved, in the range and gravity of their side effects and in their prospects of success. An example is the situation where, on one hand, there is a less dangerous form of intervention, associated however with years of reduced quality of life, and, on the other hand, a more radical and more dangerous method of treatment which, if successful, would secure a higher quality of life. Some forms of cancer therapy in particular provide examples of this.

Non-randomised clinical trials are also of this type. From a legal point of view, there are no objections to such clinical trials provided that the physician carrying out the research follows the indicated rules concerning the giving of information: that, in a situation where information is necessary regarding alternative procedures, he lets his patients themselves choose a form of therapy corresponding to their own wishes and that he compares the results obtained from the trials in his scientific work.

Randomisation and Information

Clinical trials with randomisation are also part of the problem area of alternative methods of treatment.

Discontinuation of Clinical Trials. The absolute limits to randomised clinical trials are independent of the otherwise central issue of whether trial patients must be informed of the randomisation. If during the trial the new therapy proves to be clearly superior to the old therapy, the trial itself must immediately be discontinued. All patients have to be treated from then on with the new and better methods; otherwise the physician would not be adhering to medical standards and he would face the consequences in criminal and civil law already referred to. It must be assumed that the consent given by the patient is always only to what is regarded as the optimum therapy in his case. For this reason, if dangers and risks involved in the new form of therapy come to light before the trial is ended corresponding action must also be taken.

Alternative Consent. The critical point comes, however, when the legal imperative to inform runs into conflict with the requirements of the scientific method.

An interpretation that is closely dependent on Article 1 Paragraph 1 and on Article 2 Paragraphs 1 and 2 of the Constitution (i.e. on human dignity, on the right to self-determination and on protection of the inviolability of the person) obliges physicians to inform all patients involved in a trial about two aspects. Information has to be given about the alternative forms of therapy available as well as about the assignment to a particular treatment being random. It may already be a strain for a physician to inform a patient about a possibly incurable disease, and he may be faced with a second problem. In each individual case he has to ask himself whether a patient who is seriously, or possibly fatally, ill can reasonably be expected to face the possibility that chance will determine the treatment that is actually given. There may also be reason for not informing a patient if, because of his knowledge of the randomisation, the trial might be ineffective. This might be either because too many patients refuse to be assigned treatment randomly, or because the knowledge of randomisation might destroy the design of the trial so that its scientific value will be limited or even nil.

It is no solution to give information only after randomisation and only to those patients who will be undergoing the new therapy. It is true that patients in the control group receive the standard therapy but, in my opinion, it is wrong to infer that the ignorance of these patients concerning the additional randomisation is of no importance. It disregards the fact that these patients (like all other participants in the trial) have a dual role. They are not only suffering from a disease but at the same time are taking part in scientific research. As such they are "living data carriers" for the researcher. However, this second role is by no means necessarily associated with their original role as a patient, but as a rule is based instead on an additional agreement. As a result, the right to self-determination and respect for human dignity (Article 1 Paragraph 1 and Article 2 Paragraph 1 of the Constitution), actually require the patient to be informed in advance and the physician to ask the patient whether he is at all willing to assume the role of test subject, in spite of the absence of personal advantage. If it is not permissible for patients to be left in the dark about randomisation, there is still a way of trying to maintain the validity of clinical trials: the physician must inform the patient before randomisation about all the forms of therapy included in the trial and also about the randomisation procedure itself. Then, the physician must request the patient's consent to both modes of treatment. It must be stressed that the word "random", which in emotional terms often has a negative connotation in this context, may be paraphrased in giving the information about randomisation. Although the value of clinical trials is diminished by giving the information required both legally and by professional ethical standards, this lowering of scientific standards is the unavoidable price of human dignity.

Some Critical Remarks on Randomised Trials

Thus far, I have set out in a clear framework the legal standards that must be met. Anyone working in this field must be familiar with them and observe them. However, there are other more critical ways of approaching the topic.

Individual Cases and Scientific Method

The Contrasting Positions of Patient and Doctor. Pointing to the contrast in a slightly crude fashion, we may say that the patient represents the principle of the individual case, the physician the methods employed by science. The needs of the two are widely divergent. The patient is looking for treatment planned for him alone, for him as an individual entity. To him, all that is of interest is his own life and survival with as little loss of quality of life as possible. Scientific progress is not his problem. His attitude tends towards exaggerated individualism, if not egocentricity: the whole hospital were to revolve around him alone, he would have no objections.

The position of the physician engaged in scientific work is very different. Everything which enhances the success of his investigation is naturally to be welcomed. Individual disruptive factors reduce the value of the data. Whilst for the physician, too, a patient's death is not something to be desired, it remains nevertheless a relevant "datum" for his research work: the death of the patient tells him something about the success or lack of success of one of the therapies applied. Thus the physician tends to adopt an egalitarian approach towards patients, in which they become depersonalised. This does not mean that he does not closely (frequently even intensively) observe each patient, but this is motivated not so much by the patient as a creature that is suffering and that deserves love and respect, but rather by him in his capacity as a "data carrier".

Randomisation and Reductionism. Randomisation might be said to be a peak in the rationalist-reductionist way of looking at science. It averts attention from the individual case, from all that is specific to the actual person in question. It reduces him to a response pattern with respect to two different therapies. It imposes itself upon him and makes him a "data component" of a technical medical system to which his being human is a matter of indifference - this is easily recognisable from the fact that the further course of things is left to chance. Such a manner of proceeding corresponds, however, to the prevalent scientific view point. Examine, analyse, dissect, divide - and then in the end try to put the parts back together again into a whole. This path has indeed proved its worth in many cases and led to great successes. Analytic-rational methods of this kind have been the lifeblood of the natural sciences since the Enlightenment. And they have not only been a lifeblood, but a vital source from which natural scientists have been living better and better - on soft upholstery, cushioned by their scientific methods which are now enthroned as a philosophy.

Through randomised trials the physician engaged in research reproduces this system. And he benefits from doing this, because he publishes papers which satisfy the requirements of the "scientific method". Even the patient, one may justifiably maintain, benefits from this because the research results obtained in this way are also there to be drawn on in his own case.

On the other hand, the physician is not only the beneficiary of the prevailing scientific methodology. He is at the same time its victim, for he runs the risk of no longer knowing how to remain sensitive to things outside the reduction. He may get a distorted picture of his patients, which may prevent him from seeing new features and acting accordingly - and thus possibly from being more successful without needing to depersonalise the patient. Seen thus, the patient too is not only a beneficiary but also a victim; he is treated in accordance with reductionist methods and becomes in the course of the randomised trial a research object for the benefit of future patients.

Randomisation and Our View of Man. Against the background of what we have been saying up to now, the question inevitably arises of whether the reductionist approach of randomised clinical trials is compatible with the view of man that has been moulded by 2500 years of Western philosophy and almost 2000 years of Christianity. The therapy trial approach is one-dimensional, restricted to just one aspect - the response to the therapy. The view of man is complex. The individual is viewed as a subject at the centre of things, not susceptible to any valuation, and yet at the same time shaped by many different interrelationships between himself and society.

If we rule out a collectivist duty to permit research on oneself - a duty which emphasises the priority of society and its interests - the contradiction can only be resolved by the patient himself. By making himself available for the trial of his own free will, he is consenting to the concomitant reduction of his personality. For this, however, he first needs to know about this imminent depersonalisation; he must be informed of it. To deny him this information would mean violating, via the process of reduction, the view of man embodied in this person, his dignity and also his self-determined "subject-hood". It is a matter for the patient alone to decide when and to what extent he casts off this "subject-hood". For others (such as the physician doing research) this self-determination and "subject-hood" of man is not valid without question. Science therefore is limited by the readiness to agree shown by every individual.

The Doctor-Patient Discussion as Information and Mediation

Individual cases and the scientific method have thus been recognised as basically incompatible. At the same time, however, we have already seen their point of intersection: they meet in the self-determination of the individual patient and in his willingness to make himself available for the trial. It becomes apparent, then, that the clarificatory or "informing" discussion is the mediator between the individual case and scientific method.

- Between patient and physician a *relationship of mutual trust* must develop. Without such trust the physician will hardly be able to generate in the patient a readiness to talk about participation in a trial; trust, however, cannot be achieved without discussion.
- Without discussion, the physician also does not learn anything about the patient's attitude to disease and death. Only a *discussion* can give the physician an indication of whether the patient might find a certain kind of therapy acceptable, for example, as regards its side effects. The alternative is that right from the very start, the patient cannot be considered for the trial.
- Similarly, the physician must, unless the patient has expressly foregone clarification, inform the patient of all the therapies which might be considered, since otherwise the patient who wants to choose cannot.
- Finally, it is the job of the doctor to get across to the patient the aim of the trial and to convince him that the reduction accompanying participation in the trial is meaningful in the pursuit of this aim. This, too, is impossible without an extensive, open and sympathetic *discussion.*

Discussion thus smooths the way between the individual case (the patient) and the scientific method (the randomised trial). It makes the reductionist view of science acceptable by subordinating it to the voluntary acceptance of the individual concerned. And here we have something worthy of note! Precisely this conclusion was also the result of the legal assessment conducted in the first part of this paper.

To conclude, informing the patient is not simply necessary out of respect for (or even fear of) the courts. It is above all respect for the independent personality of the patient which makes this imperative.

The Value of Small Clinical Trials

K. D. MacRae

Charing Cross and Westminster Medical School, St. Dunstan's Road,
London W6 8RP, Great Britain

Introduction

Large clinical trials and overviews which pool several clinical trials addressing substantially the same question have an important role in clinical research, viz., the detection of small or moderate differences between treatments where the outcome is an important one, such as survival. Also, large numbers give narrow confidence intervals for the estimate of the treatment effect. However, small clinical trials still have an important part to play. Firstly, pilot studies need to be carried out before a large trial is begun. Secondly, in the treatment of certain diseases, especially where treatment is aimed at relief of symptoms, it may be felt that only large differences between treatments are of interest. Thirdly, it may be difficult to carry out a large clinical trial because of ethical or other problems, but a small trial may be able to provide useful pragmatic information. The important statistical concepts are the confidence interval for the estimated treatment difference and the type-III error.

Confidence Intervals for Treatment Differences

It is widely recognised (e.g. Freiman et al. 1978; Gardner and Altman 1986) that quoting the point estimate of the treatment difference and categorising this difference as being either 'statistically significant' or 'nonsignificant' according to an arbitrary type-I error probability, such as 0.05, has limitations. Giving a confidence interval for the range of 'true' treatment differences consistent with the study data is much more informative - whether or not the treatment difference is statistically significant.

For instance, with 100 patients per group, the difference between a 'success' rate of 85% and one of 75% just fails to reach significance at the 0.05 level, an uncorrected chi-square giving $P=0.077$. The 95% confidence interval for the estimate of the 'true' treatment difference is -1.4%–21.4%. If, however the difference in the study is made 2% larger, by making the success rates 86% and 74% respectively, statistical significance is achieved (an uncorrected chi-square gives $P=0.033$). The

Recent Results in Cancer Research, Vol. 111
© Springer-Verlag Berlin · Heidelberg 1988

95% confidence interval is now 0.6%–23.4%. The confidence intervals for the non-significant and the significant differences are very similar. Both the confidence intervals convey helpful information to the clinician about what the study has shown.

If, for instance, the true difference would need to be at least 30% to be clinically important, the confidence intervals show that such a difference between the two treatments is inconsistent with the data, and therefore further trials comparing these two treatments are not indicated. Powell-Tuck et al. (1986) illustrate this use of small trials having wide confidence intervals with three gastroenterological studies in which only large differences would have justified continued research into the treatments.

On the other hand, if the treatment difference needs to be at least 5% for the difference to be clinically important, the confidence intervals show that differences smaller than 5% are consistent with the trial data, although the difference might indeed be more than 5%. This means that a larger trial would need to be carried out to obtain a more precise estimate of the difference between the treatments. Collins and Langman (1985) provide an example of this in their suggestion that the randomization of at least 10000 patients would be needed to establish whether the marginally significant reduction in deaths from acute upper gastrointestinal hemorrhage by the use of histamine H2 antagonists found from an overview of 27 trials amounted to a clinically worthwhile reduction of at least 20%.

Type-III Errors

Schwartz and Lellouch (1967) distinguished between what they termed 'explanatory' and 'pragmatic' aims in clinical trials. An explanatory study is one aimed at testing a biological hypothesis, whereas a pragmatic trial seeks to choose between two (or more) treatments. The explanatory/pragmatic distinction is relevant to several aspects of clinical trials, such as the treatments to be compared, the patients suitable for the study, the size of the trial and the assessment of results. The relevance to trial size and assessment of results will be considered here.

The explanatory approach is intended to improve understanding. The clinical trial compares two treatments chosen for their relevance to a particular biological hypothesis, and the result of the trial is used to judge whether the hypothesis is to be retained or discarded. In so doing it is important not to conclude that the treatments are different when, in fact, they are not – i.e. the results must be analysed using a suitably strict level of statistical significance to keep the probability of a type-I error small. Also, it is important to avoid concluding that the treatments do not differ when, in truth, they do – i.e. to avoid a type-II error. To make the probabilities of both the type-I and type-II errors small, a sufficiently large number of patients must be used.

A pragmatic trial is aimed at making a choice between the two treatments. The two treatments are compared in order to obtain adequate data to decide which treatment is preferable. The type-I error can be ignored, because if two treatments are exactly equivalent it is unimportant which one is used. There is no need to carry out a test of statistical significance – the apparently better treatment is chosen.

As it is never concluded that the treatments are identical, the probability of a type-II error is zero. Pragmatically, the evil to avoid is a choice in favour of the inferior treatment - i.e. it is important to have a low probability of a type-III error.

Sample size computations are usually based on three factors, viz., the desired type-I error probability, the desired type-II error probability, and the difference between treatments that is considered to be of clinical importance (e.g. Lachin 1981). If the type-I error probability is chosen to be 0.05, the Normal deviate for this error in the sample size formula is 1.96. If the type-II error probability chosen is 0.05 (i.e., the power of the trial = 95%), the Normal deviate for this error in the sample size calculation is −1.645. The sample size will therefore be calculated having 1.96 - (−1.645) = 3.605 as the total of the Normal deviates in the numerator of the formula. The total of the Normal deviates is squared in the calculation, so the study size calculation would include 12.996 in the numerator.

If, however, the type-III error is considered to be all important, the calculation of the study size needs only to include the Normal deviate for the desired probability of a type-III error. For example, for a type-III error probability of 0.001, the Normal deviate is −3.09. The square of −3.09 is 9.584, which is 73.5% of 12.996. Thus a study having 73.5% of the number of patients needed to have type-I and -II error probabilities of 0.05 has a type-III error probability of 0.001 (using the same treatment difference for the calculation, of course). For a type-III error probability of 0.01, the Normal deviate is −2.326 (squared = 5.41, 41.6% of 12.996), and for a type-III error of 0.05 the Normal deviate is −1.645 (squared = 2.706, 20.8% of 12.996). So, trials having just 41.6% and 20.8% of the number of patients needed for a trial having type-I and -II error probabilities of 0.05 will give type-III error probabilities of 0.01 and 0.05 respectively.

As an example, consider a trial to compare mastectomy and lumpectomy in the treatment of early breast cancer. Suppose a 10% difference in survival is judged to be clinically important. A trial with a power of 95% of detecting a 10% difference in survival (either way from 50% survival at some arbitrary follow-up interval) at the 0.05 level of statistical significance would need about 640 patients per treatment. If a power of 90% were considered acceptable, about 520 patients per treatment would suffice, and 385 per treatment would give a power of 80%. If, however, a pragmatic view were taken and the treatment with the better survival would be considered preferable, regardless of statistical significance, only 133 patients per treatment would be needed to have a type-III error probability of 0.05. What this means is that the probability that the inferior treatment would appear to be the superior one is less than 0.05 if the 'true' treatment difference is as large as 10%. A type-III error probability of 0.01 would be obtained with 266 patients per treatment, and a type-III error probability of 0.001 with 470 per treatment.

Concluding Comments

The use of confidence intervals to express the results of clinical trials is widely accepted to be greatly superior to merely quoting a *P*-value, and this is so whether the trial is small or large. However, the explanatory/pragmatic distinction still raises issues that clinicians and statisticians find difficult to accept. For example 'intention-to-treat' analysis of clinical trials is based on pragmatic considerations, but many clinicians find it counterintuitive to include patients who have not received treatment, or who have received the wrong treatment, in the treatment group to which they were originally allocated.

In assessing the results of a clinical trial, it would be preferable to be reasonably confident that any treatment difference seen is of clinical importance; i.e., the trial would be a 'positive' one with a statistically significant difference, and the confidence interval would have a lower limit indicating that the 'true' difference is likely to be clinically important.

On the other hand, a 'negative' trial, one not producing a statistically significant difference, is often taken to be something of a failure, unless it is very large. Detsky and Sackett (1985) and Makuch and Johnson (1986) discuss small negative trials from the standpoint of showing whether two treatments are equivalent. A pragmatic view of the negative trial is rather different, in that a small study can provide a basis for treatment choice in which the apparently superior treatment (but not statistically significantly so) is unlikely to be inferior to the alternative treatment by an amount that matters clinically. If further large clinical trials are impossible or very difficult for practical or ethical reasons, a pragmatic treatment choice based on avoidance of the type-III error would seem to be the most rational way to use the information available.

References

Collins R, Langman M (1985) Treatment with histamine H2 antagonists in acute upper gastrointestinal hemorrhage. N Engl J Med 313: 660-666

Detsky AS, Sackett DL (1985) When was a 'negative' clinical trial large enough? Arch Intern Med 145: 709-712

Freiman JA, Thomas AB, Chalmers TC, Smith H, Keubler RR (1978) The importance of beta, the type-II error and sample size in the design and interpretation of the randomized controlled trial. N Engl J Med 299: 690-694

Gardner MJ, Altman DG (1986) Confidence intervals rather than *P* values: estimation rather than hypothesis testing. Br Med J 292: 746-750

Lachin JM (1981) Introduction to sample size determination and power analysis for clinical trials. Controlled Clin Trials 2: 93-113

Makuch RW, Johnson MF (1986) Some issues in the design and interpretation of 'negative' clinical studies. Arch Intern Med 146: 986-989

Powell-Tuck J, MacRae KD, Healy MJR, Lennard-Jones JE, Parkins RA (1986) A defence of the small clinical trial: evaluation of three gastroenterological studies. Br Med J 292: 599-602

Schwartz D, Lellouch R (1967) Explanatory and pragmatic attitudes in therapeutic trials. J Chronic Dis 20: 637-648

*A Predictive Approach to Selecting the Size of a Clinical Trial, Based on Subjective Clinical Opinion**

D. J. Spiegelhalter and L. S. Freedman**

MRC Biostatics Unit, 5 Shaftesbury Road, Cambridge CB2 2BW, Great Britain

Introduction

When planning a clinical trial to compare experimental therapy against a standard treatment or placebo, the choice of sample size necessarily involves some informal trade-off between the human and monetary resources available and the precision with which the organizers would ideally like to estimate the improvement from the new treatment, denoted by δ, as measured on a primary outcome scale. The formal part of this exercise, as described in many articles and textbooks, currently consists of estimating the 'power' of a proposed trial at a specified alternative hypothesis δ_A, where 'power' is generally understood to be the probability of rejecting the null hypothesis $\delta = 0$ (but in a two-sided test may be the probability of rejecting the null hypothesis *and* drawing the correct conclusion). If this power is judged insufficient, even with the maximum sample size available, then ideally the trial should not even be attempted.

In this paper we argue that there are a number of implicit and often arbitrary judgements in this apparently formal procedure, and that by making these subjective opinions explicit a more open and rational process can be established for selecting a sample size for a trial. In reviewing the published recommendations, we emphasize the ill-defined manner in which clinical *demands* and *expectations* of the new treatment are used in the specification of δ_A, and in the following section recommend the explicit measurement of these two aspects of clinical opinion: the former, when specified as a 'minimal clinically important difference', to be used as a null hypothesis; the latter, specified as a consensus prior distribution on the treatment difference, to be used as a basis for a subjective forecast of the trial results.

---

* This article is based on Spiegelhalter DJ, Freedman LS (1986) A predictive approach to selecting the size of a clinical trial, based on subjective clinical opinion. Stat Med 5: 1-13. With permission from John Wiley and Sons Ltd.

** We thank the chairman, Mr. Brian Richards, and members of the MRC subgroup on superficial bladder cancer for their whole-hearted collaboration. Professor Michael Healy, Dr. Jørgen Hilden, and Dr. Sheila Gore provided valuable comments.

Recent Results in Cancer Research, Vol. 111
© Springer-Verlag Berlin · Heidelberg 1988

This argument is illustrated with a multicentre trial currently taking place for which relevant clinical opinion has been elicited. The problems of reliable elicitation of subjective judgements are discussed, but we conclude by suggesting that this method should be appropriate to any group, whether a pharmaceutical company or a collaborative team of clinicians, who have an interest in ensuring that patients enter trials which are judged, by a formal analytic technique, as having reasonable potential to reach clinically important conclusions.

'Textbook' Approach to Selection of Sample Size

The crucial aspect in the selection of sample size is the alternative hypothesis δ_A, conditional on which the power of the trial is fixed at some value, usually 0.9, 0.8 or 0.5, depending on the perceived disadvantage of erroneously not rejecting the null hypothesis given that δ_A is true. A bewildering array of rather ill-defined recommendations is available concerning the specification of δ_A. Traditional textbooks give little guidance, suggesting that it is a difference 'worth detecting' (Fleiss 1981) or which 'you would not wish to overlook' (Armitage 1971). Others, possibly recognizing that a concept of 'clinical importance' places no upper bound on δ_A, specify that it should be the *smallest* clinically worthwhile difference (δ_w) (Lachin 1981; Spriet and Beiler 1979), but this is clearly not appropriate if *any* improvement at all is worthwhile (Pocock 1983). Others acknowledge that an upper bound on δ_A should be set at the 'maximum envisaged improvement' (Whitehead 1983), and that δ_A should lie somewhere between δ_w and this value; this corresponds to statements that the difference should be 'possible and important' (Brown 1980), 'realistic and worthwhile' (Gore 1981) or 'biologically important and capable of achievement' (Bulpitt 1983). Sometimes δ_A is explicitly specified only in terms of belief concerning the new treatment, as an 'expected' (Halperin et al. 1982) difference or one that 'might well exist' (Peto et al. 1976). Frequently, authors do not distinguish between 'anticipated' and 'clinically important' (Donner 1984) differences and for example, state that δ_A should 'reflect realistic expectations or goals' (Pocock 1983).

Overall, there is very little explicit guidance as to how to set δ_A, and in practice it seems likely that δ_A is juggled until it is set at a value that is reasonably plausible and yet detectable, given the available patients (Feinstein 1975). The minimal clinically worthwhile difference δ_w appears to have only two minor roles within this framework: firstly, if δ_w is not even plausible, then the trial is obviously pointless, and secondly, since δ_w is the minimal difference it is worthwhile trying to detect, it sets a (rather unnecessary) maximum on the sample size. However, in the next section we argue that, if we adopt a slightly different perspective on the aims of the trial, δ_w may take over the role of the null hypothesis.

Subjective Opinion and the Specification of a Null Hypothesis

It seems reasonable to assume that a collaborative group wishes to conduct studies that are judged likely to show results of *practical* value, in terms of identifying therapies that show sufficient superiority to make them the treatments of choice in at least a range of clinical practice. This in turn implies an approach to clinical trials described as 'pragmatic' by Schwartz, Flamant and Lellouch (1980) or as 'management' by Sackett and Gent (1979), in which the primary objective of a trial is to be able to make explicit recommendations concerning the treatment of patients in the future (Healy 1978). This view may influence the design and conduct of trials in a variety of ways, but here we are interested only in the specification of the null hypothesis. In particular, if the new treatment has some associated disadvantage (perhaps in terms of toxicity, cost, patient or doctor inconvenience) the point of therapeutic equivalence should not be set at $\delta = 0$ but at $\delta = \delta_w$, the smallest clinically worthwhile improvement necessary to recommend the new treatment: δ_w is the 'handicap' of Schwartz (Schwartz et al. 1980). For example, Levine (1982) has recently argued that testing a hypothesis of exactly equivalent survival in breast cancer is inappropriate when one treatment is markedly more unpleasant for the patient. This shift of the null hypothesis to a non-zero improvement has previously been discussed with regard to clinical trials which are to test the 'equivalence of treatments' (Blackwelder 1982, Dunnett and Gent 1977). However, we believe that this concept extends to many clinical trials which seek *differences* between, rather than the *equivalence* of, treatments (for an example, see below). Indeed, once one admits the general possibility of a shift in the null hypothesis, the distinction between 'equivalence'- and 'difference'-seeking trials largely disappears. We note also that Armitage (1984) has recently followed Meier (1975, 1979) in arguing the relevance of non-zero null hypotheses in group sequential designs.

In attempting to elicit the point of clinical equivalence in the context of the choice of stopping rules in sequential trials, it has been found (Freedman et al. 1983, 1984) that clinicians frequently identify a 'range of equivalence' above which the new treatment would be routinely adopted and below which the old. In this paper we consider only a single point, δ_w, below which the new treatment would not be regarded as worthwhile. The methodology we describe here could, however, be adapted to a range of equivalence.

Let us suppose that δ_w has been identified (possibly as $\delta_w = 0$) and that a trial of a maximum of n subjects is envisaged, at the termination of which an interval for the treatment difference will be formed. (Whether this is a confidence interval adjusted for interim analyses, an interval based purely on the likelihood, or a Bayesian credible interval based on a combination of the likelihood and a prior distribution, is irrelevant to our current discussion.) Taking our point of equivalence of the treatments at δ_w gives three possible results: the interval lies wholly below δ_w and we conclude that the new treatment is inferior, the interval contains δ_w and the trial is not conclusive, and the interval lies wholly above δ_w and we conclude that the new treatment is superior. (The precise interpretation given to these conclusions may again depend on one's 'ideological' viewpoint.) Before the trial starts we may calculate the probability of any of these conclusions *conditional* on a value for δ, and, for example, the probability of concluding that the new treatment is superior may be plotted as a function of δ, representing the 'power' of a test of the null hypothesis that $\delta = \delta_w$ against a one-sided alternative that $\delta > \delta_w$. However, unless we make some judgement about the *plausibility* of particular values of δ, the power curve itself gives us no guidance as to whether the sample size is sufficient.

Subjective Opinion and the Specification of the Alternative Hypothesis

Having calculated a power curve for an intended choice of sample size, a specific value δ_A is usually chosen and the power at this single value is considered. Having used the notion of a minimum clinically worthwhile difference to define the *null* hypothesis, it becomes clear that δ_A must be chosen on the grounds of plausibility alone. Since the actual value of δ may well be greater or less than δ_A, the choice of a specific δ_A may be thought of as a summary of the *distribution* of belief about the possible benefits of the new treatment. If this prior distribution were available and based on objective evidence such as a pilot trial, two options would present themselves:

1. δ_A could be defined as a somewhat arbitrarily chosen location parameter of the distribution (for example the mean, the median or the 70th percentile)
2. The *whole* distribution could be used instead of a single summary measure

In the latter case, the *average* power would provide an overall predictive probability of obtaining a 'significant' result, where the averaging is with respect to the prior distribution. There are advantages and disadvantages to these two options; choosing a summary measure δ_A is arbitrary and does not allow for the possibility that δ might be considerably more, or less, than δ_A. However, calculations are simple and the conventional framework remains familiar. Using the whole distribution leads to the nontrivial mathematical task of calculating average power. However, it avoids the arbitrary choice of δ_A and provides, through the averages power, a measure with a more direct predictive interpretation than conditional power. Whichever method is chosen, however, there remains the principle of using solely the notion of plausibility or belief for the determination of the power of a trial. In this paper we will explore our second avenue, using the whole prior distribution to calculate average power, first because of its novelty and second because we are attracted by the advantages mentioned above.

We would argue that either of the methods above is appropriate even if the prior distribution must be based on the consensus of subjective judgements of the expert clinicians involved in the study. This clearly makes the reliability of the predictive statements dependent on the skills of the doctors at expressing their uncertainty at an interview, and the problems involved in the process of elicitation and reaching a consensus are acknowledged later. Nevertheless, it is clear that subjective clinical beliefs are *implicit* in each of the approaches described, and by making these *explicit* we would hope for a more rational approach to the planning of trials.

We note a number of other suggestions for the use of prior opinion in the analysis of clinical trials: in the use of historical controls (Pocock 1976), in the assessment of subgroups (Donner 1982) and in bioequivalence studies (Selwyn et al. 1981). A full decision-theoretic framework for trials also demands an explicit statement of prior belief (Day 1969; Thompson 1981). From a design point of view, predictions based on subjective opinion have been recommended by Herson and colleagues (Herson 1979; Atkinson et al. 1982) in deciding stopping rules in phase-II studies and by McPherson (1982) in selecting numbers of interim analyses, and we have previously suggested the use of subjective opinion in sequential trials (Freedman and Spiegelhalter 1983); however, all of these reports retain an explicit alternative δ_A and entail an entirely standard analysis with no 'averaging' of power. In practice, quantitative clinical judgement does not appear to have been routinely incorporated into trial methodology.

The next section illustrates our argument in a common design of fixed sample size and normal likelihood, which is later illustrated with an example of a multi-centre trial. The ideas carry over into more complex designs, but these are not discussed here.

Mathematical Formulation of Predictions in a Common Trial Design

Non-mathematicians may omit this section without loss of understanding. Assume that a new treatment is to be compared with a standard treatment and let δ be the unknown true difference in response. The participants are considering a trial in which n responses are to be observed, and a statistic is calculated whose distribution is approximately normal. This formulation covers many common situations. In this paper we assume that even though prior opinion is available for the design of the trial, the results for communication will be based on the trial data alone.

After the n observations have been taken it is proposed to form an interval for the true value of δ. Thus, before a trial starts, the participants acknowledge that their conclusions will be based on a symmetrical random interval $(\underline{\Delta}, \overline{\Delta})$, and that the conclusion will be 'S' (new superior) if $\delta_w < \underline{\Delta}$, 'N' (no firm conclusion) if $\delta_w \; \varepsilon \; (\underline{\Delta}, \overline{\Delta})$, and 'I' (new inferior) if $\delta_w < \overline{\Delta}$.

We note that the symmetry of the interval is not a necessary ingredient of the argument. From any particular prior distribution the joint probability of any possible conclusion and its correctness or falsity may be calculated; for example, the probability of concluding that the new treatment is superior *and* of this being correct is denoted by P_{Ss}.

The notation for the other joint probabilities appears in Table 1. The quantities in Table 1 will generally be evaluated by approximating the prior distribution as a step function.

Various quantities may be used to summarize the properties of a proposed design: for example, P_{Ss} represents the predictive probability of correctly recom-

Table 1. Joint probability distribution of trial conclusions and underlying truth, based on prior probability distribution $p(\delta)$, where $P(\delta < \delta_w) = P_{\cdot i} = 1 - P_{\cdot s}$

		Truth		Total
		New inferior (i) $(\delta < \delta_w)$	New superior (s) $(\delta > \delta_w)$	
Conclusion:	New superior (S)	P_{Si}	P_{Ss}	$P_{S\cdot}$
	Noncommital (N)	P_{Ni}	P_{Ns}	$P_{N\cdot}$
	New inferior (I)	P_{Ii}	P_{Is}	$P_{I\cdot}$
	Total	$P_{\cdot i}$	$P_{\cdot s}$	1

mending a superior treatment, $P_{Ss}/P_{\cdot s}$ represents the probability of recommending a new treatment *given* that it is superior, and $P_{s\cdot}$ is the overall probability of recommending the new treatment whether it is appropriate or not. In general, P_{Si} and P_{Is} (the probabilities of the type-III errors of actually drawing firm but incorrect conclusions) will be small, and hence $P_{S\cdot}$ and P_{Ss} will be similar. Besides the type-III error, the remaining sort of trial 'failure' is a noncommital conclusion. When type-III probabilities are small, a useful measure of the trial design is therefore the probability $P_{N\cdot}$ of no firm conclusion.

In the next section we illustrate these theoretical ideas with data from a recent multicentre collaborative trial in bladder cancer.

An Example

The UK Medical Research Council (MRC) study of thiotepa in superficial bladder cancer is designed to compare three treatment policies: surgery (transurethral resection), surgery plus one immediate instillation of the drug thiotepa, and surgery plus five instillations at 3-month intervals. We shall concentrate on the comparison of the first two policies, for which δ measures the increase in 2-year recurrence-free rate from one instillation of thiotepa.

Eighteen participating urological surgeons were individually interviewed before the start of the trial. When asked about their *demands* for the new treatment, all of them stated that δ would need to be proved greater than zero before they would use thiotepa routinely, due to the increased inconvenience to the patient and clinic. Although some demanded considerable improvement (up to 20%), the average value was $\delta_W = 5\%$, and after group discussion this was selected as the minimum improvement at which thiotepa was worth considering.

Their *expectations* about the new treatment also varied considerably. When averaged over all 18 consultants the prior opinion shown in Fig. 1 emerged.

We note the skewness towards 'optimism'. There is only a 2% belief that the true difference lies below the 'classical' null hypothesis of zero, which taken by itself would suggest that it might be unreasonable to volunteer patients for a trial. However, the point of 'clinical equivalance' lies well within the prior distribution, which seems an ethically sound position from which to embark on a randomized study.

The test statistic is the difference in observed 2-year recurrence rates after each treatment has been given to n patients. Assuming the final inference is to be based upon a standard two-sided 95% interval for δ, we may calculate the power curves assuming a proposed sample size of $n = 150$. These are shown in Fig. 2, for null hypotheses of zero and 5%. We note, for example, that were the true difference to be, say, 10%, there would be a 40% chance of rejecting H_0: $\delta = 0$ in favour of the new treatment but only a 15% chance of rejecting the 'pragmatic' null hypothesis of $\delta_W = 5\%$.

However, over the range of plausible values of δ the power of the experiment varies considerably. Averaging the power curves with respect to the prior distribution of Fig. 1 provides the 'predictive' powers shown in Tables 2 and 3.

We see, for example, that the probability P_{Ss} of the new treatment being gen-

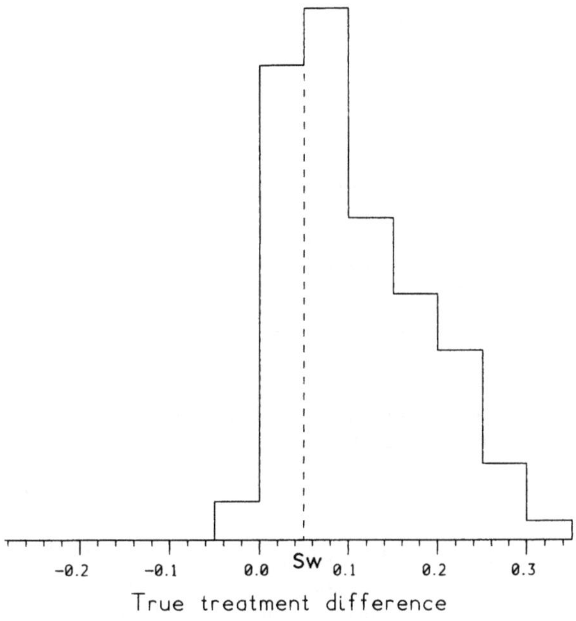

Fig. 1. Consensus prior opinion of 18 surgeons concerning the absolute improvement in 2-year recurrence-free rate over the baseline value of 50%

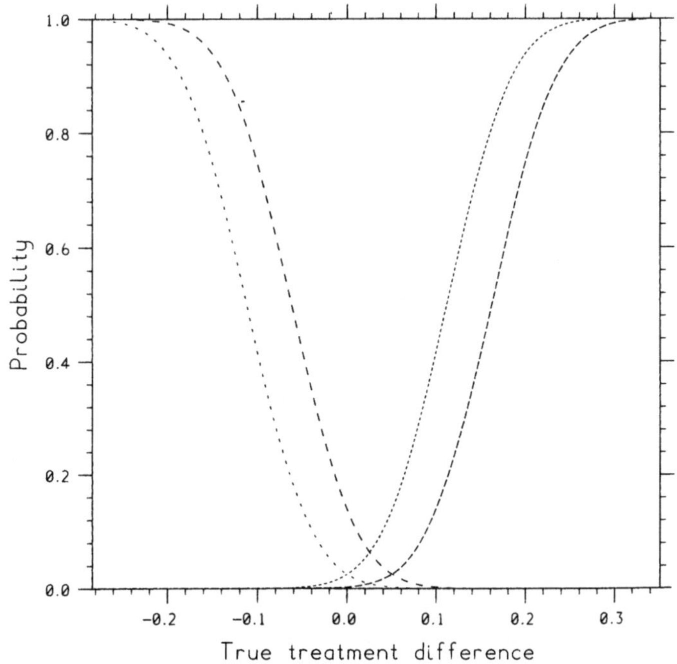

Fig. 2. Power of experiment to detect specified treatment differences ($\alpha=0.05$, $n=150$ in each group): -----, probability of concluding new is superior, H_0: $\delta=\delta_w=0.05$; ---, probability of concluding new is inferior, H_0: $\delta=\delta_w=0.05$; · · · · ·, probability of concluding new is superior, H_0: $\delta=0$; · · · · ·, probability of concluding new is inferior, H_0: $\delta=0$

Table 2. Joint probabilities of trial conclusions and the truth using a 'classical' null hypothesis of $\delta=0$, $n=150$

		Truth		
		New inferior ($\delta<0$)	New superior ($\delta>0$)	Total
Conclusion:	New superior	0.0002	0.450	0.450
	Noncommital	0.018	0.527	0.546
	New inferior	0.001	0.003	0.004
	Total	0.020	0.980	1.000

Table 3. Joint probabilities of trial conclusions and the truth using a 'pragmatic' null hypothesis of $\delta=0.05$, $n=150$

		New inferior ($\delta<0.05$)	New superior ($\delta>0.05$)	Total
Conclusion:	New superior	0.002	0.276	0.278
	Noncommital	0.245	0.451	0.696
	New inferior	0.023	0.003	0.026
	Total	0.270	0.730	1.000

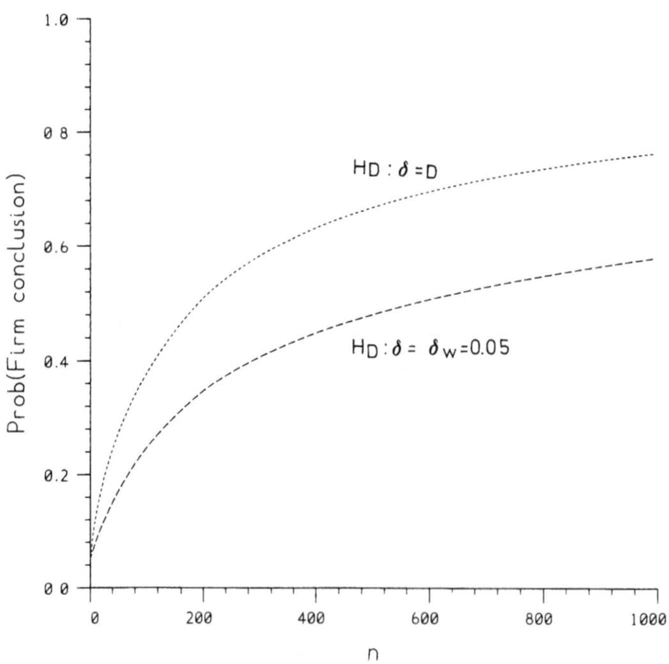

Fig. 3. Predictive probability of a trial with n in each group to reach a firm conclusion ($\alpha=0.05$, $\sigma=0.70$)

uinely clinically superior (i.e. $\delta > 0.05$) and of proving it in the trial is 0,276, whereas the probability $P_{Ss}/P_{.s}$ of asserting that the new treatment is superior *given* that this is a correct conclusion is $0.276/0.73 = 0.38$. The predicted probability of reaching no firm conclusion is 0.696. Repeating the analysis with σ set at the low value of 0.65 leads to a negligible change of this figure, to 0.67. For either choice of null hypothesis, the predictive probability of drawing a wrong conclusion (a type-III error) is extremely small.

It is useful to see how an increase in sample size affects the chance of reaching a firm conclusion. From Fig. 3 we see, for example, that given the prior opinion expressed in Fig. 1, sample sizes of 190 and 580 patients in each group are required to have a predicted probability of 50% of rejecting a hypothesis of 'no difference' and 5% difference respectively.

We may use Fig. 3 to investigate predictions of the consequences were a 'traditional' approach taken to selecting sample size. For example, taking a null hypothesis of zero and 'realistic and important' alternative hypotheses δ_A of 0.20, 0.15, and 0.10, the group sample sizes necessary to have 80% power are $n = 96$, 171, and 384 respectively, from which the clinicians would predict a probability of only 0.18, 0.25, and 0.40 of coming to a firm conclusion concerning treatment recommendations in practice.

Discussion

Our interest in this approach stems from our dissatisfaction with the currently reported procedure of setting a null and 'the arbitrary choice' (Feinstein 1975) of an alternative hypothesis, and our desire to see implicit judgements made explicit and accountable. However, in consequence we inevitably encounter the thorny problem of elicitation of individual opinion on clinical equivalence and, unless strong background evidence is available, subjective prior belief about the benefits of the new treatment.

Our techniques for eliciting a point of clinical equivalence and a prior distribution have been reported previously (Freedman and Spiegelhalter 1983) and involve a personal interview of each clinical participant lasting about 15 min. Clinical equivalence is investigated using iterative questioning and concentrates on the practical issue of whether, under varying treatment differences, the new treatment would definitely be used as routine in place of the standard. Prior opinion is assessed by eliciting a central and two outlying points of the distribution, sketching out a preliminary distribution curve and redrawing the curve in response to feedback from detailed interrogation of the clinician, in which every effort is made to prevent his 'anchoring' (Kahneman et al. 1982) to his initial opinions. The reasons the clinician provides for his opinion are also noted. After the interview, the final distribution is approximated by a step function and the group's distribution is taken to be the average of the individual clinicians' step functions. Similarly, the point of equivalence is averaged over the clinicians to give the group's consensus value.

An objection to using the point of equivalence in planning the study is that it is subjective and will vary between person, time and place. We acknowledge this but stress that using subjective information to plan a study is inevitable, since by definition adequate objective information does not exist. Our approach does not prevent the results from being reported in a 'classical' manner, using frequency or likelihood based interval estimates of the treatment difference.

There are well-known difficulties in the elicitation of realistic subjective probability distributions (Kahneman et al. 1982). In particular, a clinician may be 'overoptimistic,' in that his distribution is shifted too far towards the superiority of the innovative treatment, and 'overconfident', in that his distribution is too tight and does not reflect realistic doubt. Brown (1980) states that 'clinicians dream of spectacular new therapies, large leaps forward in efficacy,' whereas Gilbert et al. (1977) have claimed that 'although innovations in surgery and anaesthesia are successful [only] about half the time ... innovations brought to the stage of randomised trials are usually expected by the innovators to be sure winners.' In addition, since 'experienced adults are likely to overrate the preciseness of their estimates,' Gilbert and his colleagues conclude that one should 'discount the pretrial expectations or hunches of physicians and other investigators.'

Our view is not so sceptical. We agree with Hogarth (1970) that overconfidence is generally found in subjects who are naive about the subject matter, and among our experts we have found that most display considerable willingness to have wide 'unconfident' prior distributions. By careful elicitation many acknowledged biases may be avoided, but we do have the impression that some clinicians hold overoptimistic expectations of the benefits of new treatments. This potential bias is reduced by our current averaging procedure for reaching a consensus which tends to 'flatten out' the prior distribution, and hence helps to avoid undue influence by particularly optimistic or overconfident participants.

Even with these precautions, there are obviously problems with relying on formally elicited subjective prior judgement on which to base forecasts of the results of a trial. Not the least of these is the extra effort needed to formally elicit clinical opinion. In informal situations such as single-institution studies, this approach may seem overly fussy. Nevertheless, we feel that in the present climate of misunderstanding over the meaning of the alternative hypothesis, the introduction of some formality into the choice of sample size can only help to improve standards.

Once a prior distribution has been elicited, one may either choose the alternative hypothesis to be an arbitrary but well-defined summary measure of location of the distribution or use the whole distribution in a 'predictive' approach. We prefer the predictive approach for a number of reasons. Firstly, we do not see our predictive results as 'true,' but rather as an expression of implication: 'If you have a prior $p(\delta)$, then you must believe there is only an X% chance of reaching a firm recommendation from a trial of size n.' Secondly, the 'average' or predictive power is a direct measure of the chances of a trial yielding a firm recommendation and is simple to interpret.

Using either approach it would be possible, in many trials, to repeat the procedure at an interim stage of the trial when the prior distribution has been updated (and possibly overwhelmed) by 'hard' data and to make a firmer predictive statement; the use of 'average' power in this context appears preferable to the use of *conditional* power (Halperin et al. 1982; Andersen 1987; Spiegelhalter et al. 1986), if the values of δ at which the power is assessed are fixed at pretrial values which may no longer be particularly plausible given the interim results. Moreover, we hope that by repeatedly presenting our clients with comparisons between their predictions and the actual results of trials, we can slowly train at least one group of clinicians to be realistic probability assessors in their area of expertise; this has been achieved among U.S. weather forecasters (Murphy and Winkler 1977).

Finally, we have found that the process of interviewing participants about their demands and expectations has been valuable in its own right: the clinicians frequently voice the opinion that, although a difficult exercise, it made them think more deeply about the forthcoming trial than they had previously, whereas statisticians gain insight into the medical background to the trial. Conducting a series of interviews with a group of clinicians is costly in terms of the statisticians' and clinicians' time and effort. However, we believe that the benefits, both direct and indirect, will more than repay the initial outlay.

References

Andersen PK (1987) Conditional power calculations as an aid in the decision whether to continue a clinical trial. Controlled Clin Trials 8: 67-74

Armitage P (1971) Statistical methods in medical research. Blackwell, Oxford

Armitage P (1984) Controversies and achievements in clinical trials. Controlled Clin Trials 5: 67-72

Atkinson EN, Brown BW, Herson J (1987) KSTAGE: an interactive computer program for designing phase-II clinical trials using predictive probability. Comp Biomed Res 15: 220-227

Blackwelder WC (1982) Proving the null hypothesis in clinical trials. Controlled Clin Trials 3: 345-353

Brown BW (1980) Statistical controversies in the design of clinical trials - some personal views. Controlled Clin Trials 1: 13-28

Bulpitt CJ (1983) Randomised controlled clinical trials. Nijhoff, The Hague

Day NE (1969) Two-stage designs for clinical trials. Biometrics 25: 111-118

Donner A (1982) A Bayesian approach to the interpretation of subgroup results in clinical trials. Chronic Dis 35: 429-435

Donner A (1984) Approaches to sample size estimation in the design of clinical trials - a review. Stat Med 3: 199-214

Dunnett CW, Gent M (1977) Significance testing to establish equivalence between treatments, with special reference to data in the form of 2 × 2 tables. Biometrics 33: 593-602

Feinstein AR (1975) Clinical biostatistics XXXIV. The other side of statistical significance, alpha, beta, delta and the calculation of sample size. Clin Pharmacol Ther 18: 491-505

Fleiss JL (1981) Statistical methods for rates and proportions, 2nd edn. Wiley, New York

Freedman LS, Spiegelhalter DJ (1983) The assessment of subjective opinion and its use in relation to stopping rules for clinical trials. Statistician 33: 153-160

Freedman LS, Lowe D, Macaskill P (1984) Stopping rules for clinical trials incorporating clinical opinion. Biometrics 40: 575-586

Freedman LS, Lowe D, Macaskill P (1983) Stopping rules for clinical trials. Stat Med 2: 167-174

Gilbert JP, McPeek B, Mosteller F (1977) Statistics and ethics in surgery and anaesthesia. Science 198: 684-689

Gore SM (1981) Assessing clinical trials - trial size. Br Med J 282: 1687-1689

Halperin M, Lam KKG, Ware JH, Johnson NJ, DeMets PL (1982) An aid to data monitoring in long-term clinical trials. Controlled Clin Trials 3: 311-323

Healy MJR (1978) New methodology in clinical trials. Biometrics 34: 709-712

Herson J (1979) Predictive probability early termination plans for phase-II clinical trials. Biometrics 35: 775-783
Hogarth RM (1970) Cognitive processes and the assessment of subjective probability distributions. J Am Stat Assoc 70: 271-289
Kahneman D, Slovic P, Tversky A (1982) Judgement under uncertainty: heuristics and biases. Cambridge University Press, London
Lachin JM (1981) Introduction to sample size determination and power analysis for clinical trials. Controlled Clin Trials 2: 93-114
Levine RJ (1982) Ethical aspects of clinical trials. In: Mike V, Stanley KF (eds) Statistics in medical research. Wiley, New York, pp 164-168
McPherson K (1982) On choosing the number of interim analyses in clinical trials. Stat Med 1: 25-36
Meier P (1975) Statistics and medical experimentation. Biometrics 31: 511-529
Meier P (1979) Terminating a trial - the ethical problem. Clin Pharmacol Ther 25: 633-640
Murphy AH, Winkler RL (1977) Reliability of subjective probability forecasts of precipitation and temperature. Appl Stat 26: 41-47
Peto R, Pike MC, Armitage P, Breslow NE, Cox DR, Howard SV, Mantel N, McPherson K, Peto J, Smith PG (1976) Design and analysis of randomised clinical trials requiring prolonged observation of each patient. I. Introduction and design. Br J Cancer 34: 585-612
Pocock SJ (1976) The combination of randomised and historical controls in clinical trials. J Chronic Dis 29: 175-188
Pocock SJ (1983) Clinical trials: a practical approach. Wiley, Chichester
Sackett DL, Gent M (1979) Controversy in counting and attributing events in clinical trials. N Engl J Med 301: 1410-1412
Selwyn MR, Dempster AP, Hall NR (1981) A Bayesian approach to bioequivalence for the 2 × 2 changeover design. Biometrics 37: 345-353
Schwartz D, Flamant R, Lellouch J (1980) Clinical trials. Academic, London
Spiegelhalter DJ, Freedman LS, Blackburn PR (1986) Monitoring clinical trials: conditional or predictive power? Controlled Clin Trials 7: 8-17
Spriet A, Beiler D (1979) When can "nonsignificantly different" teratments be considered as "equivalent"? Br J Clin Pharmacol 7: 623-624
Thompson MS (1981) Decision-analytic determination of study size. The case of electronic fetal monitoring. Med Decis Making 1: 165-179
Whitehead J (1983) The design and analysis of sequential clinical trials. Ellis Horwood, Chichester

Statistical Properties and Use of Sequential Methods in Randomized Clinical Trials when the Response Criterion Is Censored

J. Bénichou and C. Chastang

Départment de Biostatistique et Informatique Médicale, Hôpital Saint-Louis, 1 av Claude Vellfaux, 75475 Paris Cédex 10, France

Introduction

In diseases such as cancer and more generally chronic conditions randomized clinical trials often use time to occurrence of a given event as the main response criterion. Survival time, i. e., time to death, is the most widely used of such criteria. Other examples include disease-free interval, duration of a remission period, or time to occurrence of a thrombosis. Such criteria are termed "censored' because at the time the analysis is performed the event has not been observed for each patient in the trial.

Stopping rules represent a major ethical problem in these trials, since the time to occurrence of an event is long. The fixed-sample design (George and Desu 1974; Rubinstein et al. 1981; Freedman 1982) requires that only one analysis be performed after a given number of events D is observed. This number is computed to ensure a size α, usually 5%, and a power $1\text{-}\beta$ for a given alternative hypothesis of treatment effect. This procedure delays the analysis for a long time after the beginning of the trial, usually several years. Therefore, it is common practice to perform interim analyses. Supported by ethical motivations, their objective is to stop the trial early if a treatment effect is detected or alternatively if it appears that there is no treatment effect. But such repeated testing increases the probability α of wrongly rejecting the null hypothesis: for example, this probability becomes 14% if five analyses are performed at the usual 5% level (Pocock 1978).

The use of a more conservative nominal level α has been proposed for each interim analysis to ensure an overall level of α. One still plans an analysis after D events according to the fixed-sample design, but interim analyses at a level α' are performed before D events and the conclusion is reached if a significant difference is observed. Otherwise, the trial goes on until the final analysis after D events are observed (Pocock 1983). This hybrid approach combines interim analyses at a level α' and then, if they are not conclusive, a final analysis at a level α as in the fixed-sample design. Also, it does not allow early stopping if there is no treatment difference. Finally, power calculations are made for the final analysis but not for the interim analyses.

© Springer-Verlag Berlin · Heidelberg 1988

For these reasons, it seems preferable to use truly sequential methods, which are designed to allow for repeated testing. Armitage (1975) described various methods. They are not suited to censored data because, first, they depend on response criteria being available in a short time and, second, patients need to be matched and analyzed in pairs. This implies very frequent analyses, which are not feasible in view of the practical difficulties with updating the patients' data, particularly in large multicenter trials.

Three sequential methods for which patient pairing is not necessary have been introduced more recently: group sequential analysis (Pocock 1977), the sequential probability ratio test (Whitehead 1983), and the triangular test (Whitehead 1983). They will be described in the following section. Thereafter, their properties for finite samples based on a simulation study (Bénichou and Chastang 1986a) will be recalled and the advantages of the triangular test will be underlined. Next, the application of the triangular test to three trials will be presented. The statistical properties will then be discussed, as well as the practical implementation of the triangular test in designing and analyzing randomized clinical trials with a censored response criterion.

Description of the Sequential Methods

For the three sequential methods - group sequential analysis, the sequential probability ratio test, and the triangular test - the stopping rules depend, as with the fixed-sample design, on the choice of the size α, the power $1-\beta$, and an alternative hypothesis of treatment effect. In addition, they depend on the frequency of the analyses which have to be performed after every D new events. Accrual of new patients goes on until a conclusion is reached.

Group sequential analysis (Pocock 1977) is based on repeated testing with a conservative nominal level $\alpha' < \alpha$. Full use of this method implies that the number of analyses N not be fixed in advance. Rather, the number of analyses N and the nominal level α' depend on the choice of α, β, and the alternative hypothesis. Contrary to the procedure described in the introduction, a truly sequential design is used here and there is no coexistence between interim analyses and a fixed-sample approach. Tables give α' and N for two-sided testing (Pocock 1977) and one-sided testing (DeMets and Ware 1980). This method was initially proposed for a continuous uncensored response criterion normally distributed with analyses after every group of $2n$ patients. It has been extended to other criteria such as binary criteria and exponentially distributed criteria. Pocock (1977) suggested the extension to censored criteria and Gail et al. (1982) studied it by simulation by using the log-rank test at equally spaced numbers of events (and not of patients recruited). For two-sided tests and with $N = 5$, they showed that the simple normal model leads to reliable prediction of size, power, and average number of groups examined (i.e., average number of analyses).

Both the sequential probability ratio test and the triangular test use sequential plans adapted to the log-rank statistic. Boundaries are computed when the trial is designed. Every D new events, the log-rank statistic is plotted as a function of its variance, and the conclusion is reached when the sample path crosses a boundary.

For instance, if one-sided testing is used, then the null hypothesis is rejected when the upper boundary is crossed. As the sequential probability ratio test uses an open plan, the sample size is potentially infinite, in contrast to the triangular test, which uses a closed plan. The asymptotic properties of the two methods for a continuous inspection of the data were given by Whitehead (1983), showing a reduction of the expected number of events compared with the fixed-sample design whatever the true difference between the two treatments. Simulations for simultaneous entry of the patients and using the modified Wilcoxon test showed close agreement with the asymptotic results for the sequential probability ratio test (Jones and Whitehead 1979). As for the triangular test, only the comparison of two proportions has been investigated (Whitehead and Stratton 1983) by simulation.

Simulation Study of the Three Sequential Methods

Since the extension of group sequential analysis to a censored response criterion had been studied only for two-sided testing and $N=5$, and, on the other hand, only asymptotic properties of the sequential probability ratio test and of the triangular test for a continuous inspection of the data were available, we carried out a simulation study of the three methods (Bénichou and Chastang 1986b). Our purpose was to compare them with each other and with the fixed-sample design for finite samples and a discrete inspection of the data (i.e., analyses after every D new events).

Denoting by δ the hazard ratio between the treatment groups we considered three situations in terms of the hazard ratio δ_a under the alternative hypothesis chosen to design the trial and δ *t*, the true hazard ratio, unknown of course when designing the trial: (a) $\delta_t=1$ (that is H_o is true); (b) $\delta_t\neq$ and $\delta_t=\delta_a$; (c) $\delta_t>1$ and δ_t/δ_a. We used one-sided testing. We found that the three sequential methods have the desired statistical properties. Repeated testing does not lead to an increase in α, and the power is the same as with the fixed-sample design.

Furthermore, they allow early stopping, except for group sequential analysis when δ_t is close to 1, i.e., when there is no or a minimal treatment difference. Both the sequential probability ratio test and the triangular test allow on average early stopping compared with the fixed-sample design whatever the treatment difference, but the sequential probability ratio test can lead to long duration trials because it uses open boundaries. For these reasons, the triangular test appears to be the optimal method.

Moreover, we studied the influence of the frequency of the analyses on the properties of the methods with additional simulations (Bénichou and Chastang 1986b). One can perform sequential analyses at the same frequency as the usual interim analyses without altering the statistical properties of the methods. Indeed, if one is looking for an improvement in one treatment group such that the median survival time is more than doubled ($\delta_a>2.0$), then analyses can be performed as rarely as after every 20 new events. If a smaller improvement is of interest ($\delta_a\leqslant$ 2.0), then analyses can be performed even more rarely, after up to every 40 new events. We gave tables (Bénichou and Chastang 1986b) to set the dates of the analyses depending on the expected median survival times in the two treatment groups and on the accrual rate. For instance, if one is looking for an improvement of 75% of the median survival time in one treatment group, from 1 year to 1.75 years, and if the expected accrual rate is 100 patients a year, the analyses can be performed after every 40 new events and the first four analyses should thus occur after 17, 25, 32, and 39 months.

Application of the Triangular Test to Three Trials

A trial in nonresectable lung cancer has been designed and analyzed using the triangular test (Jones et al. 1982; Whitehead et al. 1983). We will recall the main statistical findings of this trial and then apply the triangular test to the analysis of two trials, one in resected lung cancer and one in chronic lymphocytic leukemia.

Trial in Nonresectable Lung Cancer

In the trial reported by Jones and Whitehead, a standard treatment (radiotherapy alone) was compared with a new treatment (radiotherapy associated with a chemotherapy, namely Razoxane) for patients with nonresectable lung cancer. The authors chose a size α of 5% and a 90% power of detecting a 25% improvement of the median survival time from 6 to 7.5 months when designing the trial. Analyses were performed every $D=12$ new deaths. After the eighth analysis (104 deaths), the sample path crossed the lower boundary so that the null hypothesis could not be rejected. No improvement was shown with the new treatment. In this trial, the triangular test allowed a very early conclusion, since the fixed sample design would have required 688 deaths before performing the analysis.

Immunotherapy Trial in Resectable Lung Cancer

The aim of this trial was to evaluate a nonspecific adjuvant immunotherapy with a mycobacterium *(Mycobacterium smegmatis)*. After surgery, patients were randomized between this treatment (immunotherapy group) and no treatment (control group). The fixed-sample approach was used to design the trial. With $\alpha=5\%$ and to show an improvement of the 1-year survival rate with the immunotherapy from 60% to 80% with a 90% power, the analysis had to be performed after 50 deaths, i.e., the accrual of 182 patients in 2.3 years (for an accrual rate of 80 patients/year). From March 1, 1978, to April 1, 1981, 219 patients entered this trial. The analysis at the end of the accrual period showed no significant difference between the two treatment groups $\chi^2=0.03$, $P=0.43$), even though more deaths than expected (82) had been observed by that time (Decroix et al. 1984). The patients were followed-up till April 1, 1985, and by that time 132 deaths had been observed, with only two patients lost to follow-up. Again, with these data no significant difference is observed between the two groups, $\chi^2=0.25$, $P=0.31$), as shown in Fig. 1a.

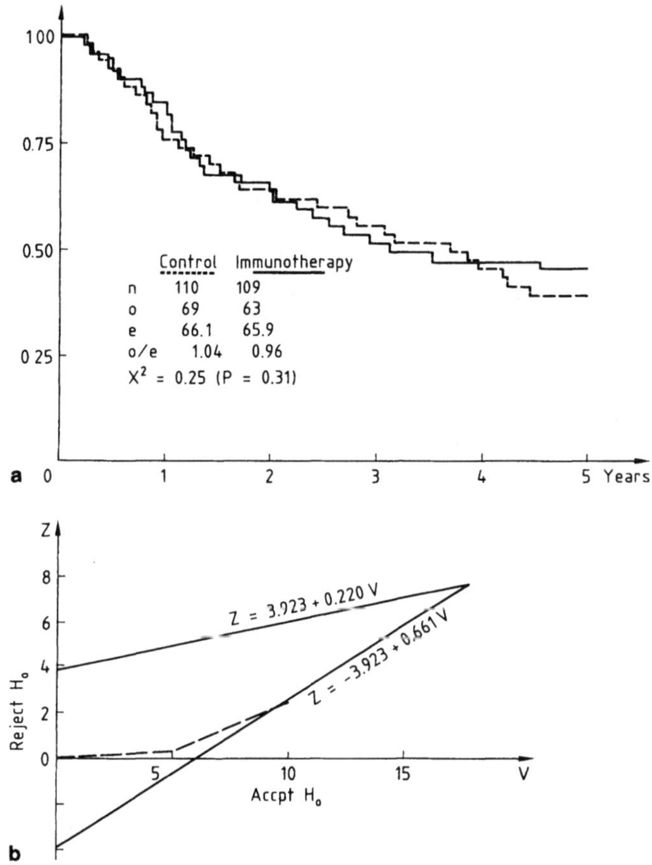

Fig. 1a, b. Trial in nonresectable lung cancer. **a** Survival curves according to treatment at the reference date of April 1, 1985. **b** Triangular test with sequential analyses performed after every 20 deaths

The triangular test can be applied to these data using the same values for α, $1\text{-}\beta$, and the treatment benefit as with the fixed-sample design. Since the treatment benefit under the alternative hypothesis corresponds to more than doubling the median survival time with the immunotherapy treatment, analyses can be performed after every 20 new deaths. If this is done, the triangular test reaches the conclusion after two analyses (40 deaths), i.e., after the entry of 162 patients in 1.7 years (Fig. 1b). Since the sample path crosses the lower boundary, the null hypothesis is not rejected; no improvement is shown with the immunotherapy treatment. This is the same conclusion as was actually reached using the fixed-sample design. But it is reached earlier and with a clear stopping rule planned in advance. It is of some interest to note that using the same hypotheses, the two other sequential methods (group sequential analysis and the sequential probability ratio test) would have reached the conclusion after three analyses (60 deaths) and the entry of 187 patients in 2.2 years.

Trial in Chronic Lymphocytic Leukemia

We applied the triangular test to the analysis of a trial in advanced-stage chronic lymphocytic leukemia (Binet et al. 1981; French Cooperative Group on Chronic Lymphocytic Leukemia 1986). For the poor-prognosis stage, i.e., stage C, the median survival time was 18 months. Two polychemotherapies, namely COP (cyclophosphamide, vincristine, prednisone) and CHOP (COP plus doxorubicin) were compared. With a size $\alpha = 5\%$ and a 90% power to observe an improvement in the 1-year survival from 60% to 80% with the CHOP regime ($\delta\ a = 2.29$), 50 deaths were required before the analyses could be performed, i.e., the accrual of 89 patients in 6.4 years, according to the George and Desu method (fixed sample design).

The protocol was activated on May 27, 1980. The first interim analysis on May 1, 1984, with only four patients lost to follow-up, dealt with 59 stage-C patients; 21 deaths were observed. A significant improvement was shown with the

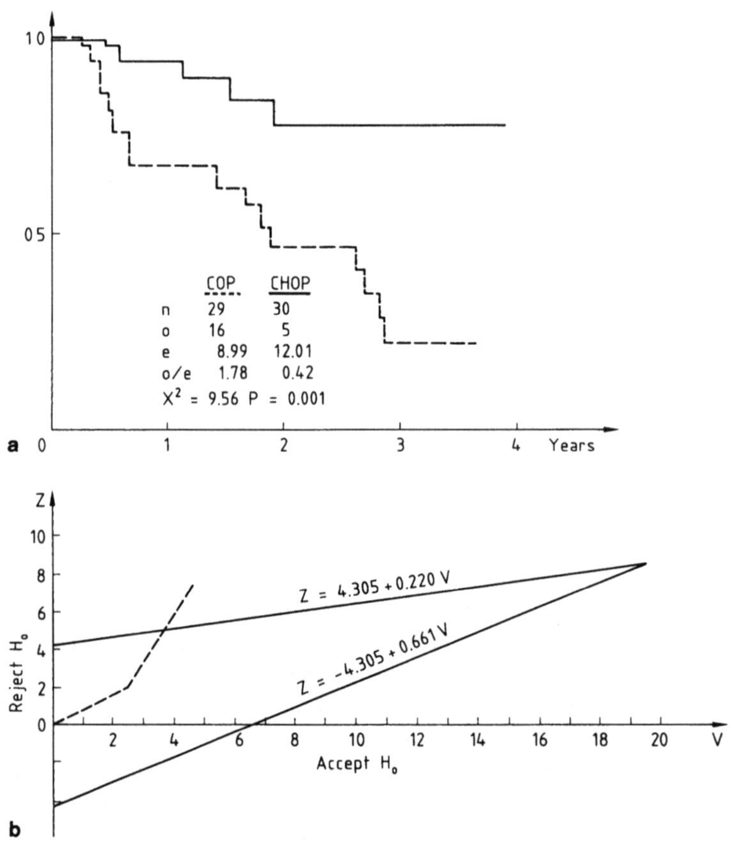

Fig. 2 a, b. Trial in chronic lymphocytic leukemia (stage C). **a** Survival curves according to treatment at the reference date of May 1, 1984. **b** Triangular test with sequential analyses performed after every ten deaths

CHOP regime ($\chi^2=9.56$, $P=0.001$), as shown in Fig. 2a. This led to an early stopping of the trial.

The triangular test can be applied to these data using the same values for α, 1-β, and the alternative hypothesis. With analyses after every ten new deaths, the conclusion in favor of the CHOP treatment would have been reached after the second analysis and the accrual of 56 patients in 3.7 years. As seen in Fig. 2b, the sample path would have crossed the higher boundary. Thus, in this situation, where the two treatments differ, the triangular test allows an early conclusion. Compared with what actually happened (conclusion after the first interim analysis), the conclusion with the triangular test would have taken place at about the same time, but with the important advantage of a rigorous planning of the analyses and of a stopping rule stated in advance and with no ambiguity.

Discussion

The sequential methods presented here are simple to implement since the stopping rules depend only on the choice of the size α, the power 1-β, an alternative hypothesis of treatment effect, and the frequency of the analyses. They use a clear stopping rule stated in advance.

The three methods have nominal size and power. The triangular test appears to be optimal, since it allows early stopping whatever the difference between the two treatment groups and without the risk of long trial duration. In addition, the frequency of the analyses does not have to be higher than for the usual interim analyses.

It must be noted that improvements of group sequential analysis have been recently proposed. They include a varying nominal significance level (O'Brien and Fleming 1979), a procedure which has recently been improved by Wang and Tsiatis (1987) to reduce the sample size under the alternative hypothesis. Other approaches to repeated testing have been used, such as Bayesian approaches (Spiegelhalter and Freedman 1986) or stochastic curtailing (Lan et al. 1982). It would be of interest to compare these procedures, as well as the "optimal" group sequential analysis of Wang and Tsiatis (1987), with the triangular test.

As to the practical use of the triangular test, two main points have to be made here. First, since the boundaries depend on the frequency of the analyses, it is important to stay close to the planned frequency in order not to alter the statistical properties. Second, the time required to update the data must be shortened as much as possible in order to maintain the advantage of early stopping. As an example, it took 20 months to update the data of the first interim analysis of the CLL 80 trial - which was not designed with a sequential method - from the reference date of May 1st, 1984. To achieve these two goals (frequency of the analyses and updating of the data) a careful follow-up of the patients has to be planned in the protocol with regular recall of the patients in the trial. This is not such an important additional effort in chemotherapy trials where patients have to come to the clinical centers on a regular basis to receive their treatment.

Other practical problems are not proper to the sequential methods; these include the use of a main response criterion to define the stopping rule and the necessary confidentiality of the sequential analyses.

In addition to performing sequential analyses after every D new events, it appears useful to plan less frequent but more extensive analyses to study other response criteria, side effects, compliance, etc. When the conclusion is reached, the terminal analysis can be more detailed, taking into account for instance prognostic information. Finally, it is of interest to follow up the patients after the formal conclusion of the trial to learn about the course of the disease and to check that a difference in favor of one treatment group does not vanish or change with time, which could be observed in case of nonproportional hazards.

References

Armitage P (1975) Sequential medical trials, 2nd edn. Blackwell, Oxford

Bénichou J, Chastang Cl (1986a) A simulation study of three sequential methods for the comparison of two treatment groups, when the response criterion is censored. Stat Med 5: 375-385

Bénichou J, Chastang Cl (1986b) Mise en oeuvre de méthodes séquentielles dans les essais thérapeutiques randomisés dont le critère de jugement est censuré. Rev Epidemiol Sante Publique 34 (3): 196-208

Binet JL, Auquier A, Dighiero G, Chastang Cl, Piguet H, Cosguen J, Vaugier G, Potron G, Colona P, Oberling F, Thomas M, Tchernia G, Jacquillat Cl, Boivin P, Lesty C, Duault MT, Monconduit M, Belabbes S, Grémy F (1981) A new prognostic classification of chronic lymphocytic leukemia derived from a multivariate analysis. Cancer 48: 198-206

Decroix G, Chastang Cl, Fichet D, Asselain B, Lebeau B, Morice V, Lepage T, Babo P, Fabre C, Rebishung JL, Accard JL, Hinault G, Sauvaget J, Rochemaure J, Soubrane Cl, Jagueux M, Toty L, Herzog P, Daumet P, Grosset J, Grémy F (1984) Adjuvant immunotherapy with nonviable *Mycobacterium smegmatis* in resected primary lung carcinoma. Cancer 53 (4): 906-912

DeMets DL, Ware JM (1980) Group sequential methods for clinical trials with a one-sided hypothesis. Biometrika 67: 651-660

Freedman LS (1982) Tables of the number of patients required in clinical trials using the log-rank test. Stat Med 1: 121-129

French Cooperative Group on Chronic Lymphocytic Leukemia (1986) Effectiveness of CHOP regimen in advanced untreated chronic lymphocytic leukemia. Lancet 1: 1346-1349

Gail MH, DeMets DL, Slud EV (1982) Simulation studies on increments of two-sample log-rank score test for survival data, with application to group sequential boundaries. In: Johnson R, Crowley J (eds) Survival analysis monograph series 2, IMS lecture notes. Hayward, CA

George SL, Desu MM (1974) Planning the size and duration of a clinical trial studying the time to some critical event. J Chronic Dis 27: 15-29

Jones DR, Whitehead J (1979) Sequential forms of the log-rank and modified Wilcoxon test for censored data. Biometrika 66: 105-113

Jones DR, Newman CE, Whitehead J (1982) The design of a sequential clinical trial for the comparison of two lung cancer treatments. Stat Med 1: 73-82

Lan KKG, Simon R, Halperin N (1982) Stochastically curtailed tests in long-term clinical trials. Commun Stat Sequential Anal 1: 207-219

O'Brien PC, Fleming TR (1979) A multiple testing procedure for clinical trials. Biometrics 35: 549-556

Pocock SJ (1977) Group sequential methods in the design and analysis of clinical trials. Biometrika 64: 191-199

Pocock SJ (1978) The size of cancer clinical trials and stopping rules. Br J Cancer 38: 757-766

Pocock SJ (1983) Clinical trials. A practical approach. Wiley, Chichester

Rubinstein LV, Gail MH, Santner TJ (1981) Planning the duration of a comparative clinical trial with loss to follow-up and a period of continued observations. J Chronic Dis 34: 469-479

Wang SK, Tsiatis AA (1987) Approximately optimal one-parameter boundaries for group sequential trials. Biometrics 43: 193-199

Whitehead J (1983) The design and analysis of sequential clinical trials. Horwood, Chichester

Whitehead J, Stratton I (1983) Group sequential clinical trials with triangular continuation regions. Biometrics 39: 227-236

Whitehead J, Jones DR, Ellis SH (1983) The analysis of a sequential clinical trial for the comparison of two lung cancer treatments. Stat Med 2: 183-190

Assessment of Quality of Life

Measurement of Quality of Life in Clinical Trials of Therapy

A. E. Fletcher

Epidemiology Research Unit, Division of Geriatrics, Royal Postgraduate Medical School, Hammersmith Hospital, Du Cane Road, London W12, Great Britain

Introduction

Over the past few years there has been an increasing interest among industrialised societies in the use of Quality-of-Life methods to evaluate therapies. With the decline of infectious diseases, and with cancer and cardiovascular diseases becoming major causes of mortality and morbidity, this interest has emerged in response to a shift in emphasis of the goals of treatment from a traditional primary curative aim.

A variety of therapeutic situations illustrate the need for a wider perspective on the impact of treatment. In the treatment of advanced cancer there is clearly a balance between small improvements in survival and the drastic sequelae of cytotoxic drugs. At the other end of the spectrum, the benefits of long-term treatment of hypertension are a balance between the costs of treatment side effects in a previously asymptomatic individual and the magnitude of the reduction in risk of a cardiovascular event. Indeed, the high dropout rates documented in many trials of mild and moderate hypertension suggest that patients withdraw from treatment because of an unacceptable level of side effects. For example, after 5 years of the Medical Research Council trial of mild-to-moderate hypertension (Medical Research Council Working Party on Mild to Moderate Hypertension 1976), 16% of patients on active treatment had withdrawn compared with less than 5% on placebo. Gout, impotence, impaired glucose tolerance, lethargy, nausea, dizziness and headache were the major reasons for withdrawal. Active treatment was discontinued in 9% of patients for definite side effects over the 5 years of the Hypertension Detection Follow-up Programme (Curb et al. 1985) and in a further 23% for possible side effects. Eight percent of all male patients discontinued treatment because of sexual problems. Lethargy, drowsiness, dizziness and minor gastrointestinal symptoms were the most common reasons for discontinuation (4%–6% of patients). Moreover, patients who discontinued treatment include those with a high risk of a cardiovascular event; 11% had a diastolic blood pressure of 115 mm Hg or greater.

It is clear, therefore, that there is a need to measure both benefits and adverse effects of treatment. Coronary artery bypass graft surgery (CABG) has not been shown to have a major impact on survival (Hampton 1984). The adverse effects of CABG include an increased risk of myocardial infarction, stroke and other neurol-

Recent Results in Cancer Research, Vol. 111
© Springer-Verlag Berlin · Heidelberg 1988

ogical morbidity. In many chronic diseases the goals of treatment are the alleviation of symptoms and the restoration of function. Traditional methods of measuring improvements in function, such as exercise stress tests in angina and congestive heart failure, may be poor proxies for the patient's daily activities in work and leisure. The Quality-of-Life approach, by considering the impact of disease and treatment on an individual's emotional, social and physical wellbeing, provides a more comprehensive assessment of treatment outcome. Quality-of-Life measurements can be used both to *describe* the quality of life of patients with a disease, and so suggest possible areas for intervention, and to *evaluate* the impact of treatment. The selection of appropriate measurements will be influenced by whether the study is descriptive or evaluative. In the former case, the measurement must be able to discriminate between patients and a control group, in order to describe differences, while an evaluative measurement must be capable of detecting change. For example, Activities of Daily Living Indices (ADLs) measure a patient's performance in various everyday activities, such as self-care and mobility, and can describe the areas of limitations for patients disabled by a stroke (Deyo 1984). The use of ADLs in studies assessing the benefit of rehabilitation for stroke patients has provided inconsistent and conflicting results (Lind 1982). It is likely that ADLs are unable to reflect changes other than gross ones.

In this article we will discuss some of the issues involved in the use of Quality-of-Life methods to *evaluate* treatment. We will consider what aspects of patients' lives should be measured and how these aspects may be measured, using examples of some available methods. We will also discuss trial design and analysis and interpretation of results.

What Should Be Measured?

The choice of aspects to measure will be influenced by many factors.

Disease State

The severity, prognosis and age distribution of patients with the disease will exclude some aspects. For example, patients with severe congestive heart failure or those who have suffered a stroke are unlikely to be working or leading physically active lives. However, performance at work would be an important choice for patients with a milder disability. Return to work has often been used to evaluate coronary artery bypass graft surgery. The results, however, have shown that this was influenced by many factors other than clinical improvement, such as preoperative employment, age and the patients' own perceptions of their limitations (Smith et al. 1983). Body image and self-esteem would be important aspects to measure in a trial of breast cancer treatment (Bransfield 1982). Sexual function is affected by many diseases or their treatments. This may be due to surgical procedures such as for gynaecological, prostate or rectal cancers (Vera 1981; Leibel et al. 1980; Williams and Johnston 1983), or to drug therapy, for example, in hypertension (Bulpitt 1982).

Psychological wellbeing should always be measured, not only as an important area in itself, but also because of its influence on response to other areas. Various symptoms have been shown to be more prevalent with either anxiety or depression (Bulpitt et al. 1974). Several studies have suggested that long-term sexual problems in patients who have recovered from a stroke may be due to depression rather than to physical incapacity (Sjogren 1983; Sjogren et al. 1983). Moreover, loss of libido after surgery in breast cancer patients may be associated more with depression than with bodily disfigurement (Fallowfield et al. 1986).

Length of the Trial

In certain areas of Quality of Life, the impact of treatment may not be apparent for several months. Major changes in behaviour are unlikely to occur for some time in patients who have already adapted their life style to a chronic disability. For example, a change in parental occupation is unlikely to occur during a 6-month trial of children with severe chronic eczema, even if a benefit of treatment results in fewer hospital visits and days off school. Conversely, a treatment may produce an immediate effect on a patient's life style which is not sustained over a longer period. For example, cardiac transplant and CABG patients showed a great improvement in various measures of Quality of Life 3 months after surgery (Wallwork and Caine 1985). The scores 1 year after the operation showed that this improvement was maintained with little change from the 3 month scores. However, 1-year scores were available for only 50% of patients. Those with deteriorating health may have been excluded.

Expected Benefits or Adverse Effects of Treatment

In many diseases, changes may be expected to occur only in certain areas of quality of life. Clearly, it is a burden on patients to include questions on aspects of their lives which will not be affected by treatment. The problem lies in deciding on relevant areas. Pilot studies, clinical experience and patients' own expectations will aid in making the choice.

Availability of Methods

Pragmatic considerations also influence the choice of areas to investigate. Questionnaires describing certain areas may not be available, or they may be unsuitable for certain diseases. Other considerations include time available for assessment and the health of the patient. Some areas, such as assessment of cognitive function, may be excluded because they require trained personnel.

How Should Quality of Life Be Measured?

In this section we will consider some issues in the choice of methods of measurement, with examples of some available instruments. Any measurement instrument needs to be *valid, reliable* and *sensitive.*

Validation

Validity may be broadly defined as the ability of an instrument to measure what it is supposed to measure. Establishment of validity is considerably more difficult in some of the areas covered by quality of life such as social isolation or life satisfaction, primarily since no gold standard exists for comparison. Evidence of validity is usually obtained by examining the relationships of the score or item to a variety of other measurements. The Nottingham Health Profile (NHP) measures perceived distress in six areas: pain, physical mobility, energy, emotions, sleep and social contacts, together with asking whether health interferes with other activities such as holidays and work (Hunt et al. 1986). The final form of the profile was developed after extensive interviewing of patients with a variety of disabilities and item reduction of 2200 statements to 45. Since the NHP describes the effects of ill health on daily life, discrimination between groups of healthy and fit subjects was the principal criterion of validity. However, the NHP has also been shown to discriminate between transplant and CABG patients before surgery, suggesting that this instrument can detect differences in the impact of moderate and severe coronary heart disease (Wallwork and Caine 1985).

The Quality-of-Life (QL) Index is a physician-rated assessment of five items on a three-point scale (Spitzer et al. 1981) developed primarily for use with cancer patients. Validation was established using a variety of approaches. Content validity was assessed by asking lay people, cancer and chronic disease patients and their relatives, and health professionals whether the items were appropriate, sufficient, important and likely to be discriminative. Seventy percent of the 34 respondents considered it completely satisfactory. Discriminative validity was assessed in a sample of healthy subjects and patients with cancer, chronic disease and serious illness; Table 1 shows the scores in each of these groups. The average score for cancer patients is much closer to that for healthy subjects than to that for the seriously ill. However, this does not imply that the QL Index would be a useful instrument in trials of cancer treatments, since patients are unlikely to be restored to a

Table 1. Mean QL scores in healthy individuals and patient groups. (Spitzer et al. 1981)

	Healthy group 1 (Sydney)	Healthy group 2 (Hunter)	Chronically diseased	Cancer patients	Seriously ill
QL Scores	8.80	9.17	7.31	7.11	3.31
SD	1.67	1.16	2.10	2.39	1.48
n	84	101	108	105	78

state of good health. For use as an evaluative instrument, a finer degree of discrimination is required.

Other measures of validity compare scores from different raters. The use of the Karnofsky Index of Performance Status (Karnofsky and Burchenal 1949), a clinician assessment of self-care, was studied with haemodialysis patients and their physicians (Hutchinson et al. 1979). Nine of 26 patients gave unscoreable answers; agreement with physicians' scores was less than one third. Clearly, the Karnofsky Index does not measure the patients' own perceptions of their capabilities.

Establishment of validity in methods measuring specific areas requires appropriate comparisons. The Symptom Rating test (SRT) is a self-rating scale of psychological distress (Kellner and Sheffield 1973). In a study of depressed patients and normals, SRT scores discriminated patients and agreed with the results of psychiatrists' ratings using the Hamilton Depression Rating Scale (Fava et al. 1982). SRT scores were also correlated with the concentration of benzodiazepam measured in the blood of anxious patients (Robin et al. 1974). Higher levels of distress were associated with lower concentrations.

The Dyspnoea Index is an interviewer assessment of the degree of functional impairment and magnitude of effort required to produce dyspnoea and gives a 12-point Baseline Index and an 18-point Transition Index (Mahler et al. 1984). Correlation coefficients of 0.6 were shown between the baseline score and both the 6- and 12-min walk tests (Mahler et al. 1984; Guyatt et al. 1985). Physiological tests (FVC and FEV_1), and cycle tests showed a weaker relationship. This illustrates the problem of deciding on an appropriate criterion for validity. Several studies have shown that stress tests and pulmonary function tests do not reflect a patients' performance in everyday activities.

Repeatability of Reliability

Repeatability is a measure of the consistency of the information and is usually established by test-retest results. These may be expressed through a variety of statistical methods, such as correlation coefficients, Kappa values, and standard deviations of repeated measurements or of differences in paired measurements. In trials, quality-of-life scores must have a high reliability when a situation is constant in order that one may be confident that changes in scores are related to treatment. The degree of variation between observers must also be measured in trials where more than one interviewer or tester is used and this error minimized by using the same observer for the same patient at various assessments during the trial.

Sensitivity

Sensitivity, as discussed above, is the ability of the methods to detect changes that occur as the result of treatment. The NHP scores showed a substantial improvement in patients surviving a cardiac transplant (Buxton et al. 1985). A similar but more comprehensive general health profile, the Sickness Impact Profile (Bergner et al. 1981), has also been shown to change in patients undergoing treatment

(Rockey and Griep 1980; Deyo and Inui 1984; MacKenzie et al. 1986). QL scores usually improve during the course of a study as a result of entry to the study. Sensitivity needs to be shown by comparison of the change in scores between control and treatment groups.

However, most trials compare two or more drugs; improvement during the trial (due to the treatment or the trial situation) may be greater than the differences between treatments. Cognitive function was evaluated in a trial of an ACE inhibitor, a centrally acting drug and a beta blocker, using the Reitan trail-making tests which measure visual motor performance (Croog et al. 1986). Improvement in speed was found in all treatment groups after 6 months in the trial, with a 17% change in the propranolol group. This was somewhat surprising, as previous work had suggested that beta blockers might produce mild cognitive impairment (Lichter et al. 1984). Patients on the centrally acting drug had the smallest improvement (11%), and this was significant only in the comparison with the ACE inhibitor (19%). This exemplifies how trial participation can overwhelm the adverse effects of a particular treatment, since clearly the antihypertensive therapies were not responsible for these dramatic improvements.

Validation of quality-of-life measurements is considered an ongoing process with continual appraisal of the performance in different diseases and study designs. Kirshner and Guyatt have discussed the different validation processes required for instruments for different uses: descriptive, predictive and evaluative (Kirshner and Guyatt 1985). Medical workers are frequently sceptical of the methods of the behavioural sciences. However, it is worth remembering that the most commonly used outcome measure in trials of congestive heart failure, the New York Heart Association functional classification (NYHA) (Harvey et al. 1974), does not fulfil the criteria of a good measurement. Patients are graded into one of four classes according to the degree of limitation of physical activity as perceived by the physician. The NYHA has high interobserver variability and a poor correlation with objective exercise testing (Guyatt et al. 1985). The broad grouping into four classes from normal to severe suggests that the NYHA will be sensitive only to treatments that produce substantial changes. Similarly, the Karnofsky Index, which has been widely used in cancer trials as a measure of quality of life, has been shown to have poor repeatability and to lack evidence of validity (Hutchinson et al. 1979).

Types of Methods

Questionnaires are the bases of most quality-of-life measurements. They may be administered by an interviewer or be self-completed. The advantages and disadvantages of either method of administration of the questionnaire are summarised in Table 2.

Self-administered Questionnaires

The choice of a self-administered method means that patients who cannot read or write for either educational, cultural or health reasons will be excluded. Question-

Table 2. Advantages and disadvantages of two forms of questionnaire administration

Self-administered	Interviewer-administered
Disadvantages	*Disadvantages*
Excludes groups of patients	Quality of interviewer may vary
Missing information	Race, sex and age of interviewer may influence results
May arouse anxiety	Expensive
	Standardisation required
Advantages	*Advantages*
Reproducible	Includes most patients
Cheap	Completeness of data assured
	Can probe to elicit unexpected information

naires should be designed to be completed by patients from differing levels of education and intelligence. Formulae are available which provide scores for different reading and comprehension abilities based on the content of the text (Ley 1973). For example, questionnaires giving scores in the upper range of the Flesch Score would be understood by 90% of the population, and the word complexity would be equivalent to that of comics. However, only 24% would comprehend the text in a typical academic journal! Instructions for completing self-administered questionnaires should be clear.

A disadvantage of self-administered questionnaires is that when they are incorrectly or inadequately completed, it is not possible to discover if this is a random error of omission, or bias due to patients not wishing to give certain information.

Self-administered questionnaires are most commonly used in large multicentre trials where training, standardizing, and deploying interviewing staff may not be feasible.

Interviewer-administered Questionnaires

The main advantage of an interviewer is that there is less restriction on who and what can be asked. This is particularly important in Quality-of-Life measurements, since little is known of the impact of disease and treatment on patients' lives. Open-ended questions allow patients the opportunity to describe their perceptions of problems, expectations and improvements. Although free text can be provided in self-administered questionnaires, our experience is that patients' answers are frequently vague and brief. An interviewer can use probes to obtain specific and detailed answers.

The quality of data obtained through an interview is highly dependent on the interviewer. Interviewers should be trained both in general techniques and specifically to administer the trial questionnaires. The main skills of interviewing are to establish a good rapport with the respondent without influencing the response, to ensure that the respondent answers the questions as truthfully and completely as possible, and to record these answers correctly without summary or distortion. Researchers and physicians often make poor interviewers, either because they have preconceptions about the data, or because they find it difficult to change from a caring to a neutral role. We have previously shown how the bias produced by physicians' expectations of treatment can influence the result of trials of antihypertensive therapies (Fletcher et al. 1987). Variability between interviewers should be reduced by joint training sessions, and inter- and intraobserver repeatability should be calculated.

Certain biases in response may be outside the control of the researcher. The age, sex and race of the interviewer has been shown to influence response (Hatchett and Schuman 1975).

Practical Problems

Place and time of completion of questionnaires should be standardized. For example, in trials of congestive heart failure, patients complete a questionnaire before a clinical examination or exercise test, as this is likely to influence response. In the outpatient and general practice settings, a quiet room should be made available.

Invitation of patients to participate in the trial should also be standardized. The aims of the study should be described and full confidentiality promised.

Cross-Cultural Issues

The results of trials of therapy should be generalisable to the patient population. Concern is often expressed that Quality-of-Life methods may not be valid in different countries. Early studies had shown differences in health-related behaviour between different nationalities, principally between immigrants in the USA of Old English or Irish descent and those of Jewish or Italian origins (Zborowski 1952). More recent work in Australia has suggested that these differences may reflect behavioural patterns due to recent immigration (Pilowsky and Spence 1977). Several Quality-of-Life instruments have been used in different Western countries, and have shown, in general, similar patterns of scores. In the Sickness Impact Profile each statement has a weighted value based on perception of its relative severity by ratings from health service professionals and from a sample of general practice patients in the USA. The SIP profile, with a few modifications to colloquial English, was used in a longitudinal study of disability in an inner-city area in London (Patrick 1981). There was very little difference between the new weights derived for the English population and the original American version. Methods used in antihypertensive trials in Europe showed a similar response in the reporting of symptoms (Fletcher et al. 1987). Westernised countries, however, probably share a cultural uniformity of life style, values and health beliefs.

Hunt and colleagues have described some of the difficulties in the application of the NHP in Egypt (Hunt et al. 1986). Although most semantic problems were overcome, the items in the profile had little meaning to the respondents. For example, the concept of enjoyment had less relevance in a culture living on the edge of poverty. Many statements were unacceptable, either because they described areas such as dressing and were considered offensive or because of differing religious perceptions of the meaning of problems.

In international trials of Quality of Life, it is particularly important to standardise methods at training sessions. Questionnaires should be translated and back-translated so that the language is acceptable to the person in the street. Sometimes it is not possible to find an equivalent meaning. For example, in our experience, the Dutch do not have vivid dreams - only nightmares, and the Germans never feel shaky!

Who Should Be Asked?

The essence of the Quality-of-Life approach is that it expresses and estimates the patients' viewpoints. There are a variety of circumstances when it is appropriate to ask for an assessment of the patient by another person involved in his or her daily life. For example, deteriorations in memory and concentration or excitable behaviour may be reported by a spouse. Severely disabled or ill patients may also be assessed by relatives, but these assessments should be validated. One study compared scores on the Sickness Impact Profile completed separately by disabled patients living at home and those taking care of them, over a period of 3 months (McCusker and Stoddard 1984). Agreement was high in all areas except sleep and rest and recreation and pastimes.

The quality of life of family members taking care of patients is also important. Higher rates of depression and an increase in health problems have been reported in families of stroke patients (Kinsella and Duffy 1979; Brockenhurst et al. 1981). A treatment which improves the patient's quality of life may also improve that of a spouse or relative. In a trial of children with severe eczema we are measuring psychological wellbeing in parents, siblings and the patient.

How Should Quality-of-Life Trials Be Designed and Analysed?

Design of Trials

Measurement of Quality of Life in double-blind randomised controlled trials offers all the usual advantages and should be the choice of design when possible. In certain treatment situations, usually surgical, trials can only be open and knowledge of the treatment is likely to influence response. Treatment comparisons should be fair; for example, the "best" alternative treatment relevant to the disease and patient should be selected. The rationale for choice and design should be explained.

Selection of Patients

Patients entering trials are inevitably a selected group, in that they are relatively fit, compliant, and willing to be randomized. A recent trial of breast surgery found a similar level of psychiatric morbidity in patients randomised to mastectomy or breast conservation (Fallowfield et al. 1986). The authors acknowledged that those women in the study who were prepared to be randomised might display different psychological characteristics from those who made choices.

Studies that have investigated patients' reasons for participating in cardiovascular trials have shown expectation of better care as the major factor (Mattson et al. 1985). The main benefits specified were extra medical monitoring due to the trial, having a "second opinion", and having "peace of mind." The actual trial treatment was not an important consideration; in fact, 50% of patients entering the Beta-Blocker Heart attack trial were "not at all sure" that the medication would prevent them having a heart attack in the next 2 years (Mattson et al. 1985).

This expectation of improved care is clearly demonstrated by the quality-of-life results showing an improvement in scores due to entry into the trial, and it presents a problem both in interpretation of results and in calculation of sample size.

Entry criteria should not bias the patient group. A trial of antihypertensive therapy (Croog et al. 1986) restricted entry to white men aged between 21 and 65 who were in full-time employment. Most work in Quality of Life has shown differences between men and women, with a higher reporting of symptoms, psychological morbidity and disruption of health to life on the part of women (Hunt et al. 1986; Fletcher et al. 1987).

Withdrawal of Patients

Dropouts reduce the power of a trial and may also constitute a selection bias. Little is known of the characteristics of patients who withdraw from trials. A higher mortality among dropouts has been shown (Committee of Principal Investigators' Clofibrate trial 1978; The Anturane Reinfarction Trial Research Group 1980). Patients who subsequently drop out have been shown to be less compliant with treatment and to have a higher symptom complaint score (Goldman et al. 1982). The implication of these studies for Quality-of-life trials is to emphasise the need to incorporate data from patients who withdraw. Questionnaires must be completed by patients at the time of exit. However, data will not be available from patients who die or enter worse states of health. A method of incorporating these states in trial results is by using a Health Index. Health Indexes include mortality and morbidity data by scoring health on a continuum, usually from 0 at death to 1 at perfect health. Different values are assigned to various states of disability along the continuum. These values may be arbitrary or derived from techniques, such as the time trade off or the standard gamble. The Quality of Well-being questionnaire (QWB) (Kaplan et al. 1976) measures mobility and physical and social activity in five levels over a period of 6 days prior to the interview. Subjects are also asked about the presence of 21 groups of symptoms and rate only the "most undesirable" one for each day. In the development of the QWB, weights were assigned to each activity level and symptom group using the method of category scaling, which is essentially a ranking of different scenarios. In order to test the validity of these scores in a disease-specific population, Balaban and colleagues (1986) undertook a similar study to rank the QWB in patients with rheumatoid arthritis. Very similar weights were obtained. Examination of these (Table 3) suggests that

Table 3. Some QWB scores in a population of rheumatoid arthritis. (Balaban et al. 1986)

Function or symptom	Score
No limitation	−0.000
In bed or wheelchair	−0.073
Not able to perform self-care	−0.126
Cough, wheezing or shortness of breath	−0.224
Taking medication	−0.130
Wearing eyeglasses	−0.135

this method produces scores which intuitively appear to deviate from accepted norms. For example, wearing glasses has a higher disability score than being in a wheelchair. Spiegelhalter (D. J. Spiegelhalter, personal communication) has shown that different methodologies for scaling produce different results and suggests that it is probably better to have an "arbitrary" index which is clinically acceptable and interpretable.

How Can the Results of Quality-of-Life Trials Be Interpreted?

Several situations can arise in the interpretation of Quality-of-Life trials; for example, all treatment groups may show an improvement, or there may be no change, or there may be deterioration in some groups. Deterioration implies either an adverse effect of treatment or a failure of the treatment to alter the prognosis. We have already discussed the beneficial effect of trial inclusion on Quality-of-Life results. An estimate of the size of the trial effect is useful, and it can be obtained in the placebo run-in period or by having a placebo control group.

In trials of antihypertensive therapies a placebo group is particularly useful. The principal aim of treatment of asymptomatic mild and moderate hypertension is to lower the blood pressure, not to improve well-being. Loss of wellbeing may result from the side effects of treatment. There is no evidence that in the mild-to-moderate range the level of blood pressure is related to well-being, though knowledge of this level and its consequences may be. Quality-of-Life results in the placebo group can act as the gold standard; an antihypertensive treatment that does better than placebo is doing something other than lowering blood pressure.

Interpretation of the meaning of changes in measurements is not unique to Quality of Life. Although in hypertension, levels of blood pressure correlate with cardiovascular mortality and morbidity risk, in other cardiovascular diseases such as congestive heart failure or angina, a change in a biological parameter such as left ventricular ejection fraction may have no prognostic significance.

In quality-of-life measurements we need to describe the size of the change in terms of its impact on the patients' experience of their daily lives. Changes in scores based on continuous measurement such as visual analogue scales are particularly difficult to interpret, since the descriptors are usually located only at the end points of the scale. In other Quality-of-Life scales, a score may be associated

Table 4. Quality of Wellbeing scores (SEM) in a trial of rheumatoid arthritis. (Bombardier et al. 1986)

	Placebo	Active
Baseline	0.600 (0.008)	0.599 (0.007)
Change	−0.001 (0.007)	0.023 (0.007)
n	149	154

with a defined state such as a diagnosis of depression. The change in score may be described in terms of the degree of change from one state to another. Usually, however, we are concerned with more subtle fluctuations of mood.

If a score based on aggregations of various Quality-of-Life components is presented, we will be unable to identify the areas in which the treatment has had an effect. The QWB was used in a trial of rheumatoid arthritis therapy (Bombardier et al. 1986). After 6 months in the trial, a significant improvement was found in active treatment compared with placebo in a variety of measures including the QWB. Table 4 shows the QWB baseline values and change at 6 months in the two groups. No change was observed in the placebo group, compared with an improvement of about 4% in the active group, i.e. from 60% of perfect health at baseline to 62% after treatment. The authors do not attempt to interpret this score, and descriptive results of areas of patients' lives influenced by therapy, such as improvements in pain, mobility and self-care, are given by other questionnaires used in this study. In fact, the QWB does provide component scores measuring mobility, physical and social activities and symptoms. Health Indexes are used to compute quality-adjusted years of survival (QALYS). These express the relationship between length and quality of survival. In the trial described above there was no survival benefit in either therapy group, so a QALYS would express only the benefit in health status. Moreover, we cannot assume that scores of 62 and 60 would be stable over a lifetime.

A similar problem of interpretation was found by the authors of a trial in hypertension. A measure of general wellbeing, The Psychological General Wellbeing Index (Dupuy 1984) showed a significant improvement of 2% in patients treated with an ACE inhibitor compared with a score decrease of 1.5% in those treated with a centrally acting drug and no change in patients on a beta blocker (Croog et al. 1986). The authors compared this benefit with data from similar scales where changes were observed due to alterations in life style. However, the life-style changes considered were of a considerable magnitude, such as losing one's job. If an antihypertensive treatment could produce the equivalent effect to a major life event, then one would have serious doubts as to what its mode of action really is. Clearly, the interpretation of data from Quality-of-Life trials is not simple, and further experience is needed of the performance of instruments in trials of different diseases and treatments.

Conclusions

We have provided a brief review of the issues involved in the measurement of quality of life in trials of treatment. It should be emphasised that Quality-of-Life trials require a positive commitment from medical and research staff. For example, extra facilities may be required, such as a quiet and private area for questionnaire completion, extra time and, sometimes, extra staff to manage the data collection. In our experience, reliable and complete data are best obtained in trials where all involved staff have been given appropriate education and training, both with respect to the general principles of measurement of quality of life and specifically to the methods to be used in the trial. Motivation of patients is far less of a problem! Patients usually welcome the opportunity to provide information on the effect of being ill on their everyday lives, especially if they are otherwise unoccupied, such as while waiting for laboratory tests and clinical examinations. However, consideration must be given to the patients' state of health and no extra burden placed on them. Measurement of quality of life in trials should not be undertaken without some degree of enthusiasm. However, a well-conducted Quality-of-Life trial can provide useful and important data, which will broaden the perspective on the outcome of treatments.

References

The Anturane Reinfarction Trial Research Group (1980) Sulfinpyrazone in the prevention of sudden death after myocardial infarction. N Engl J Med 302: 250-256

Balaban DJ, Sagi PC, Goldfarb NI, Nettler S (1986) Weights for scoring the quality of well-being instrument among rheumatoid arthritics. Med Care 24: 973-980

Bergner M, Bobbitt RA, Carter WB, Gilson BS (1981) The Sickness Impact Profile: development and final revision of a health status measure. Med Care 19: 787-805

Bombardier C, Ware J, Russell IJ, Larson M, Chalmers A, Leighton Read J, The Auranofin Cooperating Group (1986) Auranofin therapy and quality of life in patients with rheumatoid arthritis. Results of a multicenter trial. Am J Med 81: 565-578

Bransfield DD (1982) Breast cancer and sexual functioning: a review of literature and implications for future research. Int J Psychiatry Med 12: 197-211

Brockenhurst JC, Morris P, Andrews K, Richards B, Laycock P (1981) Social effects of stroke. Soc Sci Med [A] 15: 35-39

Bulpitt CJ (1982) Quality of life in hypertensive patients. In: Amery A (ed) Hypertensive cardiovascular disease: pathophysiology and treatment. Nijhoff, pp 929-948

Bulpitt CJ, Dollery CT, Carne S (1974) A symptom questionnaire for hypertensive patients. J Chronic Dis 27: 309-323

Buxton M, Acheson R, Caine N, Gibson S, O'Brien B (1985) Cost and benefits of the heart transplant programmes at Harefield and Papworth hospitals, London. Her Majesty's Stationery Office, London

Committe of Principal Investigators' Clofibrate Trial (1978) A co-operative trial in the primary prevention of ischaemic heart disease using clofibrate. Report from the Committee of Principal Investigators. Br Heart J 40: 1069-1118

Croog SH, Levine S, Testa M, Brown B, Bulpitt CJ, Jenkins CD, Klerman GL, William GW (1986) The effects of antihypertensive therapy on the quality of life. N Engl J Med 314: 1657-1664

Curb JD, Borhani NO, Blaszkanski TP, Simbaldi N, Fotiu S, Williams W (1985) Long-term surveillance for adverse effects of antihypertensive drugs. JAMA 253: 3263-3268

Deyo RA (1984) Measuring functional outcomes in therapeutic trials for chronic disease. Controlled Clin Trials 5: 223-240

Deyo RA, Inui TS (1984) Towards clinical applications of health status measures; sensitivity of scales to clinically important changes. Health Serv Res 19: 275-289

Dupuy HJ (1984) The psychological general well-being (PGWB) index: 170-183. In: Wenger NK, Mattson ME, Fuberg CP (eds) Assessment of quality of life in clinical trials of cardiovascular therapies. Le Jacq, Washington, DC

Fallowfield LF, Baum M, Maguire GP (1986) Effects of breast conservation on psychological morbidity associated with diagnosis and treatment of early breast cancer. Br Med J 293: 1331-1334

Fava GA, Kellner R, Munari F, Pavan L (1982) The Hamilton Depression Rating Scale in normals and depressives. Acta Psychiatr Scand 66: 26-32

Fletcher AE, Hunt BM, Bulpitt CJ (1987) Evaluation of quality of life in clinical trials of cardiovascular disease. J Chronic Dis 40: 557-566

Goldman AI, Holcomb R, Mitchell Perry H, Schnaper HW, Fitz AE, Frohlich E (1982) Can dropout and other noncompliance be minimized in a clinical trial? Controlled Clin Trials 3: 75-89

Guyatt GM, Thompson PJ, Berman LB, Sullivan M, Townsend M, Jones AL, Pugsley SO (1985) How should we measure function in patients with chronic heart and lung disease? J Chronic Dis 38: 517-524

Hampton JR (1984) Coronary artery bypass grafting for the reduction of mortality: an analysis of the trials. Br Med J 289: 1166-1170

Harvey RM, Doyle EF, Ellis K et al. (1974) Major changes made by the criteria committee of the New York Heart Association. Circulation 49: 390

Hatchett S, Schuman H (1975) White respondents and race of interviewer effects. Public Opinion Q 34: 523-528

Hunt SM, McEwen J, McKenna SP (1986) Measuring health status. Croom Helm, London

Hutchinson TA, Boyd NF, Feinstein AR (1979) Scientific problems in clinical scales, as demonstrated in the Karnofsky Index of performance status. J Chronic Dis 32: 661-666

Kaplan RM, Bush JW, Berry CC (1976) Health status: types of validity for an index of well-being. Health Serv Res 11: 478-507

Karnofsky DA, Burchenal JH (1949) The clinical evaluation of chemotherapeutic agents in cancer. In: Macleod CM (ed) Evaluation of chemotherapeutic agents. Symposium held at New York Academy of Medicine, New York. Columbia University Press, New York, pp 191-205

Kellner R, Sheffield BF (1973) A self-rating scale of distress. Psychol Med 3: 88-100

Kinsella GJ, Duffy F (1979) Psychosocial readjustment in the spouses of aphasic patients. Scand J Rehabil Med 11: 129-132

Kirshner B, Guyatt G (1985) A methodological framework for assessing health indices. J Chronic Dis 38: 27-36

Leibel SA, Pino Y, Torres JL, Order SE (1980) Improved quality of life following radical radiation therapy for early stage carcinoma of the prostate. Urol Clin North Am 7: 593-604

Ley P (1973) The measurement of comprehensibility. J Inst Health Educ 11: 17-20

Lichter I, Richardson PJ, Wyke MA (1984) Differential effects of atenolol and enalapril on tests of memory during treatment for essential hypertension. J Hypertens 2: 560

Lind K (1982) A synthesis of studies on stroke rehabilitation. J Chronic Dis 35: 133-149

MacKenzie CR, Charlson ME, Digioa D, Kelly K (1986) Can the Sickness Impact Profile measure change? An example of scale assessment. J Chronic Dis 39: 429-438

Mahler DA, Weinberg DM, Wells CK, Feinstein AP (1984) The measurement of dyspnoea. Contents, inter-observer agreement and physiologic correlates of two new clinical indexes. Chest 85: 751-758

Mattson ME, Curb JD, Mcardle R, The AMIS and BHAT Research Groups (1985) Participation in a clinical trial: the patient's point of view. Controlled Clin Trials 6: 156-167

McCusker J, Stoddard AM (1984) Use of a surrogate for the Sickness Impact Profile. Med Care 22: 789-795
Medical Research Council Working Party on Mild-to-Moderate Hypertension (1976) Adverse reactions to bendrofluazide and propranolol for the treatment of mild hypertension. Lancet 2: 539-543
Patrick D (1981) Standardization of comparative health status measures: using scales developed in America in an English-speaking community. In: Sudman S (ed) Health survey research methods, third biennial conference, Hyattsville, MD. National Center for Health Services Research. PHS publication no 81-3268, pp 216-220
Pilowsky I, Spence N (1977) Ethnicity and illness behaviour. Psychol Med 7: 447-452
Robin A, Curry SH, Whelpton R (1974) Clinical and biochemical comparison of chlorazepate and diazepam. Psychol Med 4: 388-392
Rockey PM, Griep JRJ (1980) Behavioural dysfunction in hyperthyroidism. Improvement with treatment. Arch Intern Med 140: 1194-1197
Sjogren K (1983) Sexuality after stroke with hemiplegia. II. With special regard to partnership adjustment and to fulfillment. Scand J Rehabil Med 15 (2): 63-69
Sjogren K, Dambe JE, Liliequist B (1983) Sexuality after stroke with hemiplegia. I. Aspects of sexual function. Scand J Rehabil Med 15 (2): 55-61
Smith HCL, Frye RL, Piehler JM (1983) Does coronary bypass surgery have a favourable influence on the quality of life? Cardiovasc Clin 13: 253-264
Spitzer WD, Dobson AJ, Hall J, Chesterman E, Levi J, Shepderd R, Battista RN, Catchlove BR (1981) Measuring the quality of life of cancer patients. A concise QL index for use by physicians. J Chronic Dis 34: 585-597
Vera MI (1981) Quality of life following pelvic exenteration. Gynecol Oncol 12: 355-366
Wallwork J, Caine N (1985) A comparison of the quality of life of cardiac transplant patients and coronary artery bypass graft patients before and after surgery. Qual Life Cardiovasc Care 1: 317-331
Williams NS, Johnston D (1983) The quality of life after rectal excision for low rectal cancer. Br J Surg 70: 460-462
Zborowski M (1952) Cultural components in response to pain. J Soc Issues 8: 16-30

*A Modular Approach to Quality-of-Life Assessment in Cancer Clinical Trials**

N. K. Aaronson, M. Bullinger, and S. Ahmedzai

The Netherlands Cancer Institute, Plesmanlaan 121, 1066 CX Amsterdam, The Netherlands

Quality of Life as Research Domain

Cancer clinical trials focus upon the evaluation of such biomedical outcomes as duration of survival, retardation of the disease process and control of major physical symptoms (Buyse et al. 1984; Friedman et al. 1985). In recent years, however, these clinical end points have been criticized for a lack of comprehensiveness (Greer 1984; Greer and Silberfarb 1982). Following the lead of the WHO in defining health as complete physical, mental and social well-being, the scope of investigation has been extended to include assessment of a range of psychosocial variables that can be subsumed under the heading "quality of life."

While the number of publications (according to a recent MEDLINE search about 3045 from 1972 to 1987) on this topic reflects the growing interest of clinicians and researchers in quality-of-life issues, the inclusion of psychosocial end points in cancer clinical trials is still rare (Bardelli and Saracci 1978; Fayers and Jones 1983). This paucity of clinical trial-based psychosocial studies reflects an array of problems at the conceptual, methodological and practical levels.

Conceptually, quality of life represents a rather abstract construct that needs to be defined and broken down into its component parts before measurement can be effectively undertaken.

Methodologically, instruments for measuring quality of life have to be developed or selected from existing scales that are reliable, valid and sensitive when applied to cancer populations (APA 1974; Nunnally 1978; Ware 1984a). In addition, decisions must be made regarding the relevance of quality-of-life end points to be

* The research described in this paper is a project of the EORTC Study Group on Quality of Life (protocol 15861). The study coordinator is N. K. Aaronson. The national coordinators are: P. B. C. Rofe (Australia), B. Pfausler (Austria), D. Razavi (Belgium), D. Osoba (Canada), M. Bullinger (Federal Republic of Germany), S. Schraub (France), S. Ahmedzai (United Kingdom), A. Filiberti (Italy), F. Takeda (Japan), J. C. J. M. de Haes (the Netherlands), S. Kaasa (Norway), J. Estape (Spain), M. Sullivan (Sweden), J. Bernhard (Switzerland), and M. Mastilica (Yugoslavia). O. Dalesio and D. Crabeels are, respectively, the EORTC Data Center statistician and data manager associated with the project.

Recent Results in Cancer Research, Vol. 111
© Springer-Verlag Berlin · Heidelberg 1988

applied in specific trials, as well as the statistical analyses most appropriate for relating psychosocial data to clinical outcomes (Kaplan and Bush 1982).

From a practical standpoint, the inclusion of quality-of-life assessments in clinical trials requires the cooperation of patients and clinicians, and the establishment of a workable organizational infrastructure via which data collection and documentation can be facilitated (Aaronson 1986).

Approaches to Assessing Quality of Life

The problems associated with quality-of-life assessment in health care research have been addressed by various workers in the field. Numerous contributions have dealt with the "who, what, how, where and why" of quality-of-life measurement (Clark and Fallowfield 1986; de Haes and van Knippenberg 1985; Fayers and Jones 1983; Van Dam et al. 1984; Ware 1984a, b; Wood-Dauphinee and Troidl 1986). While researchers have yet to reach consensus on all, or even the majority of issues surrounding quality-of-life assessment, there does appear to be some basic agreement regarding the desired content and properties of a measurement instrument for use in clinical trials. Such an instrument should be multidimensional in nature and should comprise at least four categories of variables:

1. Physical complaints (i.e., somatic sensations, disease symptoms, side effects)
2. Psychological distress (e.g., anxiety, depression)
3. Social interaction (quality and quantity of relationships with significant others)
4. Functional status (e.g., activity level, vocational activity)

Additional factors that have been proposed for inclusion in quality-of-life assessments include sexuality (Andersen 1985), body image, and satisfaction with medical care (Aaronson 1986).

The instrument should be patient based, as the patient is the best and sometimes the only logical source of information about the impact of disease and treatment on daily living (Krauth 1982). In order to be used in clinical trials, it should be administered in questionnaire rather than interview form. The instrument should be acceptable to both patients and clinicians. It should be brief, easy to understand and easy to respond to (Aaronson et al. 1987; Hutchinson et al. 1979). In addition, the instrument should possess sufficient levels of validity, reliability and sensitivity for detecting changes in patients' quality of life over time (Ware 1987).

Much discussion has been devoted to the relative merit of standard versus disease-specific measures, that is, to whether a standard quality-of-life instrument can be developed for use across a wide range of oncological research settings or whether specific questionnaires for different research situations should be constructed (Greer 1987). The primary advantage of the first approach is that it would afford the opportunity of comparing results across studies - a feature that is quite desirable in this age of meta-analysis. The advantage of the second approach is the specifity of quality-of-life problems that can be detected by the instrument.

A review of the literature indicates that the trial-specific solution has been most widely adopted in cancer research (de Haes and van Knippenberg 1985). While omnibus measures with proven psychometric robustness are available from health status research (e.g., the Sickness Impact Profile, Bergner et al. 1981; the McMaster Health Index, Chambers et al. 1983; the Nottingham Health Profile, Hunt et al. 1981; the Psychological General Well-being Index, DuPuy 1984), they were not developed or validated specifically for cancer populations.[1] In addition, these measures typically are lengthy and do not contain information on symptoms and side effects.

With regard to cancer-specific questionnaires, there is an abundance of newly developed measures. Unfortunately, the large majority of these instruments have yet to undergo sufficient field testing and have undocumented psychometric properties (Ciampi et al. 1983). Among psychometrically tested instruments, the Functional Living Index Cancer (FLIC: Schipper et al. 1984) and the cancer questionnaire of Selby and associates (1984) reflect opposing sides of the same data reduction problem. The FLIC uses an overall score reflecting the sum of the individual items, while the Selby questionnaire treats each item separately. In the former case, the total quality-of-life score is probably too coarse to be of clinical value. In the latter case, the absence of subscales that summarize the data may lead to a situation of information overload.

In order to reconcile the conflict between standard and specific quality-of-life measures, it may be possible to synthesize both approaches in one measurement strategy. Specifically, a *modular system* of quality of life may represent a reasonable compromise (Aaronson et al. 1987). Conceptually, such a system would facilitate investigations into the structure of the quality-of-life construct (i.e., the relationship between components). Methodologically, such an approach would permit comparisons across trials without loss of trial-specific data.

A Modular Approach to Quality-of-Life Assessment

Based on the various theoretical and methodological considerations outlined in the preceding section, the Study Group on Quality of Life of the European Organization for Research and Treatment of Cancer (EORTC) has developed a questionnaire consisting of both general (core QLQ; 36 items) and disease-specific modules (supplement QLQ; 9 items). The questionnaire is: (a) multidimensional, (b) cancer specific, (c) patient based and designed for self-administration, (d) intended for application across a range of cancer diagnoses, (e) relatively short, (f) intended to yield a number of multi-item scales (i.e., modules), and (h) translatable into different languages. The English version of the core QLQ is presented in Appendix A.

The following quality-of-life dimensions were identified as key elements of the core QLQ: (a) functional status, (b) physical symptoms common to many malignancies and/or treatment modalities, (c) psychological distress, (d) social interaction, (e) financial/economic impact, (f) perceived health status, and (g) overall quality of life. Each of these measurement domains will be addressed briefly in the following sections.

---

[1] It should be noted, however, that a recent study of the Sickness Impact Profile (Greenwald 1987) lends support to its potential use with cancer populations.

Functional Status

Functional status refers to the performance of (or the capacity to perform) a variety of activities that are normal for most people (often age-adjusted). Included under this heading are self-care activities, mobility, physical activity level and role activities (Katz 1987).

In the core QLQ, two Guttman scales were chosen to measure functional status. A Guttman scale is constructed from a set of items with dichotomous (i. e., yes-no) response choices representing a continuum of increasing levels of intensity, difficulty or severity. The first is a seven-item scale of personal functioning that includes items assessing self-care, mobility and physical activity (items 1-7). These items are similar to those that have been tested for scale validity and reliability in patients with arthritis (Meenan 1980) and among cancer patients (Stewart et al. 1982). The second Guttman scale is composed of two items reflecting the extent to which patients can perform their usual work or housework activities (i. e., social role functioning) (items 8 and 9).

Disease and Treatment-related Symptoms

Physical symptoms reported frequently by cancer patients, either as a result of the disease process or of treatment, include pain, breathlessness, constipation, diarrhoea, sleeplessness, cognitive disorder, nausea and vomiting, and fatigue and malaise (Linssen et al. 1981; Daut and Cleeland 1982). In the core QLQ these symptoms (items 10-22 and 31) are assessed with a series of single items (for pain, breathlessness, constipation, diarrhoea, sleeplessness and cognitive disorder) and multiple-item scales (for nausea and vomiting, and fatigue and malaise). Response categories range on a four-point Likert scale from "not at all" to "quite a bit".

Psychological Distress

A number of studies have documented elevated levels of psychological distress among cancer patients as compared with rates found among primary-care populations (Derogatis et al. 1983). The most common symptoms reported by cancer patients are depression (Endicott 1984) and anxiety (Gottschalk 1983). Even though a variety of measures are available for assessing psychological morbidity in psychiatric or general populations (ranging from lengthy, omnibus interviews to more concise unidimensional scales), these measures typically include a number of symptoms (e.g., tiredness, decreased sexual drive, appetite loss, etc.) that may result from the somatic disease process itself, rather than reflect somatic manifestations of psychological distress.

The Hospital Anxiety and Depression Scale (HADS: Zigmond and Snaith 1983), a 14-item instrument with high internal consistency and discriminant validity developed for use with physically ill patients, avoids this methodological problem by concentrating solely on anxious and depressed affect. Additionally, the wording of questions avoids allusions to psychopathology, rendering it more acceptable to cancer patients than other psychiatric scales.

Despite the brevity of the HADS, it was considered to be too long for inclusion in a multidimensional quality-of-life questionnaire. Thus, after inspection of individual item factor loadings and discussions with the scale's authors, eight of the original 14 items were retained for the core QLQ (items 23-30). Additionally, response categories were adapted to the uniform four point Likert scale.

Social Interaction

Both clinical observation and empirical research point to the importance of social contact and social support in the life of the cancer patient (Wortman 1983). Yet physical, functional and psychological problems of the patients (e.g., fear of being a burden to others), or the reaction of family and friends (e.g., feelings of awkwardness or inadequacy) may lead to social isolation (Bury 1982).

Assessment of social interaction can be seriously hampered by an underreporting bias, particularly if questions are phrased in such a way as to imply criticism of family members and friends. By focusing on the behavioural aspects of interpersonal relationships (e.g., the ability to maintain normal social contacts) rather than on their affective components (e.g., feelings of love and support), such bias may be minimized. Adopting such a strategy, the core QLQ includes two questions (items 32 and 33) that address perceived disruption of normal social activities as a result of either the patient's health condition or the medical treatment being received.

Financial/Economic Impact

Cancer can have a dramatic impact on the financial situation of a patient and his family. This includes direct and indirect costs of treatment, as well as substantial loss of income due to reduced work levels or altered work schedule of family members. A single question of the core questionnaire (item 34) asks patients to report whether their condition or treatment has resulted in financial difficulties.

Global Health and Quality-of-Life Items

In general, construction of the core QLQ has been guided by the assumption that the quality-of-life concept, in order to be of clinical use, must be broken down into component parts. However, several arguments can be forwarded for the inclusion of more globally oriented items in such a questionnaire. First, "quality of life" may be more than the sum of its component parts (de Haes and van Knippenberg 1985). Thus, a global question regarding overall health status or quality of life may capture information not covered by the more specific sets of items. Second, a global quality-of-life item may be valuable in assessing the relative value (weight) placed on specific modular components (e.g., the relative importance of physical versus psychological symptoms). Third, a global quality-of-life measure facilitates incorporating psychosocial data into medical decision-making models (Lane

1987). For these reasons, two questions were included in the core QLQ that are intended to assess, in a more global sense, the patient's perception of his or her subjective well-being. One question asks patients to rate, on a seven-point scale ranging from "very poor" to "excellent", his or her "overall physical condition" during the past week (item 35). This perceived health status question is similar to others that have been employed in studies both of the general population (Ware et al. 1978) and of chronic-disease patients (Gough et al. 1983). Using the same range of response categories, the second question asks patients to rate their "overall quality of life" during the past week (item 36).

Lung Cancer-Specific QLQ Module

While the core quality-of-life questionnaire is designed to be applicable across a range of tumour sites and treatment situations, a tumour-specific supplement was designed to provide information on problems unique to lung cancer patients (the target population for initial psychometric testing of the questionnaire; see below). Nine additional questions were included in a supplemental QLQ module that has particular relevance to lung cancer patients: (a) two questions on coughing, (b) a three-item scale assessing dyspnoea (providing more detailed information than the single breathlessness item included in the core QLQ), (c) four items tapping additional side effects of chemotherapy, and (d) four items on pain and use of pain medications (see Appendix A).

Psychometric Analysis of the Quality-of-Life Questionnaire

In order to investigate the psychometric properties of the QLQ, the EORTC Study Group on Quality of Life is currently conducting a multicenter study with participants from 15 member countries including Australia, Austria, Belgium, Canada, France, Great Britain, Italy, Japan, The Netherlands, Norway, Spain, Sweden, Switzerland, West Germany and Yugoslavia. The primary objectives of the study are to determine both the statistical and cross-cultural validity, reliability and sensitivity of the core and supplement QLQ (Aaronson 1987). The following sections will describe the design of the study and the psychometric analysis strategy.

The Study Sample

Although the proposed study is intended to yield a core questionnaire capable of assessing the quality of life of a range of patient groups, for methodological and practical reasons it was considered desirable to employ initially a study sample that is relatively homogeneous with regard to diagnosis.

Thus, the study sample will be limited to nonresectable lung cancer patients. No further restrictions will be made with regard to histological type, age, or performance status. Factors that guided our choice of this patient population include (a) the high incidence of the disease, (b) the palliative nature of available therapies (implying the need for including psychosocial end points in treatment evaluations), and (c) the paucity of research on the effects of lung cancer and its treatment on patients' quality of life. Further, from a practical standpoint, the high incidence of the disease facilitates rapid sample accrual and permits an examination of the relationship between changes in clinical and psychosocial health status within a compressed time frame. To minimize any potential bias in the sample composition, patient accrual is based on a consecutive series of patients who meet the eligibility criteria.

While, from a purely statistical standpoint, the required sample size is approximately 350 patients (i. e., ten cases per item included in the core QLQ), each participating country is asked to enter 50 patients into the study, thus yielding a total sample across countries of 750 patients. This sample size is sufficiently large to permit grouping of patients by nationality and/or language for purposes of cross-cultural comparisons.

Research Design and Study Procedures

The study design calls for administration of the QLQ at two points in time: (a) following diagnosis but prior to the start of treatment, and (b) once during the course of treatment (i. e., on the last day of the first course of radiotherapy or on the last day of the second cycle of chemotherapy). Patients are also asked to complete a debriefing form following the second QLQ administration regarding the time required to complete the questionnaire, the need for assistance in completing the questionnaire, and the presence of questionnaire items that were confusing, difficult to answer, or upsetting. Additional sociodemographic data to be collected include age, sex, marital status, household composition, education and occupation. Medical data include histology, site, measurability and evaluability of primary disease, disease stage, sites of metastases, symptomatic or asymptomatic disease, weight loss, comorbidity, treatment schedule, performance status and treatment toxicities.

Psychometric Analysis Plan

The primary objective of the study is to generate data regarding the reliability, validity and sensitivity of the core and supplement QLQ when applied in a cross-cultural clinical context. Essentially, reliability refers to the consistency of the scores derived from a set of items, or to the extent to which the scores are free of random error. Validity refers to whether the hypothesized scales measure adequately the concepts that they are intended to measure. Sensitivity refers to the instrument's ability to detect changes in quality of life induced by treatment (Ware 1987). In the current study, a range of statistical techniques will be employed to establish the psychometric properties of the QLQ modules (or scales). These analyses can be divided into three major categories:

1. Examination of the internal structure of the QLQ
2. Comparison of the QLQ with external data sources
3. Analysis of changes in QLQ scores over time

Scaling and Internal Consistency Analyses

To test whether the individual items that make up the QLQ can be combined into a more limited set of multi-item scales, either Likert's Method of Summated Ratings (Likert 1932) or Guttman's Scalogram Analysis (Guttman 1944) will be employed. The Likert method will be used to examine the psychometric robustness of the physical symptom, psychological distress, and social interaction modules of the core QLQ. For Likert scaling, item responses are first assigned numerical values. Items in a hypothesized scale are summed to form a total scale score. An item analysis is carried out, in which each item is correlated with the total scale score, but with the item score taken out of the total (i. e., the correlation is corrected for overlap). In order to be retained in the scale, each item should correlate 0.40 or greater with the total score (Nie et al. 1970).

Second, principal component analysis will be used to confirm that only one scale should be constructed from a set of items. With the use of this statistical procedure the unidimensionality of a hypothesized scale can be examined.

Third, the reliability of the Likert scales will be assessed cross-sectionally by calculating their internal consistency. The most commonly employed measure of internal consistency is Cronbach's alpha coefficient (Cronbach 1951). Internal consistency estimates are considered acceptable for group comparisons if they are of a magnitude of 0.50 or greater (Helmstadter 1964). Guttman Scalogram Analysis will be used to assess the physical functioning and social role functioning modules of the core QLQ, both of which are constructed of items with dichotomous (i. e., "yes" or "no") response choices representing a continuum of increasing levels of difficulty. Because of the cumulative nature of the items, the scale scores describe rather precisely the logical pattern of response to all of the items. Thus, for example, in the hypothesized physical functioning scale, if a patient reports being able to take a long walk, it is a logical assumption that he or she can walk a short distance, does not have to stay indoors most or all of the day, and does not need help with basic self-care activities. The two statistics used to evaluate whether a set of items meet the Guttman criteria for scalability are the coefficient of reproducibility (CR) and the coefficient of scalability (CS). Minimal standards of 0.90 and 0.60 for CR and CS, respectively, are recommended as evidence of Guttman scale structure (Nie et al. 1970).

Assessment of Construct Validity

A series of analyses will be undertaken to examine the construct validity of the scales. Construct validity refers essentially to whether the hypothesized scales are actually measuring the underlying constructs that they are intended to measure and, of equal importance, whether they are *not* measuring some other underlying construct.

Three approaches will be taken to assessing the construct validity of the hypothesized QLQ scales. First, a simultaneous factor analysis of all items of the core QLQ will be carried out. Evidence of construct validity is provided if the items representing the hypothesized scales "load" on separate factors (e.g., if items composing the fatigue/malaise scale cluster together under one factor, and the items from the psychological distress scale cluster under a second factor).

Second, multitrait scaling techniques will be used to test for item-discriminant validity (Campbell and Fiske 1959). A matrix of item-scale correlations will be created, such that each item is correlated with all of the scales being constructed, including the scale to which it is hypothesized to belong (corrected for overlap). According to the discriminant validity criterion, each item should correlate most strongly with its own scale.

Finally, a correlation matrix will be constructed including the various hypothesized scales of the QLQ. An examination of the direction and strength of relationships among the scales will provide additional evidence of construct validity. It is expected that, because they are measuring various dimensions of a more global "quality-of-life" construct, a number of the scales will correlate significantly with one other. Nevertheless, the strength of the correlation should be only moderate (e.g., $r \leq 0.35$), indicating that each scale is measuring a distinct, albeit related, quality-of-life dimension.

Assessment of Criterion Validity

In order to further examine the validity of the core QLQ, the hypothesized scales will be correlated with a number of reference or criterion variables. These variables include the physician-rated ECOG performance status ratings, the WHO toxicity scales, disease stage, weight loss, and sociodemographics. A number of hypotheses can be generated regarding the anticipated relationship between the QLQ scales and these criterion variables. For example, it is expected that the QLQ functional status measure will correlate significantly with the ECOG ratings, although the magnitude of the correlations is expected to be only moderate (e.g., $r = 0.50$ range). In general, it is expected that the core QLQ scales scores will vary as a function of external indicators of patients' health status (e.g., that patients with more advanced disease will exhibit lower quality of life).

Analysis of Scale Sensitivity and Stability Over Time

The availability of two quality-of-life questionnaires, one administered prior to the start of treatment and one at a mid-treatment point, permits (a) a preliminary examination of the sensitivity of the QLQ scales to changes in health status as reflected by clinical indicators of the disease course and treatment-induced toxicities, and (b) the stability of the QLQ structure as evidenced by the statistical relationships within and between the various QLQ scales over time.

For the sensitivity analysis, clinical changes in the health status of the patients, as determined by the physician-based performance status ratings and treatment toxicity scales, will be correlated with changes in subjective physical and psychosocial health status as reflected in the patient-based questionnaire. It is recognized that the physician-based indicators represent imperfect criteria against which to judge the sensitivity of the QLQ elements to change over time. Nevertheless, we feel that such an approach is justified, in that it is precisely these variables that are relied upon in clinical research settings to document changes in health status resulting from the disease process and/or the applied therapies.

The stability of the QLQ structure will be examined by comparing the statistical properties of the various scales, as well as the correlations among scales, for each of the two QLQ administration points. While it is expected that the magnitude of the correlations of items to scales, and scales to scales, will vary to some degree from one QLQ administration to the other, the overall pattern of results (i.e., the factor structure, internal consistency estimates, and interscale correlations) is expected to remain essentially unchanged.

While it is expected that the QLQ structure will exhibit stability over time, it will be of particular theoretical interest to examine whether the relative contribution of the specific quality-of-life dimensions (e.g., physical functioning, social functioning, symptom experience, psychological distress) to overall quality-of-life ratings (as measured by the two global questions included in the QLQ) changes from the pretreatment to mid-treatment period. Multiple linear regression techniques will be used to address this issue.

Cross-Cultural Issues

The foregoing discussion has focused on the proposed strategy for examining the properties of the QLQ from a statistical or psychometric perspective. Of equal importance is the determination of whether the QLQ can be applied successfully in an international research context, that is, whether it exhibits cross-cultural validity. While cultural differences in patient groups may have little or no impact on the measurement of biological outcomes, they can exert a significant influence when one is attempting to assess the subjective experience of the patient.

In constructing the QLQ, careful attention was paid to assuring that questions had as close to the same meaning across languages and cultures as possible. Including individuals from a range of countries in the process of questionnaire development was a first, important step toward minimizing cross-cultural problems. This led, for example, to the rejection of several candidate measures for assessing psychological distress because of the culturally idiomatic nature of their question wording. When translated into other languages, such measures either took on a distinctly different meaning than was originally intended or lost their meaning altogether.

The current version of the QLQ underwent a rigorous "forward-backward" translation process. This entailed translating the questionnaire first from its original language (English) into the various other languages (Dutch, French, German, Italian, Japanese, Norwegian, Spanish, Swedish, and Yugoslavian), and then translating it back again into English. This was an iterative process, requiring several refinements in question wording before equivalence could be best approximated.

Several strategies were considered in order to test whether the statistical properties of the scales remain constant when the QLQ is used in differing cultural settings. Ideally, this would be accomplished by replicating the full set of multivariate psychometric analyses for each national or cultural subsample. However, the sample size required for such a strategy would have been prohibitively large (approximately 350 patients per country or, minimally, per language).

As a more feasible alternative, we have chosen a mixed approach to cross-cultural validation. At the most basic level - that of examining item frequency distributions and simple correlation matrices - analyses will be replicated for each national sample. In this way it will be possible to determine if response patterns to particular questions are skewed for a given national sample.

For the more complex multivariate analyses, where a larger sample size is required, two strategies will be followed. First, the total sample will be divided into basic language groups. Thus, for example, the English, Australian, and English-speaking Canadian cases will be combined into one subgroup, the French and French-speaking Belgian, Canadian, and Swiss cases will be combined into a second subgroup, and so forth. While this strategy cannot be applied to all cases (e.g., the Japanese and Yugoslavian samples cannot be combined with others), it will nevertheless yield a number of language subgroups of sufficient size to allow replication of the requisite psychometric analyses.

The second strategy involves carrying out the full set of psychometric analyses on the total sample minus a given language group. Thus, for example, analyses will be carried out on a sample comprised of all cases minus the English-speaking subsample. The same set of analyses will then be replicated on a sample comprised of all cases minus the French-speaking subsample, and so on. By comparing the results of each of these repeated sets of analyses with those based on the total sample, it will be possible to detect significant changes in the reliability, validity and sensitivity characteristics of the QLQ subscales that are language dependent.

It should be emphasized that this analysis strategy is not intended to yield detailed information regarding cross-cultural differences in the psychosocial impact of cancer and its treatment (a substantive issue). Rather, the goal is to identify potential measurement problems related to the application of the QLQ in varying national and cultural settings.

Forecasting Future Research Directions

The QLQ development study described in the preceding sections represents the first, cross-sectional phase of a two-phase project. In order to put this first phase into proper perspective, a brief overview of the second, longitudinal phase of the study may be useful. The longitudinal study will involve, most likely, the administration of the QLQ at four points in time: (a) at the time of diagnosis, prior to the start of treatment; (b) on the last day of the first course of treatment; (c) 3 months following entry to the study; and (d) 6 months following entry to the study. This design will allow for a more detailed examination of the validity and reliability of the QLQ over time. Thus, at each measurement point, appropriate statistical analyses will be carried out to confirm the robustness of the QLQ at different points in the disease and treatment process.

An additional feature of the second phase of the research concerns the inclusion of a more comprehensive approach to instrument validation. Specifically, at the time of the second QLQ administration (i. e., at the end of the first course of therapy), an extensive validity interview will be conducted that will serve as an external validation of the QLQ. The interview will cover the same topic areas as those included in the QLQ, using questions drawn from existing interview schedules and validated questionnaires (e. g., the Sickness Impact Profile, the Spielberger State-Trait Anxiety Inventory, the CES-D Depressions Scale), as well as questions developed specifically for the study. By comparing the results obtained from the QLQ with those derived from the interview it will be possible to determine more precisely the robustness of the scales embodied in the questionnaire. For example, we would expect a high correlation between the eight-item anxiety and depression scale included in the QLQ and the more extensive measures of psychological distress employed during the interview.

Hence, it can be seen that the second phase of the research is ambitious in scope, requiring tracking of patients over time and administration of a rather extensive interview. It is for this reason that it is considered prudent to first carry out the cross-sectional study. On the basis of the data derived from the cross-sectional analysis, it will be determined whether the QLQ can be applied in the longitudinal study as originally designed, or whether certain modifications are required before moving into the second phase of the research.

Conclusions

In recent years there has been an ever increasing interest in evaluating the efficacy of cancer treatments, not only from a biological perspective, but also in terms of their impact on the daily lives of patients. Yet, to date, only a few investigational protocols have actually incorporated, in a systematic manner, psychosocial or "quality-of-life" end points as part of the evaluation package. A major barrier to the introduction of quality-of-life end points in clinical research would appear to be the absence of measurement instruments that demonstrate adequate levels of validity, reliability and sensitivity when used with cancer populations.

In this paper we have described a "modular" approach to quality-of-life assessment that has been developed, and is currently being tested, by the EORTC Study Group on Quality of Life. This approach involves disaggregating the quality-of-life construct into a number of discrete conceptual domains reflecting the physical, functional, social and psychological health of the individual. For each of these domains, one or more assessment modules (i. e., questionnaire scales) have been developed such that, when combined into a core questionnaire, they can be employed to assess the psychosocial status of a broad range of cancer patients (i. e., patients with varying diagnoses and/or undergoing varying treatments). This core instrument has been supplemented by an additional questionnaire module that addresses specific questions relevant to lung cancer patients. We hope that adoption of this assessment strategy can reconcile two of the principal requirements of quality-of-life assessment in cancer clinical trials - a sufficient degree of generalizability to allow for cross-study comparisons and a level of specificity adequate for answering those questions of particular relevance in a given trial setting.

This modular system is currently being tested on a large sample of lung cancer patients drawn from institutions in 15 countries. The results of the study will provide essential data regarding the adequacy of this approach in terms of clinical feasibility, psychometric robustness, and cross-cultural applicability. It is hoped that through this international research collaboration significant progress will be made toward establishing standardized methods of quality-of-life assessment in cancer clinical trials.

References

Aaronson NK (1986) Methodological issues in psychological oncology with special reference to clinical trials. In: Ventafridda V, van Dam FSAM, Yancik R, Tamburini M (eds) Assessment of quality of life and cancer treatment. Elsevier Science, Amsterdam, pp 29-41

Aaronson NK (study coordinator) (1987) EORTC protocol 15861: development of a core quality-of-life questionnaire for use in cancer clinical trials. EORTC Data Center, Brussels

Aaronson NK, Bakker W, Stewart Al, van Dam FSAM, van Zandwijk N, Yarnold JR, Kirkpatrick A (1987) Multidimensional approach to the measurement of quality of life in lung cancer clinical trials. In: Aaronson N, Beckmann J (eds) The quality of life of cancer patients. Raven, New York, pp 63-82

American Psychological Association (1974) Standards for educational and psychological tests. APA, Washington, DC

Andersen BL (1985) Sexual functioning morbidity among cancer survivors: current status and future research directions. Cancer 55 (8): 1835-1842

Bardelli D, Saracci R (1978) Measuring the quality of life in cancer clinical trials: a sample survey of published trials. UICC technical report series, Geneva

Bergner M, Bobbit RA, Carter WB, Gilson BS (1981) The Sickness Impact Profile: development and final revision of a health status measure. Med Care 19: 787-805

Bury M (1982) Chronic illness as biographical disruption. Sociology Health Illness 41: 167-182

Buyse ME, Staquet MJ, Sylvester RJ (eds) (1984) Cancer clinical trials. Oxford University Press, Oxford

Campbell DT, Fiske DW (1959) Convergent and discriminant validation by the multitrait-multimethod matrix. Psychol Bull 56: 81-105

Chambers LW, MacDonald LA, Tugwell P (1983) The McMaster health index questionnaire as a measure of quality of life for patients with rheumatoid arthritis. J Rheumatol 9: 780-784

Ciampi A, Silberfeld M, Till JE (1983) Health status indices: some approaches and their limitations for oncology. Int Psychol 15: 4-14

Clark A, Fallowfield LJ (1986) Quality-of-life measurements in patients with malignant disease: a review. J R Soc Med 79 (3): 165-169

Cronbach LJ (1951) Coefficient alpha and the internal structure of tests. Psychometrika 16: 297-334

Daut RL, Cleeland CS (1982) The prevalence and severity of pain in cancer. Cancer 50: 1913-1918

de Haes JCJM, van Knippenberg FCE (1985) The quality of life of cancer patients: a review of the literature. Soc Sci Med 20: 809-817

Derogatis LR, Morrow GR, Fetting J, Penman D (1983) The prevalence of psychiatric disorders among cancer patients. JAMA 249: 751-757
DuPuy HJ (1984) The psychological general well-being (PGWB) index. In: Wenger NK, Mattsen ME, Furberg CD, Ellinson J (eds) Assessment of quality of life in clinical trials of cardiovascular therapies. Le Jacq, Washington, DC, pp 170-184
Endicott J (1984) Measurement of depresssion in patients with cancer. Cancer 53: 2243-2248
Fayers PM, Jones DR (1983) Measuring and analysing quality of life in cancer clinical trials: a review. Stat Med 2: 429-446
Friedman LM, Furberg CD, DeMets DL (1985) Fundamentals of clinical trials. PSG, New York
Gottschalk LA (1983) Measurement of mood and affect in cancer patients. Cancer 53 [Suppl]: 2236-2240
Gough IR, Furnival CM, Schilder L, Grove W (1983) Assessment of the quality of life of patients with advanced cancer. Eur J Cancer Clin Oncol 19: 1161-1165
Green S, Silberfarb PM (1982) Psychological concomitants of cancer: current state of research. Psychol Med 12: 563-573
Greenwald HP (1987) The specificity of quality-of-life measures among the seriously ill. Med Care 25: 642-651
Greer DS (1987) Quality-of-life measurement in the clinical realm. J Chronic Dis 40: 629
Greer S (1984) The psychological dimension in cancer treatment. Soc Sci Med 18 (4): 345-349
Guttman LA (1944) A basis for scaling qualitative data. Am Soc Rev 9: 139-150
Helmstadter CG (1964) Principles of psychological measurement. Appleton-Century-Crofts, New York
Hunt SM, McWeen J, McKenna SP (1981) The Nottingham Health Profile: subjective health status and medical consultations. Soc Sci Med [A] 15: 221-229
Hutchinson TA, Boyd NF, Feinstein AR (1979) Scientific problems in clinical scales as demonstrated in the Karnofksy Index of performance status. J Chronic Dis 32: 661-666
Kaplan M, Bush J (1982) Health-related quality-of-life measurement for evaluation research and policy analysis. Health Psychol 1: 61-80
Katz S (1987) The science of quality of life. J Chronic Dis 40: 459
Krauth J (1982) Objective measurements of the quality of life. Experientia 41: 402-451
Lane DA (1987) Utility, decision and quality of life. J Chronic Dis 40: 585
Likert R (1932) A technique for the measurement of attitudes. Arch Psychol 140: 1-55
Linssen ACG, Hanewald G, van Dam FSAM, van Beek-Couzijn AL (1981) The development of the "complaint questionnaire" at the Netherlands Cancer Institute. In: Proc 1st EORTC study group on quality of life workshop, Amsterdam, 22-23 May 1981
Meenan RF (1980) Measuring health status in arthritis: the arthritis impact measurement scale. Arthritis Rheum 23: 146-152
Nie NH, Hull CH, Jenkins JG, Steinbrenner K, Bent DH (1970) Statistical package for the social sciences, 2nd edn. McGraw Hill, New York
Nunnally JC (1978) Psychometric theory, 2nd edn. McGraw Hill, New York
Schipper H, Clinch J, McMurray A, Levitt M (1984) Measuring the quality of life of cancer patients: the functional living index cancer. J Clin Oncol 2: 472-483
Selby PJ, Chapman JAW, Etazadi-Amoli J, Dalley D, Boyd NF (1984) The development of a method of assessing the quality of life of cancer patients. Br J Cancer 50: 13-22
Stewart Al, Ware JE, Brook RH (1982) Constructing and scoring of aggregate functional status measures, vol 1, R-2551-1-HHS. Rand Corporation, Santa Monica, CA
van Dam FSAM, Linssen CAG, Couzijn AL (1984) Evaluating quality of life in cancer clinical trials. In: Buyse et al. (eds) Cancer clinical trials: methods and practice. Oxford University Press, Oxford, pp 26-46
Ware JE (1984a) Methodology in behavioral and psychological cancer research: conceptualizing disease impact and treatment outcomes. Cancer 53 [Suppl]: 2316-2326

Ware JE (1984b) Methodological considerations in the selection of health status assessment procedures. In: Wenger NK, Mattson ME, Furberg CD, Elinson J (eds) Assessment of quality of life in cardiovascular clinical trials. Le Jacq, Washington, DC, pp 87-112
Ware JE (1987) Standards for validating health measures: definition and content. J Chronic Dis 40: 473 ff
Ware JE, Davies-Avery A, Donald CA (1978) Conceptualization and measurement of health for adults in the health insurance study, vol 5. Rand Corporation, Santa Monica, CA
Wood-Dauphinee S, Troidl H (1986) End points for surgical clinical studies: conventional and innovative variables. In: Troidl H, Spitzer WO, McPeek B, Mulder DS, McKneally MA (eds) Principles and practice of research. Springer, Berlin Heidelberg New York, pp 54-68
Wortman CB (1983) Social support and the cancer patient: conceptual and methodological issues. Cancer 53: 2217-2384
Zigmond AS, Snaith RP (1983) The hospital anxiety and depression scale. Acta Psychiatr Scand 67: 3661-370

Appendix A. The EORTC Core Quality of Life Questionnaire and Lung Cancer-Specific Questionnaire Module

Note: The EORTC Core Quality of Life Questionnaire and Lung Cancer-Specific Questionnaire Module are reproduced for informational purposes only. Use of the questionnaires outside of the context of EORTC protocol 15861 is prohibited without prior written consent of the study coordinator. The questionnaires will be made available for general use after documentation of the psychometric properties of the instrument and development of standard scoring procedures have been completed.

Questionnaire

We are interested in some things about you and your health. Please answer all the questions yourself by circling the number that best applies to you. There are no 'right' or 'wrong' answers. The information that you provide will remain strictly confidential.

Please fill in your initials: ....

Your birth date (Day, Month, Year): ....

Today's date (Day, Month, Year): ....

for administration only

1 [1|5|8|6|1]
6 [| |]
9 [| | | | |]
15 [|1|7|2|0|]

	No	Yes	
1. Can you do hard activities, like moving heavy furniture?	1	2	22 ☐
2. If you wanted to, could you run a short distance?	1	2	23 ☐
3. Do you have any trouble taking a long walk?	1	2	24 ☐

4. Do you have any trouble walking a short distance?	1	2	25 ☐
5. Are you in bed or a chair for most of the day?	1	2	26 ☐
6. Do you have to stay indoors most of the day?	1	2	27 ☐
7. Do you need help with eating, dressing, washing yourself or using the toilet?	1	2	28 ☐
8. Are you limited in any way in doing your work or household jobs?	1	2	29 ☐
9. Are you completely unable to work at a job or do household jobs?	1	2	30 ☐

During the past week:	Not at all	A little	Quite a bit	Very much	
10. Were you short of breath?	1	2	3	4	31 ☐
11. Have you had pain?	1	2	3	4	32 ☐
12. Did you need to rest?	1	2	3	4	33 ☐
13. Have you felt ill?	1	2	3	4	34 ☐
14. Have you had trouble sleeping?	1	2	3	4	35 ☐
15. Have you felt weak?	1	2	3	4	36 ☐
16. Have you lacked appetite?	1	2	3	4	37 ☐
17. Have you felt nauseated?	1	2	3	4	38 ☐
18. Have you vomited?	1	2	3	4	39 ☐
19. Have you been constipated?	1	2	3	4	40 ☐
20. Have you had diarrhea?	1	2	3	4	41 ☐
21. Were you tired?	1	2	3	4	42 ☐
22. Have you had difficulty in concentrating or remembering things?	1	2	3	4	43 ☐
23. Could you sit at ease and feel relaxed?	1	2	3	4	44 ☐

24. Have you lost interest in your appearance?	1	2	3	4	45 ☐
25. Have you felt restless as if you had to be on the move?	1	2	3	4	46 ☐
26. Did you look forward with enjoyment to things?	1	2	3	4	47 ☐
27. Did you get sudden feelings of panic?	1	2	3	4	48 ☐
28. Could you enjoy a good book or radio or television program?	1	2	3	4	49 ☐
29. Have you felt tense or 'wound up'?	1	2	3	4	50 ☐
30. Could you laugh and see the funny side of things?	1	2	3	4	51 ☐
31. Were you physically well?	1	2	3	4	52 ☐
32. Has your condition interfered with your family or social life?	1	2	3	4	53 ☐
33. Has your medical treatment interfered with your family or social life?	1	2	3	4	54 ☐
34. Has your condition or treatment caused you financial difficulties?	1	2	3	4	55 ☐

For the following questions please circle the number between 1 and 7 that best applies to you

35. How would you rate your overall physical condition during the past week?

1	2	3	4	5	6	7	
Very poor						Excellent	56 ☐

36. How would you rate your overall quality of life during the past week?

1	2	3	4	5	6	7	
Very poor						Excellent	57 ☐

Patients sometimes report that they have the following symptoms. Please indicate the extent to which you have experienced these symptoms during the past week.

During the past week:	Not at all	A little	Quite a bit	Very much	
37. How much did you cough?	1	2	3	4	58 ☐
38. Did you cough blood?	1	2	3	4	59 ☐
39. Were you short of breath when you rested?	1	2	3	4	60 ☐
40. Were you short of breath when you walked?	1	2	3	4	61 ☐
41. Were you short of breath when you climbed stairs?	1	2	3	4	62 ☐
42. Have you had a sore mouth or tongue?	1	2	3	4	63 ☐
43. Have you had trouble swallowing?	1	2	3	4	64 ☐
44. Have you had tingling hands or feet?	1	2	3	4	65 ☐
45. Have you been bothered by hair loss?	1	2	3	4	66 ☐
46. Have you had pain in your chest?	1	2	3	4	67 ☐
47. Have you had pain in your arm or shoulder?	1	2	3	4	68 ☐
48. Have you had pain in other parts of your body?	1	2	3	4	69 ☐
If yes, where? ____________________					
49. Did you take any medicine for pain?					
1 No					
2 Yes – how much did it help?	1	2	3	4	70 ☐☐

Please check to make sure that you have answered all of the questions 72 ☐☐☐☐☐☐

Please use the space below for any additional comments you may have:

*Effects of Breast Conservation on Psychological Morbidity Associated with Diagnosis and Treatment of Early Breast Cancer**

L. J. Fallowfield, M. Baum, and G. P. Maguire**

Cancer Research Campaign, Clinical Trials Centre, Rayne Institute,
London SE5 9NU, Great Britain

Introduction

There is growing evidence that in early breast cancer relapse-free intervals and survival rates are comparable in patients treated either by mastectomy or by local excision and radiotherapy (Fisher et al. 1985). These data, together with reports that women who undergo mastectomy suffer high levels of anxiety or depression, or both (Morris et al. 1977; Maguire et al. 1978), have led to an increasing trend towards more conservative surgery. In any case, many surgeons dislike performing the more mutilating operation (Ray and Baum 1985).

While most clinicians believe intuitively that breast conservation will protect women against psychiatric morbidity, there has been little systematic study of the psychosocial outcome of this treatment (Sanger and Reznikoff 1981; Schain et al. 1983; Steinberg et al. 1985; Ashcroft et al. 1985). Two reports comparing psychological outcome of lumpectomy versus mastectomy for breast cancer found no appreciable differences between, or serious problems within, treatment groups, but they were studies conducted on small samples of patients (Sanger and Reznikoff 1981; Steinberg et al. 1985). The authors of both papers also acknowledged that some emotionally distressed patients were not included. Another report described data from 38 patients randomised to treatment (Schain et al. 1983). Psychological problems were assessed using a nonstandardised postal questionnaire. The only significant difference between treatment groups on 13 psychosocial variables was a less negative reaction to body image among the conservatively treated patients.

A recent study presented preliminary data on 40 patients who were helped to discuss treatment options and make their own choice (Ashcroft et al. 1985). The authors concluded that giving the patient autonomy over her treatment or offering reconstruction when choice is not possible prevents psychiatric morbidity.

General conclusions about the relative psychological impact of different treatments are difficult to draw from these small studies, but they provide no clear evi-

---

* Reproduced with permission from: British Medical Journal (1986) 293: 1331-1334.
** We thank all the surgeons and radiotherapists who permitted access to their patients and the Cancer Research Campaign for financial support.

© Springer-Verlag Berlin · Heidelberg 1988

dence that lumpectomy rather than mastectomy necessarily lessens the likelihood of psychological problems. Possibly, the advantages of conserving the breast are outweighed by greater worries about cancer (Senescu 1963) and the adverse effects of radiotherapy (Peck and Boland 1977; Forester et al. 1978; Holland et al. 1979). The Cancer Research Campaign's breast conservation trial (Peckham 1982) provided a unique opportunity to investigate these issues.

Subjects and Methods

Sample

Patients came from ten of the 11 different centres participating in the Cancer Research Campaign's breast conservation trial. One centre chose to conduct its own psychological study. The protocol required participants to ascertain whether suitable patients - that is, women under 70 with early breast cancer - had a strong preference for mastectomy or breast conservation. If no preference was expressed, the patient was randomly allocated to treatment by a telephone call to the clinical trials coordinator. The randomisation lists were generated by computer for individual participants, optimising the probability of a balanced treatment allocation for each participating clinician. All patients had a confirmed diagnosis of "early" stage-I or -II breast cancer - that is, tumours of 5 cm diameter or less with or without palpable axillary nodes and no evidence of distant metastases - and were judged by the surgeon to be eligible for either treatment strategy before randomisation.

The proportion of suitable patients who were not entered into the trial will not be known until a full audit of the main study is done in every centre.

The original protocol envisaged a *prospective* parallel psychological arm to the main breast conservation trial, but the study of psychosocial sequelae began 24 months after the start of the main trial. As empirical work comparing psychological outcome of the different treatments was so sparse, and no study of patients randomised to treatment had been published, we decided to initiate a *retrospective* study of all the patients already recruited.

There were 127 patients in the conservation trial potentially available for the psychological study; of these, seven died before interview, one was deemed physically too sick with recurrent disease to participate, nine refused or failed to reply to an invitation to join the study, and nine filled in questionnaires but declined to be interviewed. One hundred and one patients therefore took part in the retrospective study, of whom 48 were treated by local excision and radiotherapy and 53 underwent mastectomy; 34 of the patients given mastectomy also had radiotherapy. Four of the patients treated by lumpectomy and one treated by mastectomy had adjuvant chemotherapy.

Method

Psychiatric morbidity, sexual functioning, and social adjustment were determined postoperatively. A trained interviewer (LJF) first administered a semistructured interview schedule designed to elicit information about the patient's marital state, key relationships, and use and availability of social support. The women were asked about their feelings on discovering the breast lump and their reaction to the diagnosis. They also recalled what doctors had told them about their diagnosis and treatment and whether the information was perceived as adequate. The interviewer then used the present state examination (Wing et al. 1974), minus the questions about psychotic symptoms, to determine the nature, frequency, and severity of symptoms of anxiety and depression in the 4 weeks before the interview. DSM III diagnostic criteria (American Psychiatric Association 1980) were then applied to establish if there had been sufficient mood disturbance and other symptoms to justify a diagnosis of depressive illness or anxiety state. For example, to rate as a case of anxiety state a woman had to have had persistent feelings of tension and apprehension or inability to relax for at least 4 weeks plus four other symptoms, such as sleep disturbance, impaired concentration, fatigability, somatic symptoms (headaches, sweating, palpitations, tremor), panic attacks, or irritability. Likewise, to rate as depressed a woman had to have had persistent, unremitting unhappiness or lowering of mood for at least 4 weeks plus four other symptoms, such as sleep disturbance, impaired concentration, loss of self-esteem, feelings of guilt, suicidal ideation, loss of energy, retardation or agitation, changes in appetite, weight loss or gain, or loss of libido.

Interviews were conducted in the patient's home, which permitted more intimate discussion than was possible on a busy ward and furthermore allowed the interviewer to assess the social environment, which might have contributed to problems experienced by the patient. All interviews lasted roughly 45 min (range 30–90 min) and were tape recorded. Rate-rerate reliability checks were performed on 30% of the tapes and showed ratings to have been consistent, with little drift. An independent rater checked the reliability of ratings for 10% of the interviews and found an overall agreement of 90%.

Interviewing patients is time consuming and expensive and requires a trained interviewer. Another important part of this project was the validation of sound research tools that are cheap and easy to administer routinely to patients by paramedical personnel. Hence, after the interview the women were given two self-assessment questionnaires, the hospital anxiety and depression scale (Zigmund and Snaith 1983) and the Rotterdam symptom check list (Pruyn et al. 1981). They completed these after the interviewer had left and returned them in a postage-prepaid envelope to the trials centre. Compliance was 100% and a full analysis of the performance of these new questionnaires will be reported separately.

Comparability of Groups

Table 1 shows the demographic characteristics of patients in the two treatment groups. Social class distributions and mean ages were similar. The times from operation to assessment of psychiatric morbidity varied in this retrospective study, but both the ranges and the mean times from operation to interview were similar in the two groups. Marital state differed between the two groups, more single and widowed women having been treated by mastectomy. This random imbalance should therefore have favoured the breast-conservation group slightly, as widowed and single people are more prone to depressive illness.

Table 1. Demographic characteristics

	Mastectomy group ($n=53$)	Lumpectomy group ($n=48$)
Mean age in years (SD) [range]	56 (10) [32–72]	58 (8) [32–71]
Marital state:		
Married	35	38
Single/widowed	14	6
Separated/divorced	4	4
Social class:		
I	8	5
II	16	15
III (a)	11	13
III (b)	11	9
IV	7	6
V	0	0
Mean time from operation to interview in months (SD) [range]	16.7 (7.9) [4–32]	15.2 (6.6) [4–31]

Table 2. Psychiatric morbidity. Figures are numbers (percentages) of patients

	Anxiety state	Depressive illness	Anxiety state and depressive illness	Either or both affective disorders
Mastectomy group ($n=53$)	14 (26)	11 (21)	8 (15)	17 (32)
Lumpectomy group ($n=48$)	15 (31)	13 (27)	10 (21)	18 (38)

Results and Discussion

Psychiatric Morbidity

Table 2 shows that, according to our diagnostic criteria, 11 (21%) of the patients with mastectomy had a depressive illness and 14 (26%) an anxiety state. Among the breast-conservation patients 13 (27%) were experiencing a depressive illness and 15 (31%) an anxiety state. Some women (eight [15%] in the mastectomy group, [21%] in the lumpectomy group) had both affective disorders. These figures mean that overall, an anxiety state or depressive illness, or both, was evident in 17 (33%) of the patients with mastectomy and 18 (38%) of those treated by lumpectomy. Table 3 shows the level of sexual interest experienced by the women in the different treatment groups. On self-assessment, 18 of 48 of the patients with mastectomy (38%) and 15 of 39 treated by lumpectomy (38%) reported a lack of sexual interest. Five patients in the mastectomy group and nine in the lumpectomy group who were elderly or single did not answer the question. We could not assess accurately the degree to which treatment might have been responsible for the decline in sexual interest, as we had no preoperative measure of sexual activity.

Table 3. Self-report on Rotterdam symptom check list assessing lack of sexual interest. Figures are numbers (percentages) of patients

	"Not at all" to "a little"	"Somewhat" to "very much"
Mastectomy group ($n=48$)[a]	30 (62)	18 (38)
Lumpectomy group ($n=39$)[a]	24 (62)	15 (38)

[a] Fourteen elderly or single women in the two groups without sexual partners did not answer the question.

Table 4. Perception of information received. Figures are numbers (percentages) of patients

	"Do you feel that the information that you received at the hospital was adequate?"		
	Yes	No	Total
Mastectomy group	26 (50)	26 (50)	52 (100)[a]
Lumpectomy group	22 (46)	26 (54)	48 (100)
Total	48	52	100

[a] One patient did not answer the question.

Information

There are consistent reports that hospital patients feel inadequately informed about their diagnosis and treatment (Ley 1982). One study of patients with mastectomy found that 21% were dissatisfied with the information given (Morris et al. 1977). Most of the ethical committees of the centres participating in our study required surgeons to obtain informed consent from patients before randomisation. It would therefore be reasonable to hope that patients in this trial would have had more information about their illness and surgical options than is perhaps always possible in a busy outpatient department. Table 4 shows that in answer to the question: "Do you feel that the information that you received at the hospital was adequate?" over half of the women (52%) said "no." There was no significant difference in this perception of information received between patients in the mastectomy and lumpectomy groups. We had hypothesised that the incidence of anxiety states and depressive illness would be less for patients who perceived information to have been good. This appeared to be so, cases of anxiety or depression, or both, being recorded in 11 of 48 women (23%) who reported the level of information to have been good as compared with 24 of 52 women (46%) who were poorly informed. This difference was significant (χ^2 test; $P<0.03$). Unfortunately, we cannot tell whether these data mean that anxious patients are less satisfied with their information or that well-informed patients are less anxious. This direction of causality is an important issue to address to improve communication between doctors and patients with breast cancer and demands further investigation in a prospective study.

While the proportions of women suffering from an affective disorder were similar in the two groups, their problems seemed to be qualitatively different.

Anxiety

The anxiety exhibited by women treated by lumpectomy seemed to stem from a feeling of uncertainty about the prognosis and the constant awareness of possible recurrence or metastatic disease. Some of these patients admitted to compulsive checking of their breasts for other lumps; five said that they examined themselves more than once a day. The following extracts are from the taped interviews of two patients:

"Do you know, if I get pain in my stomach now it's got to be cancer; if I've got a pain in my back I'm going to get lung cancer; get a bad head, I'm getting a tumour on the brain. I just can't get it out of may head."

"I just cannot keep my hand off [my breast]. It's something that I've never ever done. I spend hours just lying there feeling, and when I touch I feel as if I've got lumps all over."

Anxious patients with mastectomy obviously shared those uncertainties but expressed more overt concern about the effect of their surgery on relationships and a heightened self-consciousness about appearance. None of the patients with mastectomy admitted to daily self-examination, though three said that they checked their remaining breast at least weekly. An item in the Rotterdam symptom check list questionnaire asked how dissatisfied patients felt about the appearance of their scars; seven of the patients with mastectomy were very or somewhat dissatisfied, compared with one of the patients treated by lumpectomy ($P = 0.04$). Many of the women who had had breast conservation seemed less certain than the patients in the mastectomy group that they had received the right operation, though this is difficult to quantify directly. Possibly, the surgeons themselves still had a subthreshold doubt, which unwittingly they were communicating to the patient.

Depression

There were also differences between the groups in the reasons given for becoming depressed. Patients treated by lumpectomy complained about the particularly unpleasant and enervating fatigue that persisted after radiotherapy. Only two reported suffering no side effects. They felt dispirited at their slow return to health and normal activity after such a seemingly small operation. Conversely, many of the patients with mastectomy had had less expectation of a rapid return to work and normal functioning, and some therefore reported surprise that the treatment had not been quite as bad as they had feared. Of the 34 patients in the mastectomy group who had to have radiotherapy, seven were depressed. One patient in our study had great difficulty in adjusting to her mastectomy. Her intractable depression necessitated admission to a psychiatric hospital for electroconvulsive therapy.

Sexual Problems

While rejection by a spouse or partner is not uncommon after mastectomy, this happened to only one patient in our sample. We have no preoperative measures of the level of sexual activity of patients in this retrospective study, but over one third of the women in both groups reported a loss of sexual interest since their diagnosis and treatment for breast cancer. Loss of libido is a common symptom of depressive illness (American Psychiatric Association 1980), but many people have assumed that the severe assault on body image and self-esteem produced by amputation of the breast is in itself sufficient cause for the deterioration of sexual activity (Bransfield 1982). As the patients treated by lumpectomy in our study had just as severe a decline in their desire for love-making as the patients in the mastectomy group, possibly such assumptions need rethinking. Three of the 11 depressed patients with mastectomy reported loss of libido, compared with seven of the 13 depressed patients treated by lumpectomy. Such numbers were not significantly different, but there was a suggestion that loss of libido was symptomatic of depression in the lumpectomy-treated patients but more linked with inhibitions, loss of femininity, self-esteem, and body image concomitant with breast loss in the more radically treated group.

Choice of Treatment

Possibly, the women in this study who were prepared to be randomised to treatment displayed rather different psychological characteristics from patients who prefer to participate in the decision-making process. Women with a greater sense of autonomy might well adapt more readily to the consequences of a treatment policy that they have chosen. Evidence from a very small sample of women suggests that careful preoperative assessment and help with decision-making reduce the levels of psychiatric morbidity that we have reported (Ashcroft 1985).

Conclusions

This retrospective study suggests that the suppositions that *(a)* all women with breast cancer wish to retain their breast and *(b)* breast conservation prevents psychiatric morbidity might well be misplaced. It was not unusual at interview for patients in the lumpectomy group to express deep concern that they had received the "wrong" operation and to comment that they felt constantly worried that the surgeon might not have removed all the cancer and that it would return. If, so far as survival and local control of disease are concerned, it really makes no difference which treatment is offered in early breast cancer, then it becomes of paramount importance to consider the psychological impact of the treatment to be offered.

The degree of psychosocial morbidity among the patients treated by local excision and radiotherapy was a disappointing finding, but one which cannot be ignored. These women clearly need just as much counselling support as patients who undergo mastectomy.

As more surgeons start to advocate breast conservation, it is important that we have more basic research into the causal factors of the psychiatric morbidity experienced by women who receive this treatment.

References

American Psychiatric Association (1980) Diagnostic and statistical manual of mental disorder, 3rd edn. APA, Washington, DC

Ashcroft JJ, Leinster SJ, Slade PD (1985) Breast cancer - patient choice of treatment: preliminary communication. JR Soc Med 78: 43-46

Bransfield DD (1982) Breast cancer and sexual functioning: a review of the literature and implications for future research. Int J Psychiatry Med 12 (3): 197-211

Fisher B, Bauer M, Margolese R (1985) Five-year results of a randomised clinical trial comparing total mastectomy and segmental mastectomy with or without radiation in the treatment of breast cancer. N Engl J Med 312: 665-673

Forester BM, Kornfield RS, Fleiss J (1978) Psychiatric aspects of radiotherapy. Am J Psychiatry 135: 960-963

Holland JC, Rowland J, Lebovits A, Rusalem R (1979) Reactions to cancer treatment: assessment of emotional response to adjuvant radiotherapy as a guide to planned intervention. Psychiatr Clin North Am 2: 347-358

Ley P (1982) Giving information to patients. In: Eiser JR (ed) Social psychology and behavioral science. Wiley, Chichester, pp 339-371

Maguire GP, Lee EG, Bevington DJ et al. (1978) Psychiatric problems in the year after mastectomy. Br Med J 1: 963-965

Morris T, Steven-Greer H, White P (1977) Psychological and social adjustment to mastectomy (a 2-year follow-up study). Cancer 40: 2381-2387

Peck A, Boland J (1977) Emotional reactions to radiation treatment. Cancer 40: 180-184

Peckham MJ (1982) Protocol for a collaborative trial to evaluate the need for mastectomy in the management of early breast cancer. Cancer Research Campaign Clinical Trials Centre, London

Pruyn JFA, Maguire P, De Haes JCJM (1981) Two methods of measuring some aspects of quality of life. In: Quality of life methods of measurement and related areas. Proceedings of the second EORTC quality of life workshop, Copenhagen. European Organization for the Research and Treatment of Cancer, pp 52-55

Ray C, Baum M (1985) Psychological aspects of early breast cancer. Springer, Berlin Heidelberg New York Tokyo

Sanger CK, Reznikoff M (1981) A comparison of the psychological effects of breast-saving procedures with the modified mastectomy. Cancer 48: 2341-2346

Schain W, Edwards BK, Gorrell CR et al. (1983) Psychosocial and physical outcomes of stage-I breast cancer therapy: mastectomy v excisional biopsy and irradiation. Breast Cancer Res Treat 3: 377-382

Senescu RA (1963) The development of emotional complications in the patient with cancer. J Chronic Dis 16: 813-832

Steinberg MD, Juliano MA, Wise L (1985) Psychological outcome of lumpectomy versus mastectomy in the treatment of breast cancer. Am J Psychiatry 142: 34-39

Wing JK, Cooper JE, Sartorious N (1974) Measurement and classification of psychiatric symptoms. Cambridge University Press, Cambridge

Zigmund AS, Snaith RP (1983) The hospital anxiety and depression scale. Acta Psychiatr Scand 67: 370

*Evaluation of Psychosocial Aspects in a Breast Preservation Trial**

M. Olschewski, R. Verres, H. Scheurlen, and H. Rauschecker

Institut für Medizinische Biometrie und Informatik der Universität Freiburg,
Stefan-Meier-Straße 26, 7800 Freiburg, FRG

Introduction

The aim of a controlled clinical trial is usually to compare the efficacy of an innovative treatment with that of an established standard therapy. In cancer clinical trials the survival time of patients, i.e., the time from entry into the trial until death or recurrence, is the most important end point. This variable gives an objective description of what happens to the patient. However, both the disease and the treatment also have a subjective impact on the patient. To combine both objective and subjective viewpoints for a comprehensive appreciation of treatment effects we must take psychosocial factors into consideration - the latter are commonly referred to as the "quality of life" (QOL).

In this paper we will outline our approach of including QOL measurements in an ongoing clinical trial in breast cancer. We will first discuss the trial and the QOL measurement, and then present some preliminary results with regard to the patient population, the factor structure, and a comparison of treatments.

The Breast Preservation Trial

The Bundesministerium für Forschung und Technologie (BMFT) breast preservation trial is a government-funded, multicenter clinical trial. Patients are clinically examined for suspected breast cancer. When primary tumor excision and axillary dissection have proven a $pT_1pN_0M_0$ lesion and other eligibility criteria are fulfilled, informed consent is sought. The patient must decide whether to accept or reject randomization.

This decision process leads to three groups of patients within the trial:

---

* See Appendix A for a list of institutions and principal investigators participating in the BMFT study Breast Preserving Treatment in Early Breast Cancer.

Recent Results in Cancer Research, Vol. 111
© Springer-Verlag Berlin · Heidelberg 1988

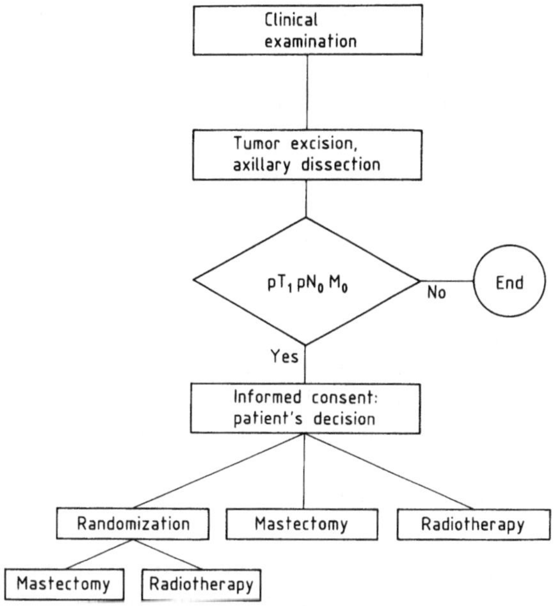

Fig. 1. Design of the BMFT breast preservation trial

1. Patients with no definite treatment preference accepting randomization
2. Patients preferring and choosing the standard therapy mastectomy
3. Patients preferring and choosing the breast preserving radiotherapy

This trial uses the methodology of a so-called comprehensive cohort study, combining randomized and nonrandomized patients in the analysis (Scheurlen et al. 1984).

The BMFT breast preservation trial started recruitment of patients in November 1983 with a scheduled end in December 1988. By February 1987 patients had been recruited in 66 participating centers all over the Federal Republic of Germany. Of these, 25% randomized at least one patient, while 75% reported that all their patients had a clear treatment preference either before or after informed consent was sought. Further heterogeneity with regard to centers is due to the fact that of those centers entering at least three patients, 25% are monotherapeutic, giving radiotherapy only. As these are inappropriate for comparisons, a detailed analysis should compare results with these centers included and excluded.

Of the 650 patients entered so far about 10% have been randomized, while 90% had a preference either for mastectomy (30%) or for radiotherapy (60%). Further results are too preliminary to be reported.

The QOL Questionnaire and its Development

We consider QOL to be multifactorial, subjective, and time-dependent. For evaluation purposes we decided to subdivide the set of questions to be asked into three main areas: physical, emotional, and social well-being.

On the basis of a survey of published and unpublished QOL questionnaires we first had several discussions to select items relevant for a woman with early breast cancer. After this first "face-and-content" selection the chosen items were conceptualized in the following way:

1. All items were formulated in the first person.
2. It was decided not to ask for symptoms, but to use bipolar self-rating scales with a range from positive to negative and a neutral point in the middle; e.g., if we were to ask about the patient's anxiety, the question would be worded "Are you concerned about your health?" in order not to stimulate negative aspects in the patient by naming them.
3. The possible answers are preformulated on five-point scales.
4. Since physical, emotional, and social well-being may change during the coping process following diagnosis and primary therapy we ask the patient to recall the last 4 weeks in order to try to avoid overemphasis on the momentary condition.
5. By asking the patient to concentrate on her reflections on the disease and the sequelae of treatment we try to adjust for other events that might interfere with her well-being.

A preliminary 32-item version of the QOL questionnaire was given to 50 patients who had had breast cancer in the aftercare units of the university surgical clinics in Heidelberg and Göttingen. Patients were asked to fill out the questionnaire and to comment on the understandability and personal relevance of each item.

The results of item analyses and exploratory factor analyses led to the elimination and reformulation of several items after further discussions. Only those items were retained that:

1. Were highly relevant to the patient and were not ambiguous
2. Had a high degree of differentiability
3. Had a response rate of over 80% through being easily unterstood and not controversial
4. Had a significant factor loading in the factor analyses

The final questionnaire then ended up with 25 items passing the selection process (see Appendix B).

An open question was appended giving the patient the opportunity to make additional comments. The patients are asked to complete the questionnaire three times, 9, 18, and 36 months after treatment, to enable changes of their well-being over time to be detected. The QOL questionnaire has proven to be a simple tool, being easy to administer to patients without assistance or training and having a mean completion time of less than 15 min.

Results

The results presented here are based on the 246 questionnaires currently available; they were completed at the first measurement point 9 months after treatment and 67% of the questionnaires due. It should be noted that these results are very preliminary and are intended only to demonstrate the kind of statements to be expected from a final analysis.

Table 1. Comparison of prognostic factors of patients who completed the first questionnaire and those that did not

Prognostic factor (mean ± percentage)	Completers of QOL questionnaire ($n=246$)	Noncompleters of QOL questionnaire ($n=111$)
Age (years)	53.3 ± 12.1	52.8 ± 13.4
Tumor size (mm)	13.9 ± 4.5	13.6 ± 4.3
Number of inspected lymph nodes	10.9 ± 3.6	11.8 ± 4.8
Postmenopausal	56.1	55.0
Lateral tumor site	63.0	69.4
Estrogen-receptor positive	68.7	54.0
Progesterone-receptor positive	67.5	54.8
Tumor grading		
1	36.9	33.0
2	51.1	52.8
3	12.0	14.3
Randomized	13.8	5.4
Breast preservation	72.8	71.2
Married	71.5	65.8
Living with significant other	73.6	77.8
Professionally active	35.0	36.0

Representativeness of the Patients

The study protocol provides for an assessment of prognostic and sociodemographic factors. These can be used to compare patients completing the questionnaire with those who do not.

Table 1 shows that the only marked differences occur with regard to randomization status and hormone receptor status. While it is plausible that randomized patients are more willing to take part in the additional QOL evaluation, the reasons for the higher proportion of patients whose tumors were receptor positive among the responders than among the nonresponders are not abvious.

In addition, as shown in Fig. 2, the response rate varied between hospitals; a few centers that entered the larger numbers of patients are responsible for more than 50% of the missing QOL questionnaires. We do not think, however, that this obvious bias of some hospitals against the QOL assessment has any serious impact on the comparability of responders and nonresponders. At present it looks as though the responders do not differ too much from the nonresponders with respect to prognostic and sociodemographic factors.

Factor Structure of the QOL Questionnaire

The 246 completed questionnaires available were analyzed by factor-analytic techniques first to reduce the dimension of the QOL measuring instrument and secondly to prove its validity. The results presented here are from a principal components analysis adequate for detecting an underlying pattern of relationship between the original items. To achieve a structure as simple as possible, we per-

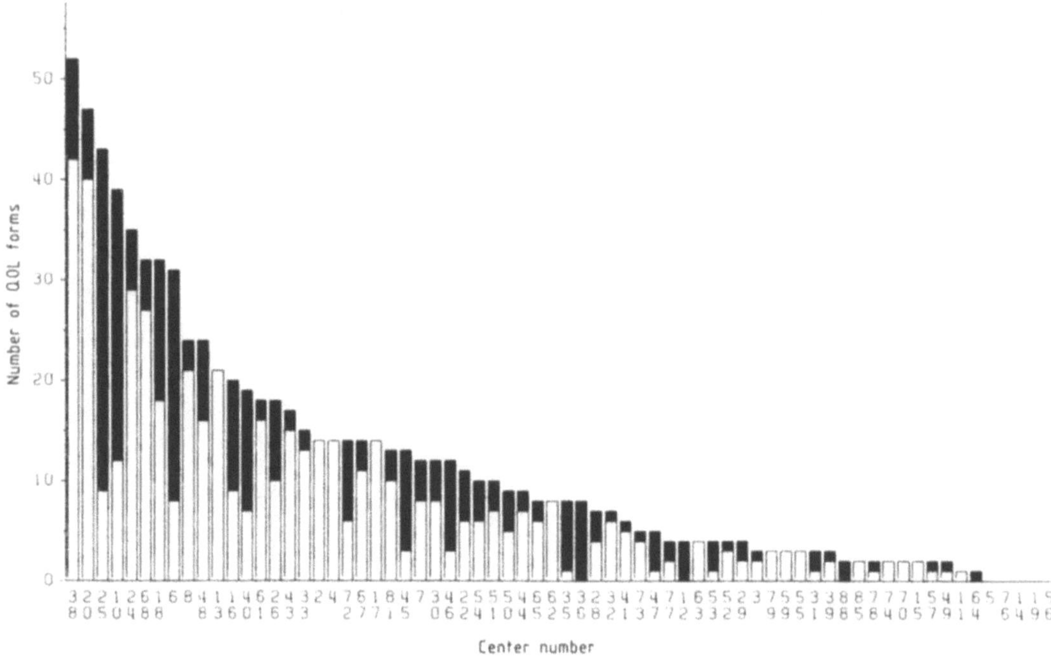

Fig. 2. Completion of QOL questionnaires across participating centers. □, Completed; ■, missing

formed a promax rotation of the factors. This twofold rotation improves the results of a first orthogonal rotation by using a nonsingular oblique transformation.

Using the criterion of number of eigenvalues greater than 1, we extracted five factors that together accounted for 60% of the variance of all items. The complete factor structure can be found in Table 2.

The first factor, which accounted for 41% of the variance, can be interpreted as a general factor of *emotional well-being* with a high loading on about half of all items. These items ask about general aspects of emotional well-being. The second factor we define as *psychosocial mobility,* showing how aspects of psychosocial well-being correlate with aspects of performance. The third factor can be interpreted straightforwardly as the dimension of *physical well-being.* In the context of the breast cancer trial this means the patients' coping with the typical side effects of treatment. The fourth factor can be explained as the dimension of *social well-being* with high-loading items dominated by social interactions. The last factor of importance can be described as one of *emotional security.* Here only the item asking about the desire for tenderness has a major loading.

Together, these results correspond quite well with our hypothesized concept of the three dimensions, physical, emotional, and social well-being. It is worth noting that the first factor by itself might be used as a one-dimensional global QOL measurement, because it explains nearly half of the variance of the items and it has an extremely high correlation of 0.93 with the ad hoc QOL score one would obtain by just calculating the mean score of all 25 items.

Table 2. Factor structure of the QOL questionnaire (loadings with an absolute value less than 0.33 are omitted)

	Factors				
	1	2	3	4	5
25 Enterprise	0.79				
22 Energy	0.76				
20 Disposition	0.76				
4 Feeling healthy	0.72				
2 Feeling strong	0.69				
15 Worries about health	0.67		0.37		
8 Satisfaction with life	0.67				
18 Hope for the future	0.65				
21 Handling free time	0.65				
6 Doing the day's work	0.55				
9 Joyfulness	0.55	0.40			
1 Sleeping	0.53				
19 Ability to make decisions	0.46	0.33			
12 Appetite		0.79			
7 Confidence in the company of men		0.69			
3 Getting on out of the house		0.54			
5 Trouble with arm on operated side			0.72		
17 Pain in region of operated breast			0.69		
10 Looking after herself at home			0.65		
23 Satisfaction with the scar			0.55		
11 Feeling of support by fellow men				0.80	0.34
24 Satisfaction in contact with relatives				0.63	
14 Social contacts		0.42		0.51	
13 Satisfaction with physical appearance	0.38			0.43	
16 Desire for tenderness					0.82
Variance explained by factors	41%	6%	5%	5%	4%

Preliminary Treatment Comparisons

The results of the factor analysis can be used for a further analysis. With the help of the factor scores we can calculate five factor values for each patient from the 25 items. These values can be interpreted as the patient's score within each factor. The factor values are standardized variates with a mean of zero and unit variance. In the original item coding a low score corresponded to a positive rating on that item and vice versa; the values for the theoretical factors can be interpreted in the same way, i.e., the smaller the factor value, the better the patient's score on that factor. The factor values can now be used for comparisons of groups of patients.

Table 3 shows the mean factor values for patient groups divided according to the treatment they received. From this it can be seen that radiotherapy looks favorable regarding factors 2, 3, and 5, while the opposite is true for factors 1 and 4. Comparing randomized and nonrandomized patients shows nonrandomized patients to be better off with respect to all five factors (Table 4).

In addition to using factor values, which represent the hypothetical underlying QOL dimensions, the original items can be used to represent specific aspects in a

Table 3. Mean factor values for patients grouped by treatment given

	Mastectomy ($n=67$)	Radiotherapy ($n=178$)
Factor 1	−0.012	0.005
Factor 2	0.144	−0.054
Factor 3	0.072	−0.027
Factor 4	−0.160	0.060
Factor 5	0.188	−0.071

Table 4. Mean factor values for patients grouped by randomization status

	Randomized ($n=34$)	Nonrandomized ($n=211$)
Factor 1	0.030	−0.005
Factor 2	0.050	−0.008
Factor 3	0.096	−0.015
Factor 4	0.003	−0.001
Factor 5	0.265	−0.043

comparison of patient groups. Again, when comparing treatment received, Wilcoxon tests yield exploratory p values of less than 0.10 for six items. Radiotherapy fares better with respect to items 3 ("getting on out of the house"), 6 ("handling the day's work"), 23 ("satisfaction with the scar"), and 1 ("sleeping well"), while the opposite is true for items 11 ("feeling of support by fellow men") and 17 ("pain in the operated breast").

Our results using both categories of variables (factor values, and original items), although only preliminary, seem to support recent findings of Schain et al. (1983), Fallowfield et al. (1986), and Lasry et al. (1987); each treatment tends to be superior with regard to some aspects of QOL, but the differences vanish when global QOL is examined.

Summary

Our preliminary and exploratory data analysis of the current state of QOL assessment in the ongoing BMFT breast preservation trial indicates that our questionnaire meets criteria of validity, differentiability, and practicability in the context of a large multi-center trial. The results of treatment comparisons tend towards accordance with those of comparable studies, in that they do not show the often-postulated global superiority of breast-preserving therapy over mastectomy with respect to QOL. The special study concept of combining patients with and without treatment preference gives rise to a lot of methodological issues but is the only way to find out whether participation in the therapeutic decision-making process is beneficial to the patient or not.

References

Fallowfield LJ, Baum M, Maguire GP (1986) Effects of breast conservation on psychological morbidity associated with diagnosis and treatment of early breast cancer. Br Med J 293: 1331-1334

Lasry JCM et al. (1987) Depression and body image following mastectomy and lumpectomy. J Chronic Dis 40: 529-534

Schain W et al. (1983) Psychosocial and physical outcomes of primary breast cancer therapy: mastectomy vs excisional biopsy and irradiation. Breast Cancer Res Treat 3: 377-382

Scheurlen H, Olschewski M, Leibbrand D (1984) Zur Methodologie kontrollierter klinischer Studien über die Primärbehandlung des operablen Mammakarzinoms. Strahlentherapie 160: 459-468

Appendix 1

List of institutions and principal investigators participating in the Bundesministerium für Forschung und Technologie (BMFT) trial Breast Preserving Treatment in Early Breast Cancer:

Study Committee:

H. Rauschecker, University Surgical Clinic and Reference Center Surgery, Göttingen (Chairman)

R. Sauer, Radiotherapeutic Clinic and Reference Center Radiology, Erlangen

A. Schauer, Pathological Institute and Reference Center Pathology, Göttingen

M. Schumacher, Institute of Medical Biometry and Methodological Center, Freiburg

Clinical Centers and Principal Investigators:

Kreiskrankenhaus Albstadt	Dr. Geier
Klinikum Bamberg	Dr. Krone
St. Josefs-Hospital Bochum	Dr. Zumtobel
Herzogin-Elisabeth-Heim Braunschweig	Dr. Kurz
Zentralkrankenhaus Links der Weser Bremen	Dr. Schuette
Zentralkrankenhaus Frauenklinik Bremen	Dr. Braun
Kreiskrankenhaus Donaueschingen	Dr. Eberl
Knappschaftskrankenhaus Dortmund	Dr. Wuestenberg
Franz-Hospital Duelmen/Westf.	Dr. Gross
Städt. Krankenhaus Düsseldorf	Dr. Broßmann
Städt. Kliniken Duisburg	Dr. Schulte-Overberg
Kreiskrankenhaus Ebersberg	Dr. Bergauer
Kreiskrankenhaus Eckernfoerde	Dr. Besch
Marienhospital Essen-Altenessen	Dr. Huth
Städt. Krankenanstalten Eßlingen/Neckar	Dr. Barth
Universitäts-Frauenklinik Frankfurt	Dr. Vering
St. Katharinen-Hospital Frechen	Dr. Pulheim
Städt. Krankenhaus Friedrichshafen	Dr. Unbehaun
Zentrum für Chirurgie Gießen	Dr. Kunze

Chirurgische Univ.-Klinik Göttingen	Dr. Rauschecker
Krankenhaus Neu-Mariahilf Göttingen	Dr. Moorthi
Ev. Krankenhaus Göttingen-Weende	Dr. Sauer
Allgem. Krankenhaus Harburg-Hamburg	Dr. Ekue
Kreiskrankenhaus St. Marienberg Helmstedt	Dr. Stolte
Marienhospital Herne	Dr. Schlenkhoff
Universitätsfrauenklinik Homburg/Saar	Dr. Breitbach
Chir. Univ.-Klinik II Innsbruck	Dr. Mueller
Krankenhaus St. Elisabeth Jülich	Dr. Scheidt
Städt. Krankenhaus Kaiserslautern	Dr. Assmus
St. Vincentius-Krankenhäuser Karlsruhe	Dr. Haase, Dr. Seger
Städt. Frauenklinik Karlsruhe	Dr. Schermann
Diakonissen-Krankenhaus Karlsruhe	Dr. Stosiek
Chir. Univ.-Klinik Kiel	Dr. Sellschopp
Univ.-Frauenklinik Kiel	Dr. Gent
Univ.-Frauenklinik Köln	Dr. Kusche
Krankenanstalten Konstanz	Dr. Siekmann
Kreiskrankenhaus Kronach	Dr. Beyerle
Kreiskrankenhaus Lahr	Dr. Fricke
Kreiskrankenhaus Landshut	Dr. Heinz
Kreiskrankenhaus Lich	Dr. Debus-Tiller
St. Vincenz-Krankenhaus Limburg	Dr. Neumann
Klinik f. Chirurgie Med. Hochschule Lübeck	Dr. Kifner
Klinikum Mannheim Chirurgie	Dr. Winter
Klinikum Mannheim Gynäkologie	Dr. Ziegler
Diakonie-Krankenhaus Marburg	Dr. Scharsich
Elisabeth-Krankenhaus Mönchengladbach	Dr. Massenkeil
Chirurgische Klinik und Poliklinik München	Dr. Richter-Turtur
Kreiskrankenhaus München-Pasing	Dr. Foeckersperger
Klinikum Großhadern München	Dr. Eiermann
Städt. Krankenhaus München-Neuperlach	Dr. Hall
Krankenhaus Hetzelstift Neustadt/Weinstraße	Dr. Sievers
Ev. Krankenhaus Oberhausen	Dr. von Wrese
St. Josefs-Hospital Oberhausen-Sterkrade	Dr. Ott
Städt. Krankenhaus Passau	Dr. Fischer
Städt. Krankenhaus Pirmasens	Dr. Steinebrei
Kreiskrankenhaus Rinteln	Dr. Baltzer
Kreiskrankenhaus Rotthalmünster	Dr. Kronpass
Städt. Krankenhaus Salzgitter-Lebenstedt	Dr. Gundelsheimer
Krankenhaus Siegburg	Dr. Horeyseck
Elisabeth-Krankenhaus Straubing	Dr. Zahn
Krankenhaus Feuerbach Stuttgart	Dr. Scheibe
Mutterhaus Trier	Dr. Dornoff
Univ.-Frauenklinik Ulm/Donau	Dr. Pfeiffer
Kreiskrankenhaus St. Elisabeth Wittlich	Dr. Saalfrank
Stadtkrankenhaus Wolfsburg	Dr. Bothmann
Knappschaftskrankenhaus Bardenberg Wuerselen	Dr. Postulka

Appendix 2

The Heidelberg Questionnaire (Scheurlen H, Olschewski M, Verres R, Zoller A, 1983)
Assessment of quality of life in a breast preservation trial (original version in German)

Dear Patient,

We doctors would like to improve our treatment methods so as to better meet the needs of our patients. You could help us in this by telling us how you have felt and how you have come to grips with your life since the treatment of your breast disease. Please answer all of the following questions, concentrating on the period of the LAST FOUR WEEKS. Your reply will be treated in strict confidence. We guarantee to observe strictly data-protection regulations.

For each question please mark the answer which best applies to you by drawing a circle around it. Please give the completed questionnaire back to the doctor from whom you received it.

Many thanks for your help.

Lately, I have slept generally:

very well	*well*	*neither well nor badly*	*badly*	*very badly*

Lately, I have felt:

very strong	*strong*	*neither strong nor weak*	*weak*	*very weak*

Out of the house (shopping, going to church, etc.) I have lately got on:

very well	*well*	*moderately*	*badly*	*very badly*

Lately, I have felt:

very healthy	*healthy*	*neither healthy nor sick*	*sick*	*very sick*

The arm on the side that was operated on has lately caused me trouble:

not at all	*seldom*	*a little*	*fairly often*	*often*

Lately, I have done my day's work:

very well	*well*	*averagely*	*badly*	*very badly*

Lately, in the company of men, I felt:

very confident	*confident*	*partly confident, partly unsure*	*unsure*	*very unsure*

Lately, with myself and my life I have been:

very satisfied	*satisfied*	*neither satisfied nor dissatisfied*	*dissatisfied*	*very dissatisfied*

Lately, I could be joyful:

often	*sometimes*	*seldom*	*almost never*	*not at all*

Lately, I have been able to look after myself at home:

fully	*in essentials*	*partly*	*hardly*	*not at all*

Lately, from my fellow men I have felt:

very much supported	*supported*	*neither supported nor left alone*	*left alone*	*left very much alone*

My appetite has lately been:

very good	*good*	*changeable*	*poor*	*very poor*

With my physical appearance I have lately been:

very satisfied	*satisfied*	*neither satisfied nor dissatisfied*	*dissatisfied*	*very dissatisfied*

My contact to friends, work colleagues, and neighbors has lately been:

very good	*good*	*neither good nor bad*	*bad*	*very bad*

About my health I have lately had:

no worries at all	*few worries*	*some worries*	*considerable worries*	*very many worries*

Lately, I have wanted tenderness:

very much	*sometimes*	*seldom*	*almost never*	*not at all*

Pains or other problems in the region of the operated breast have lately given me trouble:

not at all	*seldom*	*sometimes*	*fairly often*	*often*

Lately, I have seen the future as:

very hopeful	*hopeful*	*with changeable feelings*	*hopeless*	*totally hopeless*

Making decisions has lately been:

very easy	*easy*	*neither easy nor difficult*	*difficult*	*very difficult*

My disposition has lately been:

very good	*good*	*changeable*	*poor*	*very poor*

In my free time I have lately been able to do:

very much	*a consider-able amount*	*at least something*	*little*	*nothing at all*

As far as energy is concerned, I have lately felt:

very lively	*lively*	*neither lively nor tired*	*tired*	*very tired*

With the scar from my operation I have lately been:

very satisfied	*satisfied*	*neither satisfied nor dissatisfied*	*dissatisfied*	*very dissatisfied*

With my closest relatives I have lately felt:

very satisfied	*satisfied*	*neither satisfied nor dissatisfied*	*dissatisfied*	*very dissatisfied*

Lately I have been:

very enter-prising	*enter-prising*	*changeable*	*lethargic*	*very lethargic*

Perhaps you think that we have forgotten some important questions. If you would like to tell us something more then do so here:

Subject Index

MIX
Papier aus verantwortungsvollen Quellen
Paper from responsible sources
FSC® C105338

If you have any concerns about our products,
you can contact us on
ProductSafety@springernature.com

In case Publisher is established outside the EU,
the EU authorized representative is:
Springer Nature Customer Service Center GmbH
Europaplatz 3, 69115 Heidelberg, Germany

Printed by Libri Plureos GmbH
in Hamburg, Germany